Challenges and Opportunities in Application of Cochlear Implantation

Challenges and Opportunities in Application of Cochlear Implantation

Editor

Nicolas Guevara

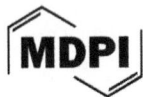

Basel • Beijing • Wuhan • Barcelona • Belgrade • Novi Sad • Cluj • Manchester

Editor
Nicolas Guevara
Université Côte d'Azur
Nice, France

Editorial Office
MDPI
St. Alban-Anlage 66
4052 Basel, Switzerland

This is a reprint of articles from the Special Issue published online in the open access journal *Journal of Clinical Medicine* (ISSN 2077-0383) (available at: https://www.mdpi.com/journal/jcm/special_issues/Challenges_and_Opportunities_in_Application_of_Cochlear_Implantation).

For citation purposes, cite each article independently as indicated on the article page online and as indicated below:

Lastname, A.A.; Lastname, B.B. Article Title. *Journal Name* **Year**, *Volume Number*, Page Range.

ISBN 978-3-0365-9534-4 (Hbk)
ISBN 978-3-0365-9535-1 (PDF)
doi.org/10.3390/books978-3-0365-9535-1

© 2023 by the authors. Articles in this book are Open Access and distributed under the Creative Commons Attribution (CC BY) license. The book as a whole is distributed by MDPI under the terms and conditions of the Creative Commons Attribution-NonCommercial-NoDerivs (CC BY-NC-ND) license.

Contents

Manon Baranger, Valeria Manera, Chloé Sérignac, Alexandre Derreumaux, Elisa Cancian, Clair Vandersteen, et al.
Evaluation of the Cognitive Function of Adults with Severe Hearing Loss Pre- and Post-Cochlear Implantation Using Verbal Fluency Testing
Reprinted from: *J. Clin. Med.* **2023**, *12*, 3792, doi:10.3390/jcm12113792 . . . . **1**

Raabid Hussain, Attila Frater, Roger Calixto, Chadlia Karoui, Jan Margeta, Zihao Wang, et al.
Anatomical Variations of the Human Cochlea Using an Image Analysis Tool
Reprinted from: *J. Clin. Med.* **2023**, *12*, 509, doi:10.3390/jcm12020509 . . . . **11**

Jan Margeta, Raabid Hussain, Paula López Diez, Anika Morgenstern, Thomas Demarcy, Zihao Wang, et al.
A Web-Based Automated Image Processing Research Platform for Cochlear Implantation-Related Studies
Reprinted from: *J. Clin. Med.* **2022**, *11*, 6640, doi:10.3390/jcm11226640 . . . . **23**

Samar A. Idriss, Pierre Reynard, Mathieu Marx, Albane Mainguy, Charles-Alexandre Joly, Eugen Constant Ionescu, et al.
Short- and Long-Term Effect of Cochlear Implantation on Disabling Tinnitus in Single-Sided Deafness Patients: A Systematic Review
Reprinted from: *J. Clin. Med.* **2022**, *11*, 5664, doi:10.3390/jcm11195664 . . . . **45**

Pierre Reynard, Virginie Attina, Samar Idriss, Ruben Hermann, Claire Barilly, Evelyne Veuillet, et al.
Effect of Serious Gaming on Speech-in-Noise Intelligibility in Adult Cochlear Implantees: A Randomized Controlled Study
Reprinted from: *J. Clin. Med.* **2022**, *11*, 2880, doi:10.3390/jcm11102880 . . . . **63**

Matthias Hey, Adam A. Hersbach, Thomas Hocke, Stefan J. Mauger, Britta Böhnke and Alexander Mewes
Ecological Momentary Assessment to Obtain Signal Processing Technology Preference in Cochlear Implant Users
Reprinted from: *J. Clin. Med.* **2022**, *11*, 2941, doi:10.3390/jcm11102941 . . . . **77**

Fabian Blanc, Catherine Blanchet, Marielle Sicard, Fanny Merklen, Frederic Venail and Michel Mondain
Audiological Outcomes and Associated Factors after Pediatric Cochlear Reimplantation
Reprinted from: *J. Clin. Med.* **2022**, *11*, 3148, doi:10.3390/jcm11113148 . . . . **87**

Gaëlle Leterme, Caroline Guigou, Geoffrey Guenser, Emmanuel Bigand and Alexis Bozorg Grayeli
Effect of Sound Coding Strategies on Music Perception with a Cochlear Implant
Reprinted from: *J. Clin. Med.* **2022**, *11*, 4425, doi:10.3390/jcm11154425 . . . . **95**

Julia Anna Christine Hoffmann, Athanasia Warnecke, Max Eike Timm, Eugen Kludt, Nils Kristian Prenzler, Lutz Gärtner, et al.
Cochlear Implantation in Obliterated Cochlea: A Retrospective Analysis and Comparison between the IES Stiff Custom-Made Device and the Split-Array and Regular Electrodes
Reprinted from: *J. Clin. Med.* **2022**, *11*, 6090, doi:10.3390/jcm11206090 . . . . **115**

Filip Asp, Eva Karltorp and Erik Berninger
Development of Sound Localization in Infants and Young Children with Cochlear Implants
Reprinted from: *J. Clin. Med.* **2022**, *11*, 6758, doi:10.3390/jcm11226758 . . . . **131**

Wojciech Gawęcki, Andrzej Balcerowiak, Paulina Podlawska, Patrycja Borowska, Renata Gibasiewicz, Witold Szyfter and Małgorzata Wierzbicka
Robot-Assisted Electrode Insertion in Cochlear Implantation Controlled by Intraoperative Electrocochleography— A Pilot Study
Reprinted from: *J. Clin. Med.* **2022**, *11*, 7045, doi:10.3390/jcm11237045 . . . . **141**

Lutz Gärtner, Bradford C. Backus, Nicolas Le Goff, Anika Morgenstern, Thomas Lenarz and Andreas Büchner
Cochlear Implant Stimulation Parameters Play a Key Role in Reducing Facial Nerve Stimulation
Reprinted from: *J. Clin. Med.* **2023**, *12*, 6194, doi:10.3390/jcm12196194 . . . . **155**

Fabiana Danieli, Miguel Angelo Hyppolito, Raabid Hussain, Michel Hoen, Chadlia Karoui and Ana Cláudia Mirândola Barbosa Reis
The Effects of Multi-Mode Monophasic Stimulation with Capacitive Discharge on the Facial Nerve Stimulation Reduction in Young Children with Cochlear Implants: Intraoperative Recordings
Reprinted from: *J. Clin. Med.* **2023**, *12*, 534, doi:10.3390/jcm12020534 . . . . **167**

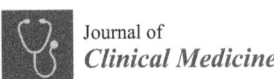

Article

Evaluation of the Cognitive Function of Adults with Severe Hearing Loss Pre- and Post-Cochlear Implantation Using Verbal Fluency Testing

Manon Baranger [1,2,*], Valeria Manera [1,2], Chloé Sérignac [3], Alexandre Derreumaux [2,4], Elisa Cancian [3], Clair Vandersteen [3], Auriane Gros [1,2,4] and Nicolas Guevara [3]

1. Département d'Orthophonie de Nice (DON), UFR Médecine, Université Côte d'Azur, 06107 Nice, France; valeria.manera@univ-cotedazur.fr (V.M.); auriane.gros@univ-cotedazur.fr (A.G.)
2. Laboratoire CobTeK, Université Côte d'Azur, 06100 Nice, France; derreumaux.a@chu-nice.fr
3. Institut Universitaire de la Face et du Cou, Centre Hospitalier Universitaire, Université Côte d'Azur, 31 Avenue de Valombrose, 06100 Nice, France; chloemarieserignac@gmail.com (C.S.); elisa.cancian.ortho@gmail.com (E.C.); vandersteen.c@chu-nice.fr (C.V.); guevara.n@chu-nice.fr (N.G.)
4. Université Côte d'Azur, Centre Hospitalier Universitaire de Nice (University Hospital of Nice), Service Clinique Gériatrique du Cerveau et du Mouvement, Centre Mémoire Ressources et Recherche (Geriatric Brain and Movement Clinic, Memory Resources and Research Centre), 06100 Nice, France
* Correspondence: manon.baranger10@gmail.com

Abstract: Hearing loss is a major public health problem with significant evidence correlating it with cognitive performance. Verbal fluency tests are commonly used to assess lexical access. They provide a great deal of information about a subject's cognitive function. The aim of our study was to evaluate phonemic and semantic lexical access abilities in adults with bilateral severe to profound hearing loss and then to re-evaluate a cohort after cochlear implantation. 103 adult subjects underwent phonemic and semantic fluency tests during a cochlear implant candidacy evaluation. Of the total 103 subjects, 43 subjects underwent the same tests at 3 months post-implantation. Our results showed superior performance in phonemic fluency compared to semantic fluency in subjects prior to implantation. Phonemic fluency was positively correlated with semantic fluency. Similarly, individuals with congenital deafness had better semantic lexical access than individuals with acquired deafness. Results at 3 months post-implantation showed an improvement in phonemic fluency. No correlation was found between the evolution of pre- and post-implant fluency and the auditory gain of the cochlear implant, and we found no significant difference between congenital and acquired deafness. Our study shows an improvement in global cognitive function after cochlear implantation without differentiation of the phonemic-semantic pathway.

Keywords: hearing loss; verbal fluency; cochlear implant; phonemic pathway; semantic pathway

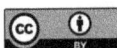

1. Introduction

Approximately 25% of French adults are affected by hearing loss, of which 4% are at a disabling level [1]. A weak but significant correlation between hearing loss and cognitive performance has been reported [2]. Elderly people with hearing loss show an accelerated cognitive decline compared to their peers without hearing impairment [3–6] and thus a higher risk of dementia. In fact, according to the Lancet Commission, hearing loss is the largest potentially modifiable risk factor for dementia [7]. Several studies have shown promising results on the positive effects of hearing aid use on cognitive decline [8–10]. However, in cases of severe to profound hearing loss, the only reliable option for auditory rehabilitation is cochlear implantation [11].

At the cognitive level, cochlear implantation leads to improved performance in attention, memory [12,13] and inhibition [13]. Improvements in executive function tasks are greater in patients with lower baseline cognitive abilities [14].

Verbal fluency tests are regularly used to assess lexical access [15,16]. They provide information on memory storage capacity, the ability to retrieve stored information, the ability to organize thought and the strategies used to search for words [17]. These tests require that the participant produces as many words as possible from a specific category/condition in a limited period of time. Verbal fluency tests are performed under two main types of conditions: the phonemic condition (the subject is asked to produce words beginning with a certain given letter) and the semantic condition (the subject is asked to produce words from a certain given category). Verbal fluency tests reflect multiple high and low level cognitive abilities [16]. Both fluency tests require the integrity of lexical and semantic representations and of executive functions [15].

Semantic and phonemic fluencies depend on distinct neural systems. For phonemic verbal fluency, it can be seen with Functional Magnetic Resonance Imagining (fMRI) that the posterior regions of the left inferior frontal gyrus are more activated. On the other hand, for semantic fluency there is greater activation of the more anterior regions of the frontal and posterior regions of the temporal cortex [18,19].

Adults with severe to profound post-lingual hearing loss have a deterioration of phonological memory and its dorsal (fronto-parietal) pathway. The longer the subjects are exposed to this hearing loss, the more they use the ventral semantic (occipitotemporal) pathway to compensate for the lack of elementary phonological decomposition [20]. Phonological decomposition is an initial auditory step that enables secondary semantic analysis. Individuals who fail phonological decomposition lack linguistic analysis and correspondence between perceived and memorized phonology. This then limits the extraction of meaning from speech.

These difficulties with internal phonological representations and the degradation of auditory information worsen with the duration of auditory deprivation [21]. For postlingual cochlear implant recipients, phonemic reconstruction is a more difficult cognitive task than semantic processing because of the degradation of auditory information delivered by the cochlear implant [22].

This study aims, firstly, to establish the phonemic and semantic lexical access abilities of adult subjects with bilateral severe to profound hearing loss and, secondly, to evaluate the impact of the cochlear implantation on phonemic and semantic lexical access.

2. Study 1

2.1. Materials and Methods

2.1.1. Population

One hundred and three subjects participated in the present study (N = 103). The group consisted of 43 males and 55 females (mean age: 61.8 years; minimum 20 years; maximum 89 years). 15 subjects had primary school education, 36 subjects had secondary school education, and 49 had higher education. Data on education level was missing for 3 subjects. The origin of the hearing loss was variable: acquired hearing loss ($n = 83$), congenital hearing loss ($n = 20$). The etiologies are described in Table 1. The category "other" includes hearing loss from otitis associated with another context, head trauma, ototoxicity, toxic shock associated with progressive deafness, drug overdose, drug treatment, sepsis, as well as idiopathic deafness, and fragile X syndrome.

Subjects were recruited from a panel of patients with severe to profound hearing loss at the Institut Universitaire de la Face et du Cou de Nice during a pre-cochlear implant assessment. All subjects included had bilateral severe to profound hearing loss and were native French speakers. This study was approved by the Recherches Non Interventionnelles de l'Université Côte d'Azur (CERNI) AVIS number 2020-62. All participants signed an informed consent form before the start of the study.

Table 1. Etiologies of hearing loss in the population ranked by frequency.

Etiologies	N
Presbycusis	15
Meniere's disease	10
Otosclerosis	8
Congenital bilateral profound deafness	5
Meningitis	3
Malformation	3
Chronic otitis	3
Hereditary	3
Genetic	3
Meniere's disease with chronic otitis	2
Infection	2
Congenital deafness with sudden aggravation	2
Autoimmune	2
Pendred's syndrome associated with malformation	2
Other	10
Unknown data	30

2.1.2. Materials and Procedure

We used Cardebat's fluencies [23] to assess phonemic and semantic lexical access. The phonemic fluencies [P] and [R] and the semantic fluencies "animals" and "fruit" were used. Each subject took a phonemic fluency test and a semantic fluency test in a randomized fashion. For each fluency test, the participant had to produce as many words as possible within 2 min. The verbal fluency tests were given to the patients during the pre-cochlear implant assessment session.

2.1.3. Statistical Analyses

The Z-score was calculated using Cardebat's fluency calibration [23]. This calibration takes into account the type of fluency as well as the gender, age and education level of the participants. The Z-score is the standard deviation. The closer the Z-score is to 0, the closer it is to the norm. A negative Z-score shows below average performance, and a positive Z-score shows above average performance. The Shapiro-Wilk test was used to check the normal distribution of the data. Since the data is normally distributed, a paired-sample t-test was used to compare the Z-scores of phonemic and semantic fluency. In order to compare the phonemic and semantic fluency Z-scores between acquired and congenital deafness, we used an independent samples t-test and a Mann Whitney test according to the distribution of the data. The Pearson correlation was used to establish the correlation between the phonemic and semantic fluency Z-scores. Significant results are reported as $p < 0.05$ ($p < 0.05$ *, $p < 0.01$ **, $p < 0.001$ ***).

2.2. Results

Of the 103 participants, 2 individuals were below the pathology threshold ($Z = -2$) in phonemic fluency and 6 individuals in semantic fluency. Table 2 shows the results of the Z-scores for phonemic and semantic fluency.

Table 2. Phonemic and semantic fluency results by Z-score.

	Z-Score Phonemic Fluency (N = 103)	Z-Score Semantic Fluency (N = 103)
Mean	−0.0446	−0.256
Standard deviation	1.25	1.18
Minimum	−2.43	−2.98
Maximum	3.14	2.49
p-value		0.043 *

The mean Z-score for phonemic fluency is higher than that for semantic fluency. The p-value shows that this result is significant ($p = 0.043$ *). In addition, there is a significant positive correlation between the phonemic fluency Z-score and the semantic fluency Z-score ($r = 0.630$, $p < 0.001$ ***). Figure 1 shows the distribution of phonemic and semantic fluency Z-scores.

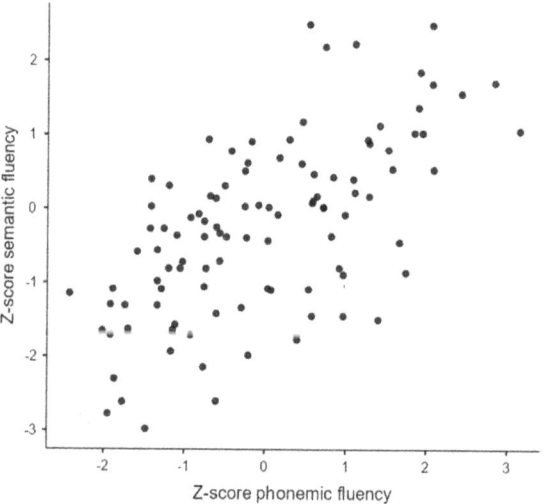

Figure 1. Distribution of Z-scores in the two fluency conditions.

The results of the phonemic and semantic fluency Z-scores according to the origin of the participants' deafness (acquired deafness or congenital deafness) are described in Table 3.

Table 3. Phonemic and semantic fluency Z-scores according to the origin of the deafness.

	Acquired Deafness (N = 81)/Congenital Deafness (N = 22)	Z-Score Phonemic Fluency	Z-Score Semantic Fluency
Mean	Acquired	−0.109	−0.379
	Congenital	0.191	0.194
Standard deviation	Acquired	1.26	1.21
	Congenital	1.22	0.974
Minimum	Acquired	−2.43	−2.98
	Congenital	−1.43	−1.50
Maximum	Acquired	3.14	2.49
	Congenital	2.06	2.48
p-value	/	0.330	0.043 *

The results show higher Z-scores in phonemic and semantic fluency for participants with congenital deafness. The p-value is significant for the Z-score in semantic fluency ($p = 0.043$ *). The p-value is not significant for the phonemic fluency Z-score.

3. Study 2

3.1. Materials and Methods

3.1.1. Population

The subjects included in study 2 (N = 43) were from study 1. The group consisted of 19 males and 24 females (mean age: 55.7 years; minimum 20 years; maximum 85 years). 4 subjects (9%) had primary school education, 13 (30%) subjects had secondary school education and 25 (58%) had higher education. Data on the educational level of 1 (2%) subject was missing. The origin of the hearing loss was variable: acquired hearing loss ($n = 31$), congenital hearing loss ($n = 12$). The etiologies were diverse: 11 subjects had presbycusis, 5 subjects had congenital bilateral profound hearing loss, 3 subjects had otosclerosis-related hearing loss, 3 subjects had genetic hearing loss, 2 subjects had Pendred's syndrome, 2 subjects had Meniere's disease, 2 subjects had Meniere's disease associated with chronic otitis, 2 subjects had hearing loss due to inner ear malformations, and 2 subjects had congenital deafness with abrupt worsening. 11 subjects had other etiologies: fragile X syndrome, autoimmune, idiopathic, meningitis, chronic ear infections, ototoxicity, sepsis.

At the end of the pre-implant assessment in Study 1, some participants had no indication for cochlear implantation. For other participants, data on verbal fluency at 3 months post-implantation were missing. These reasons explain the difference in participants between Study 1 and Study 2.

3.1.2. Materials and Procedure

Different brands of cochlear implants were used: Medel ($n = 15$), Cochlear ($n = 16$), Advanced Bionics ($n = 7$) and Oticon Medical ($n = 7$).

Subjects were reviewed at a post-cochlear implant assessment session approximately 3 months after surgery. During this assessment, they were randomly retested for semantic and phonemic fluencies.

3.1.3. Statistical Analyses

The Z-score was calculated following the fluency calibration of Cardebat [23]. This calibration takes into account the type of fluency as well as the gender, age and education level of the participants. Cochlear implant auditory gain was calculated as the difference between post-implant Pure Tone Audiometry (PTA) and pre-implant PTA. The Shapiro-Wilk test was used to check the normal distribution of the data. Since the data followed the normal distribution, a paired-sample t-test was used to compare the Z-score of pre- and post-implantation fluencies. In order to compare the differences in Z-scores of post-implantation and pre-cochlear implantation phonemic fluencies and post-implantation and pre-cochlear implantation semantic fluencies between acquired and congenital deafness, we used an independent samples t-test and a Mann Whitney test according to the distribution of the data. Pearson correlations were performed to analyse the relationship between differences in fluency scores and implant gain. Significant results are reported as $p < 0.05$ ($p < 0.05$ *, $p < 0.01$ **, $p < 0.001$ ***).

3.2. Results

Of the 43 subjects, one subject was below the pathological threshold ($Z = -2$) in phonemic fluency post cochlear implantation. For semantic fluency, 2 subjects were below the pathological threshold pre- and post-cochlear implantation. One participant went from a non-pathological to a pathological Z-score after implantation. One participant went from a pathological to a non-pathological Z-score after implantation.

Table 4 shows the results of the pre- and post-cochlear implantation Z-scores in the two fluency conditions (phonemic and semantic).

Table 4. Phonemic and semantic fluency Z-score results pre and post cochlear implantation.

	Z-Score Phonemic Fluency Pre-CI	Z-Score Phonemic Fluency Post CI	Z-Score Semantic Fluency Pre-CI	Z-Score Semantic Fluency Post CI
Mean	0.00116	0.302	−0.0635	−0.0342
Standard deviation	1.30	1.15	1.16	1.41
Minimum	−1.95	−2.25	−2.77	−2.27
Maximum	2.83	2.46	2.23	4.00
p-value		0.024 *		0.863

The results show a higher Z-score for post-implantation phonemic fluency than for pre-implantation phonemic fluency. The p-value shows that the result is significant ($p = 0.024$ *). In semantic fluency, the post-implantation Z-score is slightly higher than the pre-implantation Z-score, but this value is not significant ($p = 0.863$).

Table 5 describes the results of the differences in the post and pre cochlear implantation Z-scores according to the origin of the deafness (acquired deafness or congenital deafness).

Table 5. Results of Z-score differences in post- and pre-cochlear implant phonemic fluency and post- and pre-cochlear implant semantic fluency between acquired and congenital deafness.

	Acquired Deafness (N = 29)/Congenital Deafness (N = 14)	Z-Score Difference Phonemic Fluency Post CI- Z-Score Phonemic Fluency Pre-CI	Z-Score Difference Semantic Fluency Post CI- Z-Score Semantic Fluency Pre-CI
Mean	Acquired	0.329	0.0766
	Congenital	0.241	−0.0686
Standard deviance	Acquired	0.843	0.971
	Congenital	0.873	1.38
Minimum	Acquired	−1.27	−1.92
	Congenital	−1.04	−1.82
Maximum	Acquired	2.51	2.63
	Congenital	2.17	2.42
p-value	/	0.751	0.692

The differences in phonemic fluency Z-scores post implant and pre implant show a gain for both groups. The mean is higher in the group of subjects with acquired hearing loss than in the group with congenital hearing loss.

The difference in semantic fluency Z-scores post implant and pre implant shows a small gain for the group of subjects with an acquired hearing loss. For subjects with congenital hearing loss the difference in semantic fluency Z-scores post implantation and pre cochlear implantation shows a small loss. No significant difference was found between the two groups in the post-implantation condition in either fluency ($p = 0.751$ and $p = 0.692$).

Figure 2 shows the distribution of the differences in Z-scores (in phonemic and semantic fluency) post and pre-implant and implant gain.

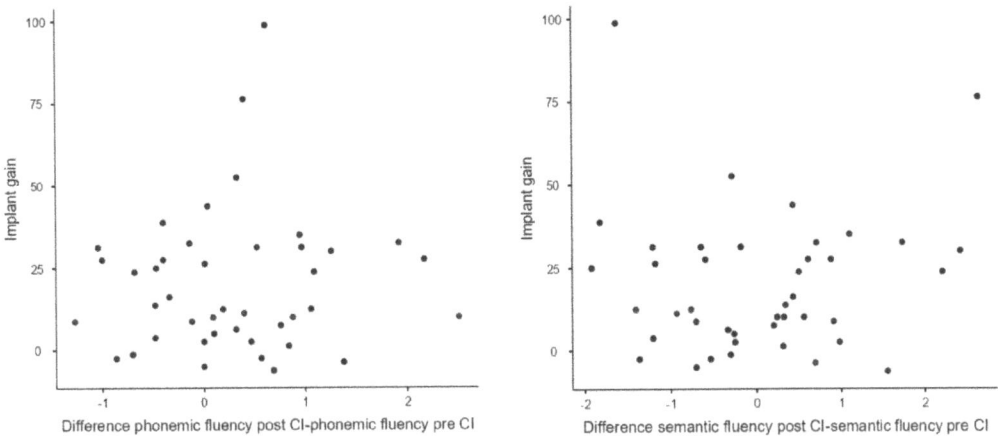

Figure 2. Distribution of post- and pre-implantation Z-score differences and implant gain.

Figure 3 shows the distribution of pre-implantation phonemic and semantic Z-score differences and implant gain.

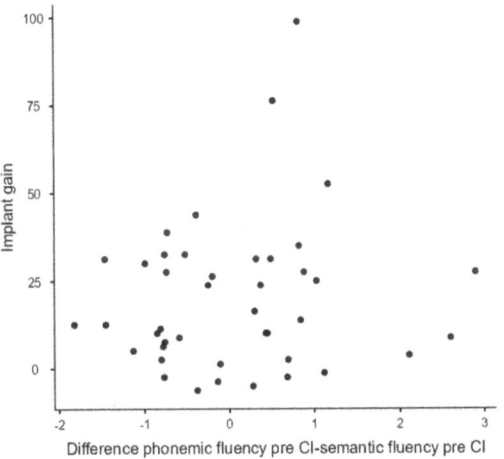

Figure 3. Distribution of pre-implant phonemic and semantic Z-score differences and implant gain.

The results show no correlation between pre-implantation phonemic and semantic Z-score differences and implant gain ($r = 0.119$, $p > 0.05$).

4. Discussion

The first aim of this study was to establish the lexical access abilities of adult subjects with bilateral severe to profound hearing loss. Study 1 showed superior performance on phonemic fluency compared to semantic fluency in the subjects included. This result is in contrast with the Santos study which showed superior performance on semantic fluency in adults with hearing impairment [24]. However, our study and Santos' study were not conducted in the same language (French vs. Brazilian Portuguese). The time allotted to measure the fluencies was also different (2 min vs. 1 min). It has been shown that semantic fluency is an indicator of a deficit in executive function [25]. Similarly, it is known that hearing impairment affects executive functions [26]. The results of this study could, therefore, demonstrate an executive function deficit more pronounced than the phonological deficit in adults with severe to profound hearing loss. Furthermore, the maintenance of this dorsal phonemic pathway in subjects with post-lingual hearing loss predicts a favourable outcome with a cochlear implant [21].

A positive correlation was observed between the phonemic and semantic Z-scores. Therefore, there is a link between success in phonemic and semantic fluencies, even though phonemic and semantic fluencies involve separate distinct systems. Semantic fluency involves the inferior longitudinal fasciculus, the unciform fasciculus, the temporal part of the inferior fronto-occipital fasciculus and the superior temporal gyrus. Phonemic fluency involves the ascending frontal tract, the frontal part of the inferior fronto-occipital bundle and the superior frontal gyrus [27]. The results of our study suggest a close link between these two pathways and that they can work together.

People with congenital hearing loss have better semantic lexical access than people with acquired hearing loss. This can be explained by the fact that people with congenital hearing loss have insufficient phonological decomposition dating to the prelingual period. Therefore, they would preferentially use the ventral (occipito-temporal) semantic pathway [20].

Secondly, we assessed the impact of cochlear implantation on phonemic and semantic lexical access. Study 2 showed a positive impact of the cochlear implant on phonemic fluency as early as 3 months post implant. Thus, cochlear implantation allowed for better phonological representation and better access to the dorsal pathway. This benefit of the cochlear implant appears relatively early after surgery. These results are important because most studies have highlighted cognitive changes at six months or one year but not so early. Indeed, since ten years the clinical research on the cognitive improvement by cochlear implantation has become increasingly recognized. Especially, studies have showed improvements in different cognitive functions as processing speed, cognitive flexibility and working memory [28–30]. These studies have conducted prospective longitudinal studies as early as 6 months after cochlear implantation but never as early as 3 months. So, our results suggest that verbal fluency improvement start since 3 months after implantation.

Study 2 showed no significant difference in pre- and post-cochlear implantation fluency between groups based on the origin of the hearing loss. The contribution of the cochlear implant on phonemic and semantic fluency is as effective for an acquired hearing loss as for a congenital one at 3 months post-implant. No correlation was found between differences in post- and pre-implant fluency and implant auditory gain. At 3 months post-implantation, the benefit of the cochlear implant is not specific to the phonemic and semantic pathways. The distribution between the pathways is not determined.

Finally, the improvement in participants verbal fluency, even elderly, and this very quickly, adds proof of the interest of cochlear implantation for cognitive stimulation and the prevention of cognitive decline as suggested by other studies [31].

It would be interesting to continue this study with a longer post cochlear implantation observation time to see if a correlation could be obtained between implant gain and the difference in phonemic and semantic fluency. It might also be interesting to analyse clustering (retrieval of words by phonemic or semantic subcategory) and switching (moving from one subcategory to another) in verbal fluency tasks in people with hearing impairment.

Study Limitations

A major limitation of our study is the short post-implantation interval. We observed verbal fluency only 3 months after implantation whereas most studies analyse cognition 1 year after implantation. Indeed, activation of the auditory associative cortex continues to increase even years after cochlear implantation for stimuli containing speech [32]. Another limitation of this study is the calibration used. The Cardebat fluencies are calibrated for age, gender and education level. The age norms range from 30 to 85 years. However, in this study, participants under 30 and over 85 years of age were included. The calibration used for these participants was the one closest in age respecting gender and education.

5. Conclusions

Our study showed higher phonemic fluency than semantic fluency, in contrast to previous studies. At 3 months after surgery, we observed a benefit of the cochlear implant in adults without differentiation between the phonemic and semantic pathways and regardless of the origin of the hearing loss. This study could be continued over a longer period of observation post cochlear implantation. It might be relevant to compare the impairment of phonemic and semantic pathways with that of executive functions in adults with hearing impairment.

Author Contributions: Conceptualization, A.G., N.G. and V.M.; methodology, V.M. and A.G.; software, A.D.; validation, A.G. and V.M.; formal analysis, M.B. and V.M.; investigation, N.G., A.G., C.S. and E.C.; data curation, C.S. and E.C.; writing—original draft preparation, M.B., V.M., A.G., C.S., A.D., E.C., C.V. and N.G.; writing—review and editing, M.B., V.M., A.G., C.S., A.D., E.C., C.V. and N.G.; supervision, A.G., N.G., C.V. and V.M. All authors have read and agreed to the published version of the manuscript.

Funding: This project was financed by the GIRCI Méditerranée in the context of the "AAP GIRCI ValoData 2022—recherche paramédicale", project acronym "ModelCo".

Institutional Review Board Statement: This study was approved by the Recherches Non Interventionnelles de l'Université Côte d'Azur (CERNI) AVIS number 2020-62.

Informed Consent Statement: All participants signed an informed consent form before the start of the study.

Data Availability Statement: Data will be provided upon the request to researchers.

Acknowledgments: The authors thank Abdallah Alshukry for advice and help in translating the text into English.

Conflicts of Interest: The authors declare no conflict of interest.

References

1. Lisan, Q.; Goldberg, M.; Lahlou, G.; Ozguler, A.; Lemonnier, S.; Jouven, X.; Zins, M.; Empana, J.-P. Prevalence of Hearing Loss and Hearing Aid Use Among Adults in France in the CONSTANCES Study. *JAMA Netw. Open* **2022**, *5*, e2217633. [CrossRef] [PubMed]
2. Loughrey, D.G.; Kelly, M.E.; Kelley, G.A.; Brennan, S.; Lawlor, B.A. Association of age-related hearing loss with cognitive function, cognitive impairment, and dementia: A systematic review and meta-analysis. *JAMA Otolaryngol. Head Neck Surg.* **2018**, *144*, 115–126. [CrossRef] [PubMed]
3. Gallacher, J.; Ilubaera, V.; Ben-Shlomo, Y.; Bayer, A.; Fish, M.; Babisch, W.; Elwood, P. Auditory threshold, phonologic demand, and incident dementia. *Neurology* **2012**, *79*, 1583–1590. [CrossRef] [PubMed]
4. Lin, F.R.; Metter, E.J.; O'brien, R.J.; Resnick, S.M.; Zonderman, A.B.; Ferrucci, L. Hearing Loss and Incident Dementia. *Arch. Neurol.* **2011**, *68*, 214–220. [CrossRef]
5. Lin, F.R.; Yaffe, K.; Xia, J.; Xue, Q.-L.; Harris, T.B.; Purchase-Helzner, E.; Satterfield, S.; Ayonayon, H.N.; Ferrucci, L.; Simonsick, E.M.; et al. Hearing Loss and Cognitive Decline in Older Adults. *JAMA Intern. Med.* **2013**, *173*, 293–299. [CrossRef]
6. Mosnier, I.; Vanier, A.; Bonnard, D.; Lina-Granade, G.; Truy, E.; Bordure, P.; Godey, B.; Marx, M.; Lescanne, E.; Venail, F.; et al. Long-Term Cognitive Prognosis of Profoundly Deaf Older Adults After Hearing Rehabilitation Using Cochlear Implants. *J. Am. Geriatr. Soc.* **2018**, *66*, 1553–1561. [CrossRef]
7. Livingston, G.; Huntley, J.; Sommerlad, A.; Ames, D.; Ballard, C.; Banerjee, S.; Brayne, C.; Burns, A.; Cohen-Mansfield, J.; Cooper, C.; et al. Dementia prevention, intervention, and care: 2020 report of the Lancet Commission. *Lancet* **2020**, *396*, 413–446. [CrossRef] [PubMed]
8. Acar, B.; Yurekli, M.F.; Babademez, M.A.; Karabulut, H.; Karasen, R.M. Effects of hearing aids on cognitive functions and depressive signs in elderly people. *Arch. Gerontol. Geriatr.* **2011**, *52*, 250–252. [CrossRef]
9. Amieva, H.; Ouvrard, C.; Giulioli, C.; Meillon, C.; Rullier, L.; Dartigues, J.-F. Self-Reported Hearing Loss, Hearing Aids, and Cognitive Decline in Elderly Adults: A 25-Year Study. *J. Am. Geriatr. Soc.* **2015**, *63*, 2099–2104. [CrossRef]
10. Mahmoudi, E.; Basu, T.; Langa, K.; McKee, M.; Zazove, P.; Alexander, N.; Kamdar, N. Can Hearing Aids Delay Time to Diagnosis of Dementia, Depression, or Falls in Older Adults? *J. Am. Geriatr. Soc.* **2019**, *67*, 2362–2369. [CrossRef]
11. Roche, J.P.; Hansen, M.R. On the Horizon: Cochlear Implant Technology. *Otolaryngol. Clin. North Am.* **2015**, *48*, 1097–1116. [CrossRef] [PubMed]

12. Mertens, G.; Andries, E.; Claes, A.J.; Topsakal, V.; Van de Heyning, P.; Van Rompaey, V.; Calvino, M.; Cuadrado, I.S.; Muñoz, E.; Gavilán, J.; et al. Cognitive Improvement After Cochlear Implantation in Older Adults With Severe or Profound Hearing Impairment: A Prospective, Longitudinal, Controlled, Multicenter Study. *Ear Hear.* **2021**, *42*, 606–614. [CrossRef] [PubMed]
13. Völter, C.; Götze, L.; Haubitz, I.; Müther, J.; Dazert, S.; Thomas, J.P. Impact of Cochlear Implantation on Neurocognitive Subdomains in Adult Cochlear Implant Recipients. *Audiol. Neurotol.* **2021**, *26*, 236–245. [CrossRef] [PubMed]
14. Zhan, K.Y.; Lewis, J.H.; Vasil, K.J.; Tamati, T.N.; Harris, M.S.; Pisoni, D.B.; Kronenberger, W.G.; Ray, C.; Moberly, A.C. Cognitive Functions in Adults Receiving Cochlear Implants: Predictors of Speech Recognition and Changes After Implantation. *Otol. Neurotol.* **2020**, *41*, e322–e329. [CrossRef]
15. Henry, J.D.; Crawford, J.R.; Phillips, L.H. Verbal fluency performance in dementia of the Alzheimer's type: A meta-analysis. *Neuropsychologia* **2004**, *42*, 1212–1222. [CrossRef]
16. Stolwyk, R.; Bannirchelvam, B.; Kraan, C.; Simpson, K. The cognitive abilities associated with verbal fluency task performance differ across fluency variants and age groups in healthy young and old adults. *J. Clin. Exp. Neuropsychol.* **2015**, *37*, 70–83. [CrossRef]
17. Costa, A.; Bagoj, E.; Monaco, M.; Zabberoni, S.; De Rosa, S.; Papantonio, A.M.; Mundi, C.; Caltagirone, C.; Carlesimo, G.A. Standardization and normative data obtained in the Italian population for a new verbal fluency instrument, the phonemic/semantic alternate fluency test. *Neurol. Sci.* **2014**, *35*, 365–372. [CrossRef]
18. Birn, R.M.; Kenworthy, L.; Case, L.; Caravella, R.; Jones, T.B.; Bandettini, P.A.; Martin, A. Neural systems supporting lexical search guided by letter and semantic category cues: A self-paced overt response fMRI study of verbal fluency. *Neuroimage* **2010**, *49*, 1099–1107. [CrossRef]
19. Costafreda, S.G.; Fu, C.; Lee, L.; Everitt, B.; Brammer, M.J.; David, A.S. A systematic review and quantitative appraisal of fMRI studies of verbal fluency: Role of the left inferior frontal gyrus. *Hum. Brain Mapp.* **2006**, *27*, 799–810. [CrossRef]
20. Lazard, D.S.; Giraud, A.L.; Gnansia, D.; Meyer, B.; Sterkers, O. Comprendre le cerveau sourd, implications dans la réhabilitation par implant cochléaire. *Ann. Françaises D'oto-Rhino-Laryngol. Pathol. Cervico-Faciale* **2012**, *129*, 122–128. [CrossRef]
21. Lazard, D.; Lee, H.; Gaebler, M.; Kell, C.; Truy, E.; Giraud, A. Phonological processing in post-lingual deafness and cochlear implant outcome. *Neuroimage* **2010**, *49*, 3443–3451. [CrossRef]
22. Giraud, A.-L.; Truy, E.; Frackowiak, R.S.J.; Grégoire, M.-C.; Pujol, J.-F.; Collet, L. Differential recruitment of the speech processing system in healthy subjects and rehabilitated cochlear implant patients. *Brain* **2000**, *123*, 1391–1402. [CrossRef]
23. Cardebat, D.; Doyon, B.; Puel, M.; Goulet, P.; Joanette, Y. Formal and semantic lexical evocation in normal subjects. Performance and dynamics of production as a function of sex, age and educational level. *Acta Neurol. Belg.* **1990**, *90*, 207–217. [PubMed]
24. Santos, I.M.M.D.; Chiossi, J.S.C.; Soares, A.D.; Oliveira, L.N.D.; Chiari, B.M. Phonological and semantic verbal fluency: A comparative study in hearing-impaired and normal-hearing people. *Codas* **2014**, *26*, 434–438. [CrossRef]
25. Kave, G.; Heled, E.; Vakil, E.; Agranov, E. Which verbal fluency measure is most useful in demonstrating executive deficits after traumatic brain injury? *J. Clin. Exp. Neuropsychol.* **2011**, *33*, 358–365. [CrossRef]
26. Ren, F.; Ma, W.; Li, M.; Sun, H.; Xin, Q.; Zong, W.; Chen, W.; Wang, G.; Gao, F.; Zhao, B. Gray Matter Atrophy Is Associated With Cognitive Impairment in Patients With Presbycusis: A Comprehensive Morphometric Study. *Front. Neurosci.* **2018**, *12*, 744. [CrossRef] [PubMed]
27. Zigiotto, L.; Vavassori, L.; Annicchiarico, L.; Corsini, F.; Avesani, P.; Rozzanigo, U.; Sarubbo, S.; Papagno, C. Segregated circuits for phonemic and semantic fluency: A novel patient-tailored disconnection study. *NeuroImage Clin.* **2022**, *36*, 103149. [CrossRef]
28. Cosetti, M.K.; Pinkston, J.B.; Flores, J.M.; Friedmann, D.R.; Jones, C.B.; Roland, J.J.; Waltzman, S.B. Neurocognitive testing and cochlear implantation: Insights into performance in older adults. *Clin. Interv. Aging* **2016**, *11*, 603–613. [CrossRef]
29. Gurgel, R.K.; Duff, K.; Foster, N.L.; Urano, K.A.; Detorres, A. Evaluating the Impact of Cochlear Implantation on Cognitive Function in Older Adults. *Laryngoscope* **2022**, *132*, S1–S15. [CrossRef] [PubMed]
30. Mosnier, I.; Bebear, J.-P.; Marx, M.; Fraysse, B.; Truy, E.; Lina-Granade, G.; Mondain, M.; Sterkers-Artières, F.; Bordure, P.; Robier, A.; et al. Improvement of Cognitive Function After Cochlear Implantation in Elderly Patients. *JAMA Otolaryngol. Neck Surg.* **2015**, *141*, 442–450. [CrossRef]
31. Babajanian, E.E.; Patel, N.S.; Gurgel, R.K. The Impact of Cochlear Implantation: Cognitive Function, Quality of Life, and Frailty in Older Adults. *Semin. Hear.* **2021**, *42*, 342–351. [CrossRef] [PubMed]
32. Giraud, A.-L.; Price, C.; Graham, J.M.; Truy, E.; Frackowiak, R. Cross-Modal Plasticity Underpins Language Recovery after Cochlear Implantation. *Neuron* **2001**, *30*, 657–664. [CrossRef] [PubMed]

Disclaimer/Publisher's Note: The statements, opinions and data contained in all publications are solely those of the individual author(s) and contributor(s) and not of MDPI and/or the editor(s). MDPI and/or the editor(s) disclaim responsibility for any injury to people or property resulting from any ideas, methods, instructions or products referred to in the content.

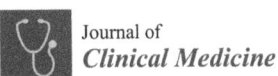

Article

Anatomical Variations of the Human Cochlea Using an Image Analysis Tool

Raabid Hussain [1,*], Attila Frater [1], Roger Calixto [1], Chadlia Karoui [2], Jan Margeta [3], Zihao Wang [4], Michel Hoen [2], Herve Delingette [4], François Patou [1], Charles Raffaelli [5], Clair Vandersteen [5] and Nicolas Guevara [5]

1. Research & Technology, Oticon Medical, 06220 Vallauris, France
2. Clinical Evidence Department, Oticon Medical, 06220 Vallauris, France
3. Research and Development, KardioMe, 01851 Nova Dubnica, Slovakia
4. Epione Team, Inria, Université Côte d'Azur, 06902 Sophia Antipolis, France
5. Institut Universitaire de la Face et du Cou, Nice, Centre Hospitalier Universitaire de Nice, Université Côte d'Azur, 06100 Nice, France
* Correspondence: raui@oticonmedical.com

Abstract: Understanding cochlear anatomy is crucial for developing less traumatic electrode arrays and insertion guidance for cochlear implantation. The human cochlea shows considerable variability in size and morphology. This study analyses 1000+ clinical temporal bone CT images using a web-based image analysis tool. Cochlear size and shape parameters were obtained to determine population statistics and perform regression and correlation analysis. The analysis revealed that cochlear morphology follows Gaussian distribution, while cochlear dimensions A and B are not well-correlated to each other. Additionally, dimension B is more correlated to duct lengths, the wrapping factor and volume than dimension A. The scala tympani size varies considerably among the population, with the size generally decreasing along insertion depth with dimensional jumps through the trajectory. The mean scala tympani radius was 0.32 mm near the 720° insertion angle. Inter-individual variability was four times that of intra-individual variation. On average, the dimensions of both ears are similar. However, statistically significant differences in clinical dimensions were observed between ears of the same patient, suggesting that size and shape are not the same. Harnessing deep learning-based, automated image analysis tools, our results yielded important insights into cochlear morphology and implant development, helping to reduce insertion trauma and preserving residual hearing.

Keywords: cochlear morphology; cochlear implantation; statistical analysis

Citation: Hussain, R.; Frater, A.; Calixto, R.; Karoui, C.; Margeta, J.; Wang, Z.; Hoen, M.; Delingette, H.; Patou, F.; Raffaelli, C.; et al. Anatomical Variations of the Human Cochlea Using an Image Analysis Tool. *J. Clin. Med.* **2023**, *12*, 509. https://doi.org/10.3390/jcm12020509

Academic Editor: Christof Röösli

Received: 14 December 2022
Revised: 30 December 2022
Accepted: 4 January 2023
Published: 8 January 2023

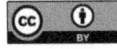

Copyright: © 2023 by the authors. Licensee MDPI, Basel, Switzerland. This article is an open access article distributed under the terms and conditions of the Creative Commons Attribution (CC BY) license (https://creativecommons.org/licenses/by/4.0/).

1. Introduction

Cochlear implants (CI) are the most successful neural prosthetic devices to date that provide hearing to profoundly hearing-impaired people around the world. CIs work by bypassing hair cell functionality and applying electrical stimulation to the auditory nerve fibers directly via a multichannel electrode array ideally implanted in the scala tympani (ST). Among other factors, CIs were shown to provide better hearing outcomes, e.g., word recognition scores for patients with greater neural survival [1,2]. In recent years, patients with low-frequency residual hearing also became eligible for CIs [3,4], and the CIs have shown a superior performance compared to those in profoundly deaf users [5–9]. Preservation of neural structures and residual hearing is therefore of high importance as it can provide additional auditory cues and improve speech understanding. There are several factors that can affect the preservation of residual hearing during cochlear implant surgery. These include the surgical approach, the type of cochlear implant being used and the skill of the surgeon. Soft surgery, with its smaller incisions and less invasive approach, may be more likely to preserve residual hearing compared to traditional surgery [10]. However, each patient's situation is unique, and the best approach for preserving residual hearing will depend on the individual's specific needs and circumstances. The delicate process of CI electrode insertion is nevertheless prone to introducing damage to cochlear structures [11–13]. Cochlear damage was shown to relate to long-term neural degeneration [14,15] and was also associated with the loss of residual hearing [16–19].

Cochlear damage due to electrode insertion may be mitigated by less traumatic surgical procedures [20,21] and by the improvement of CI electrode array designs [22–24]. Manufacturers may offer electrode arrays that best match the needs of individuals by providing electrodes with different dimensions that are the most suitable for the candidates. However, cochlear size and morphology are known to have large inter-individual variability [25–27]. To guide electrode development, detailed information is required about the variability of parameters that describe the cochlear size and shape [27]. These parameters can be obtained from computed tomography (CT) images, which are routinely available from CI candidates [28].

Recent studies relating cochlear morphology to CI electrode insertion focused on the establishment of normative datasets and reliable cochlear size measures [28], quantification of internal cochlear dimensions with high precision [27], evaluation of electrode mechanical properties in relation to induced cochlear trauma [29] or the establishment of a mathematical model that describes the shape of the cochlea [30]. In this study, variability and correlation of cochlear parameters, extracted via 3D reconstruction by the Oticon Medical Nautilus software [31], are investigated in a large set of 1099 cochleae. Additionally, intra-patient, inter-patient and inter-sex similarities are also analyzed.

2. Materials and Methods

2.1. Dataset

A total of 590 patients undergoing various treatments at the Institut Universitaire de la Face et du Cou, Nice, France, from 2008 to 2013 were included in this retrospective study. Preoperative temporal bone CT scans were obtained for each patient, constituting a dataset of 1099 CT images comprising 560 right and 539 left scans. The acquired images were of varying quality, with voxel resolutions ranging from $0.187 \times 0.187 \times 0.250$ to $0.316 \times 0.316 \times 0.312$ mm^3. In accordance with the data agreement, EU General Data Protection Regulation (GDPR) and local regulations on data privacy and processing, the dataset was fully pseudonymized before further processing. Therefore, the correspondence between the identifying metadata and the pseudonyms used to identify individual datasets was not available, with the exception of patients' sex. Analysis related to patients' demographics such as origin, age, etc., was beyond the scope of this study.

2.2. Image Analysis

A cooperative multi-agent reinforcement learning framework (C-MARL) as described in [32] was used to automatically detect the cochlear apex, center and round window landmarks for each image. Although only the cochlear center landmark was required for further processing, using a three landmark C-MARL approach ensured better detection of the landmark [33]. CT image-detected cochlear center landmark coordinates, cochlear side and operative status for each CT image were compiled and uploaded to Nautilus (v20220801; Oticon Medical, Vallauris, France)—a web-based cochlear image analysis tool [31].

Nautilus processed the images automatically, generating the cochlear view, intracochlear segmentations and various clinically relevant cochlear parameters. Figure 1 depicts different parameters that Nautilus extracts from each image. Once all the images had been processed, an export bundle was prepared with the following characteristics for analysis: cochlear and ST models, cochlear size, shape, duct lengths and cross-sectional measurements. Nautilus' output confidence scores were also exported and used to filter out any processing failures.

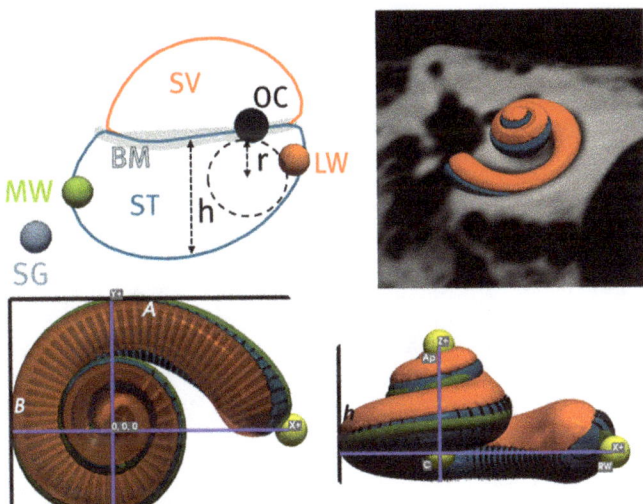

Figure 1. Description of clinical metrics computed by Nautilus. A: maximum length between round window and lateral wall; B: maximum perpendicular length to A. h: height of cochlea; h: maximum vertical ST height; r: radius of maximum circle that can fit in ST; ST: scala tympani; SV: scala vestibuli; BM: basilar membrane; OC: organ of corti; LW: lateral wall; MW: modiolar wall.

2.3. Statistical Analysis

A histogram of the cochlear parameters extracted by Nautilus such as volume, A, B, height, lateral wall (LW) length, the wrapping factor and roller coaster height was generated using 50 bins. Based on the mean and the standard deviation of the parameters, Gaussian curves were plotted on top of the histograms. Correlation analysis was performed via visual inspection of scatter plots and the calculation of the Pearson correlation coefficient between the aforementioned parameters, as well as between parameters A, B and the LW length at various cochlear angles. A regression curve was fitted to the correlation data by the ordinary least squares method. For the correlation and regression analysis, the relevant functions from the SciPy and Scikit-learn python packages were used [34,35].

Analysis of ST height, area and radius was performed up to a cochlear angle of 705°. The mean, standard deviation, 10th and 90th percentile of the ST angular data were calculated based on the data points falling within ±15° of every 30° ST angle, e.g., the metadata at 90° were based on individual data points between 75° and 105°.

Additionally, an intra-patient analysis was conducted to determine the similarity between contralateral ears. Four hundred fifty-eight patients for whom CT imaging was conducted for both ears were selected for the analysis. The ears were assessed with respect to both imaging and clinical metrics. For imaging analysis, the 3D left–right segmentation meshes were registered together based on landmarks [36,37]. Intra-patient Dice coefficients, Hausdorff distances and average symmetric surface distances were computed [38]. An inter-patient analysis was also conducted in which 18 patients were uniformly and randomly selected from the dataset and compared with all other patients ($n = 440$) in the dataset. Global metrics defining cochlear size and shape such as A, B, volume and duct lengths were also evaluated. Statistical *t*-tests with Holm–Sidak correction were performed to analyze the results. A *p*-value of <0.05 was considered significant. A correlation analysis was also performed to determine the relationship between different parameters.

Inter-sex comparison was also carried out based on the cochlear parameters generated by Nautilus. Both size and shape parameters were analyzed to gain insights into whether a distinction could be observed between both sexes. An independent two-sample *t*-test was conducted to determine whether the difference was significant. A *p*-value of <0.05 was considered significant.

3. Results

3.1. Population Statistics and Correlation Analysis

Figure 2 shows a matrix of correlations and histograms of the cochlear parameters where the histograms can be seen to follow a normal distribution [30]. Strong correlations were found between the cochlear volume and all other parameters (B ($\rho = 0.82$, $p < 0.05$), height ($\rho = 0.58$, $p < 0.05$), cochlear duct length ($\rho = 0.74$, $p < 0.05$) and roller coaster height ($\rho = 0.53$, $p < 0.05$)), except for A ($\rho = 0.41$, $p < 0.05$) and the wrapping factor ($\rho = -0.45$, $p < 0.05$). Cochlear volume was negatively correlated with the wrapping factor. In addition to the strong correlation with the cochlear volume, cochlear B also showed a strong positive correlation with LW length ($\rho = 0.74$, $p < 0.05$) and strong negative correlation with the wrapping factor ($\rho = -0.62$, $p < 0.05$). Unsurprisingly, cochlear B was only weakly correlated to cochlear height ($\rho = 0.39$, $p < 0.05$) and roller coaster parameter ($\rho = 0.43$, $p < 0.05$), as these parameters are related to a dimension orthogonal to the plane where cochlear B was measured. In addition to the strong correlation between cochlear height and volume, cochlear height was also strongly correlated with the roller coaster parameter ($\rho = 0.74$, $p < 0.05$), which was measured in the same dimension. Cochlear A did not show any strong correlation with the other parameters. The correlation between cochlear B and A was also weak ($\rho = 0.39$, $p < 0.05$). Figure 3 shows the correlation plots between parameters A, B and the LW length at different cochlear angles (90°, 180°, 270°, 360°, 450°, 540°). In general, B shows a stronger correlation to the LW length than A at all angular insertion depths.

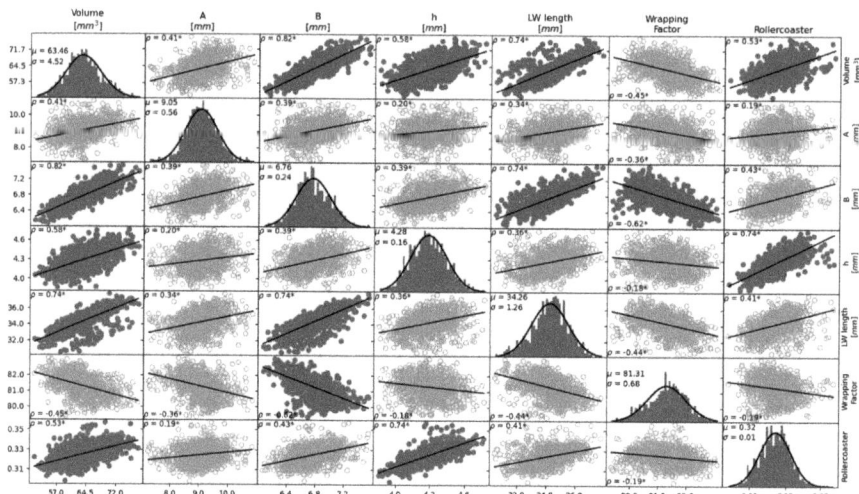

Figure 2. Population statistics and correlation plots between anatomical features of the cochlea. Histograms of the parameters with fitted Gaussian curves are shown in the diagonal of the matrix. Scatter plots show the correlation between the parameter indicated in the column titles and the parameter in the row titles. A strong correlation ($\rho > |0.50|$) between parameters is represented by scatter plots with filled circles and a weak correlation is shown by empty circles. Solid lines indicate the linear regression curves. Note that the scales of the y-axes do not apply to the histograms. ρ: Pearson correlation coefficient; μ: mean; σ: standard deviation; * depicts a significant correlation (*p*-value < 0.05).

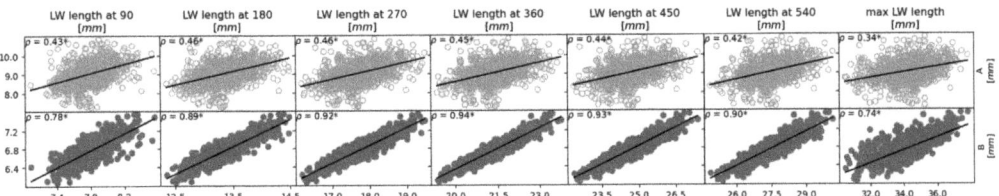

Figure 3. Correlation plots between cochlear duct lengths and cochlear size. A strong correlation ($\rho > |0.50|$) between parameters is represented by scatter plots with filled circles and a weak correlation is shown by empty circles. Solid lines indicate the linear regression curves. ρ: Pearson correlation coefficient, * depicts significant correlation (p-value < 0.05).

Figure 4 shows the evolution of the ST height, area and radius parameters along the cochlea. All investigated ST parameters show a non-monotonic decrease between 0 and 570° followed by an approximately linear decrease up to 690°. Between 0 and 570°, all ST parameters display notches around 150°, 360° and 510°, and local peaks around 270° and 420°. These could be due to the presence of the porous bone surrounding the common cochlear artery [39].

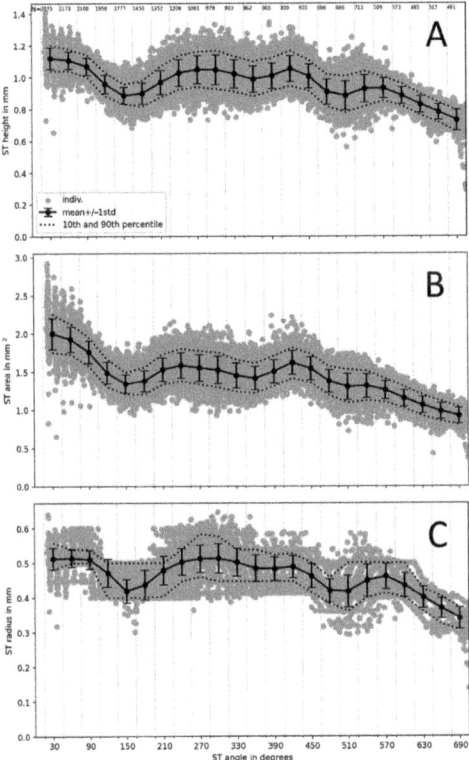

Figure 4. Scala tympani maximum vertical height (**A**), area (**B**) and radius of largest fitted circle (**C**) as a function of the angular distance. Dots represent individual measurement points. Error bars represent the mean and ±1 standard deviation; dotted lines show the 10th and 90th percentiles. Vertical dotted grid lines indicate the angular distance bands that were used to select the N measurement points indicated at the top of panel A to calculate the statistics.

3.2. Inter-Sex Analysis

Figure 5 shows the inter-sex differences between each cochlear parameter. For the male population, the following dimensional characteristics were observed: A (mean: 9.11 ± 0.58 mm, median: 9.13 mm, inter-quartile range (IQR): 0.81 mm), B (6.85 ± 0.25 mm, median: 6.83 mm, IQR: 0.37 mm), height (4.32 ± 0.15 mm, median: 4.31 mm, IQR: 0.22 mm), volume (64.93 ± 4.40 mm3, median: 64.70 mm3, IQR: 5.99 mm^3), cochlear duct length (41.48 ± 1.06 mm, median: 41.56 mm, IQR: 1.61 mm) and the wrapping factor (81.20 ± 0.69°, median: 81.19^0, IQR: 0.97^0). By comparison, the following dimensions were observed for the female population: A (8.97 ± 0.52 mm, median: 8.92 mm, IQR: 0.63 mm), B (6.73 ± 0.21 mm, median: 6.71 mm, IQR: 0.28 mm), height (4.25 ± 0.15 mm, median: 4.24 mm, IQR: 0.21 mm), volume (62.04 ± 3.91 mm^3, median: 41.90 mm^3, IQR: 4.70 mm^3), cochlear duct length (41.07 ± 0.91 mm, median: 40.96 mm, IQR: 1.13 mm) and the wrapping factor (81.30 ± 0.71°, median: 81.36^0, IQR: 0.85^0). An independent *t*-test revealed statistically significant differences for all parameters except the wrapping factor. Generally, female cochleae seem to be smaller and more tightly wound around the modiolus than male cochleae. However, all parameters showed a significant overlap between the two populations.

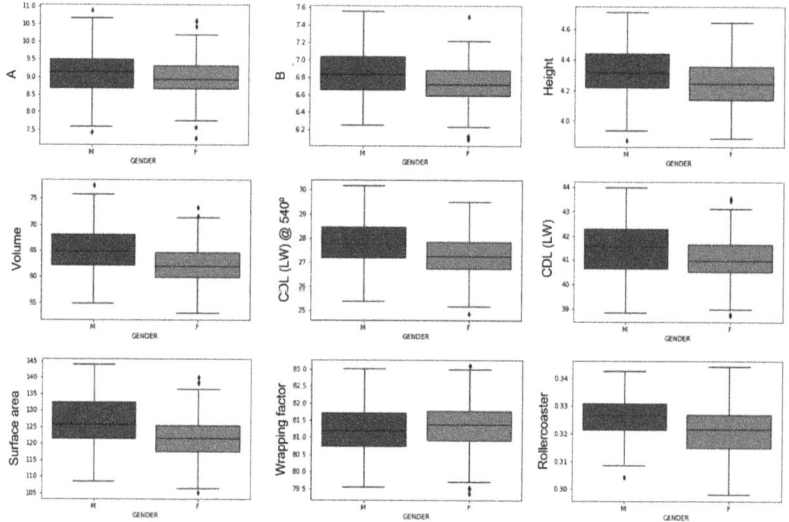

Figure 5. Inter-sex population comparison depicting that female ears are generally smaller and more tightly wound than male ears. CDL (LW): lateral wall cochlear duct length.

3.3. Intra- and Inter-Patient Analysis

The intra-patient analysis yielded mean Dice coefficients of 94.15 ± 0.01% and 91.51 ± 0.02% for cochlea and ST, respectively, indicating high congruency. Similarly, strong correlations were also observed for surface distance metrics (Table 1). The similarity between the cochlea and ST was also high ($\rho > 0.97$, $p < 0.05$), wherein a strong negative correlation was observed between surface distance errors and Dice coefficients ($\rho < -0.99$, $p < 0.05$) (Figure 6).

Table 1. Intra-patient analysis of imaging and clinical parameters. Positive values in the mean column represent a larger right cochlea and vice versa. ASSD: average symmetric surface distance; HD: Hausdorff distance; CDL: cochlear duct length; LW: lateral wall.

Left vs. Right (n = 458)	Absolute Mean	Standard Deviation	Mean	Maximum	Minimum
Dice (ST)	91.51	0.02	-	96.34	81.91
ASSD (ST)	0.05	0.01	-	0.11	0.03
HD (ST)	0.34	0.11	-	1.17	0.14
Dice (CO)	94.15	0.01	-	97.17	85.74
ASSD (CO)	0.07	0.01	-	0.15	0.04
HD (CO)	0.39	0.12	-	1.20	0.16
A (ST)	0.50	0.44	−0.03	2.38	−2.32
A (CO)	0.51	0.44	−0.01	2.21	−2.31
B (CO)	0.08	0.05	0.05	0.30	−0.29
Height	0.07	0.05	0.01	0.29	−0.27
Volume	0.95	0.76	−0.06	5.38	−4.85
Surface area	1.66	1.21	0.63	8.39	−5.26
Wrapping factor	0.31	0.29	−0.08	1.58	−2.22
Wrapping ratio	0.44	0.57	−0.01	3.09	−3.31
Roller coaster	0.004	0.004	−0.001	0.01	−0.03
CDL_LW@90°	0.08	0.07	−0.02	0.36	−0.58
CDL_LW@180°	0.10	0.10	0.01	0.63	−0.64
CDL_LW@270°	0.17	0.13	0.06	0.80	−0.73
CDL_LW@360°	0.22	0.17	0.09	0.97	−0.96
CDL_LW@450°	0.25	0.18	0.11	1.14	−1.15
CDL_LW@540°	0.25	0.20	0.08	1.42	−1.19
CDL_LW	0.56	0.66	0.09	3.86	−3.6
CDL@540° approx. [28]	1.61	1.40	−0.05	6.92	−7.23
CDL approx. [40]	0.71	0.61	0.068	3.08	−3.02
Insertion angle@17 mm	3.33	2.70	−1.15	15.32	−14.88
Insertion angle@19 mm	4.57	3.56	−1.81	20.79	−18.81
Insertion angle@21 mm	5.37	4.10	−2.26	24.50	−20.83
Insertion angle@23 mm	6.35	4.75	−2.77	28.17	−26.46
Insertion angle@25 mm	7.53	5.58	−3.11	34.74	−29.05
Insertion angle@27 mm	8.17	6.27	−2.85	35.87	−35.41

Interestingly, inter-patient analysis also yielded high similarity indexes in terms of imaging analysis, with cochlear and ST Dice coefficients of 93.90 ± 0.05 and 91.04 ± 0.06%, respectively. Statistical analysis revealed no significant difference ($p > 0.05$), even when subdivided into groups based on cochlear size and shape (A, B, wrapping factor). However, the inter-patient variability was four times the intra-patient variability. Another interesting observation was that there was no correlation between imaging and clinical intra-patient metrics (Figure 6). The only correlations observed were with the roller coaster factor ($\rho = 0.45$, $p < 0.05$), B ($\rho = -0.17$, $p < 0.05$) and the wrapping factor ($\rho = 0.14$, $p < 0.05$).

Concerning the clinical metrics defining the size and shape of the cochlea, intra-patient analysis revealed a mean difference of 0.01 and 0.05 mm for dimensions A and B, respectively, suggesting that neither of the sides is generally larger than the other. By contrast, a mean absolute difference of 0.50 and 0.08 mm was observed for the same parameters. The t-test revealed a statistical difference ($p < 0.05$) for most of the clinical metrics, suggesting that size and shape of contralateral ears are not the same. Interestingly, the well-known size metrics A, CDL and volume did not reveal a significant difference (Figure 6).

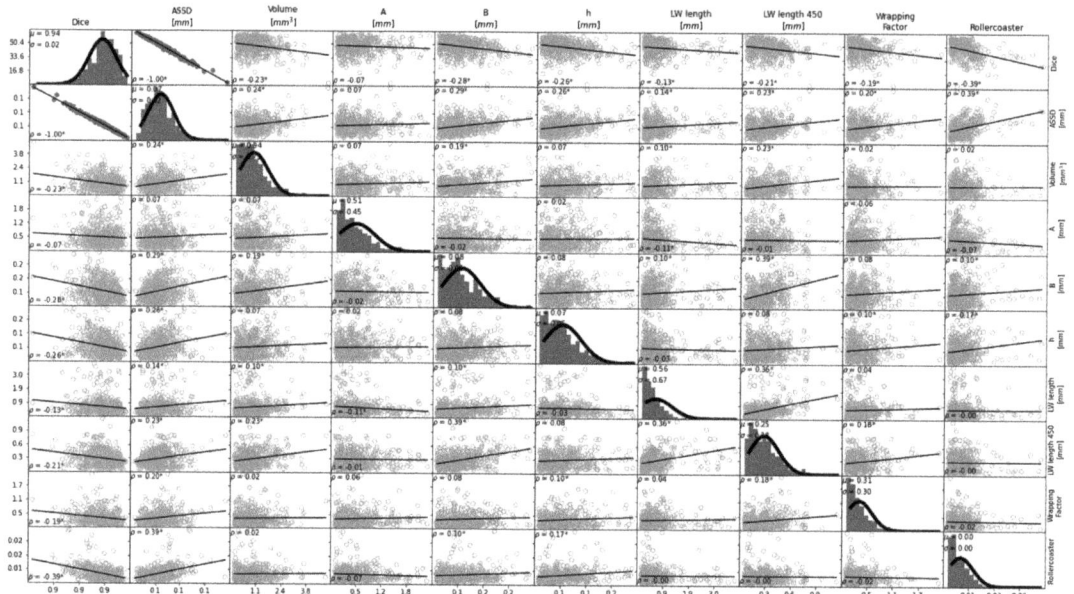

Figure 6. Intra-patient population and comparative correlation plots for imaging and clinical parameters. Strong correlations ($\rho > |0.50|$) between parameters are represented by scatter plots with filled circles and weak correlations are shown by empty circles. P: Pearson correlation coefficient; μ: mean; σ: standard deviation; * depicts significant relation (p-value < 0.05).

The difference in B showed medium correlations with differences in cochlear duct lengths ($\rho = 0.28$–0.54, $p < 0.05$), wrapping factor ($\rho = -0.2$, $p < 0.05$), volume ($\rho = 0.49$, $p < 0.05$) and surface area ($\rho = 0.56$, $p < 0.05$), whereas A only showed weak correlations with cochlear duct length ($\rho = 0.12$–0.15, $p < 0.05$) and the wrapping factor ($\rho = -0.10$, $p < 0.05$). The roller coaster factor correlated with the height of the cochlea ($\rho = 0.463$, $p < 0.05$), whereas the discretized duct lengths showed medium and low correlations with most metrics ($\rho < 0.66$, $p < 0.05$).

4. Discussion

There is a need for large, automated population studies on cochlear anatomy to improve our understanding of the structure and its implications for CI surgery. The goal of this study was to better understand the anatomy of the cochlea and its variability in size and shape, which is important for developing less traumatic electrode arrays and insertion guidance for cochlear implantation surgery. The shape and size of the cochlea can also influence the choice of cochlear implant electrode, with flexible electrode arrays being preferred for more complex cochlear shapes, whilst rigid electrodes are more suitable for cochleae with a more straightforward shape and ossifications. Knowledge of the density and location of spiral ganglion cells can help surgeons choose an electrode array that is most likely to provide good electrical contact with the spiral ganglion cells coupled with minimal frequency mismatch and therefore exhibiting the best hearing outcomes for the patient [41]. In addition, knowledge of cochlear morphology can help surgeons in identifying any abnormalities or variations in the anatomy of the cochlea that may impact on the placement or function of the cochlear implant electrode. By understanding these variations, surgeons can tailor their surgical approach to the specific needs of each patient.

Previous studies have mostly focused on the size, rather than the shape and other parameters, and have only been able to analyze a small number of temporal bones due to the time-consuming nature of manual measurements which limits the scope of the analysis.

The use of automated analysis is particularly important in the context of cochlear implant surgery, as manual measurements can be time-consuming and inconsistent. For example, a recent study found that manual measurements of cochlear duct length (CDL) had a maximum absolute intra-rater difference of 3.2 mm and the intra-rater reliability between the two radiological methods used in the study was only 0.65–0.84 [42], indicating that manual measurements may not be reliable. Furthermore, manual measurements were deemed reliable only up to 720 degrees in both CT and MRI scans.

Recent advances in automated analysis tools such as CoreSlicer 2.0 (CoreSlicer, Montreal, QC, Canada), Innersight 3D (Innersight Labs, London, UK), Arterys (Arterys Inc., Redwood Shores, CA, USA), etc., have made it possible to conduct larger studies with more robust and reliable results, as demonstrated in a recent study on cardiac anatomy which showed the feasibility and reliability of using automated analysis tools for population studies [43]; thus, similar approaches can be applied to cochlear anatomy. This study analyzed a large number of clinical temporal bone CT images using Nautilus (v20220801; Oticon Medical [31]) to determine cochlear morphology and characteristics, making it more efficient and robust than manual measurements. Nautilus is a web-based image analysis tool that supports the automatic analysis of pre-operative surgical planning and post-operative assessment for cochlear implant procedures; additionally, it has the potential to influence the intraoperative workflow in an augmented reality setup and to control insertion forces and trajectories.

The analysis showed that cochlear morphology follows a Gaussian distribution, meaning that most cochleae fall within a typical range of sizes and shapes, with relatively few individuals falling outside of this range. Multiple recent studies have drafted cochlear duct-length prediction models based mainly on dimension A or a combination and dimensions A and B [28,40,44]. Another advantage of using AI-based automatic segmentation tools is that duct lengths can be easily computed in the original image space, decreasing dependence on such mathematical models.

Cochlear dimensions A and B were observed not to be well-correlated with each other. The study also suggests that dimension B is more correlated with cochlear duct lengths, the wrapping factor and volume than dimension A, contrary to popular belief. This suggests that cochlear B may be a more important factor in determining the optimum diameter and length of the electrode array. Moreover, the correlation between cochlear dimensions and discretized duct length increases as the cochlear angle increases, further supporting this observation.

Additionally, the study found that cochleae in female populations tend to be smaller and more tightly wound around the modiolus than male cochleae, but there is a significant overlap between the two populations. There is also a need to study the inter- and intra-individual variability of cochlear anatomy, as this can impact on the reliability of population statistics and the generalizability of findings. Some studies have suggested using contralateral ear CT images when a preoperative CT image for the target ear is not available [45]. However, more research is needed to confirm this and determine the extent of the variability addressed in this study. On average, the dimensions of both ears are similar, but there are statistically significant intra-individual differences in clinically relevant dimensions. This suggests that, while the average size and shape of the cochlea may be similar between the left and right ears, there can be significant differences between the two ears of an individual. However, the results showed that inter-individual variability is four times greater than intra-individual variability, suggesting that contralateral ear CT may be used for analysis only as a last resort if preoperative imaging is not available.

The study also found that the scala tympani size varies considerably among the population, generally decreasing along the insertion depth with dimensional jumps along the trajectory (also observed in a previous study on μCT images [27]). This means that the size of the scala tympani can change significantly as the electrode array is inserted. These findings can help reduce insertion trauma and preserve residual hearing, which, in turn, may impact on the performance of the implant.

In conclusion, the results of the study suggest that certain cochlear parameters are strongly correlated and there are sex-based differences in cochlear dimensions. The results also suggest that it may be necessary to use individualized cochlear models to accurately predict surgical outcomes and optimize implant design. The implications of this research are significant for CI surgery. The size and shape of the cochlea can affect residual hearing, as well as the translocation and tip foldovers/buckling of the electrode array. The mean size and shape of the cochlea, as well as its cross-sectional analysis along the spiral, can provide important information for determining the optimum diameter and length of the electrode array, leading to better hearing outcomes for patients.

Author Contributions: Conceptualization, H.D., F.P., C.R., C.V. and N.G.; methodology, R.H., A.F. and J.M.; software, R.H., A.F., J.M. and Z.W.; validation, R.H. and A.F.; formal analysis, R.H., A.F. and C.K.; investigation, R.H., A.F., R.C., C.V. and N.G.; resources, R.C., H.D., F.P. and N.G.; data curation, Z.W., C.R. and C.V.; writing—original draft preparation, R.H., A.F. and C.K.; writing—review and editing, R.H., A.F., R.C., C.K., J.M., Z.W., M.H., H.D., F.P., C.R., C.V. and N.G.; visualization, R.H., A.F. and J.M.; supervision, R.C., M.H., H.D., F.P. and N.G.; project administration, R.C., H.D., F.P. and N.G.; funding acquisition, H.D., F.P. and N.G. All authors have read and agreed to the published version of the manuscript.

Funding: This research received no external funding.

Institutional Review Board Statement: The study was conducted in accordance with the data agreement, EU General Data Protection Regulation (GDPR) and local regulations on data privacy and processing that govern the use of anonymized data provided under an agreement between CHU Nice, INRIA and Oticon Medical.

Informed Consent Statement: Informed consent was obtained from all patients, and all experiments were performed in accordance with relevant guidelines, regulations and in accordance with the Declaration of Helsinki.

Data Availability Statement: The dataset analyzed within the scope of the current study cannot be made publicly available, as it has been made available to the authors under the specific authorization of CHU Nice. This authorization does not extend to the public publication and distribution of the data. Access to the Nautilus tool is, however, available upon reasonable request at raui@oticonmedical.com.

Acknowledgments: The authors would like to thank Stephane Hlavacek for assistance during data processing.

Conflicts of Interest: R.H., A.F., R.C., C.K., M.H. and F.P. are employed at Oticon Medical, France, developers of the Nautilus tool. J.M. works as a consultant for the same company. The remaining authors declare no conflict of interest.

References

1. Seyyedi, M.; Viana, L.M.; Nadol, J.B., Jr. Within-Subject Comparison of Word Recognition and Spiral Ganglion Cell Count in Bilateral Cochlear Implant Recipients. *Otol. Neurotol.* **2014**, *35*, 1446–1450. [CrossRef] [PubMed]
2. Pfingst, B.E.; Zhou, N.; Colesa, D.J.; Watts, M.M.; Strahl, S.B.; Garadat, S.N.; Schvartz-Leyzac, K.C.; Budenz, C.L.; Raphael, Y.; Zwolan, T.A. Importance of Cochlear Health for Implant Function. *Hear. Res.* **2015**, *322*, 77–88. [CrossRef]
3. Gstöttner, W.; Kiefer, J.; Baumgartner, W.D.; Pok, S.; Peters, S.; Adunka, O.F. Hearing Preservation in Cochlear Implantation for Electric Acoustic Stimulation. *Acta Oto-Laryngol.* **2004**, *124*, 348–352. [CrossRef] [PubMed]
4. Sampaio, A.L.L.; Araújo, M.F.S.; Oliveira, C.A.C.P. New Criteria of Indication and Selection of Patients to Cochlear Implant. *Int. J. Otolaryngol.* **2011**, *2011*, 573968. [CrossRef]
5. Adunka, O.F.; Dillon, M.T.; Adunka, M.C.; King, E.R.; Pillsbury, H.C.; Buchman, C.A. Hearing Preservation and Speech Perception Outcomes with Electric-Acoustic Stimulation after 12 Months of Listening Experience. *Laryngoscope* **2013**, *123*, 2509–2515. [CrossRef] [PubMed]
6. Büchner, A.; Schüssler, M.; Battmer, R.D.; Stöver, T.; Lesinski-Schiedat, A.; Lenarz, T. Impact of Low-Frequency Hearing. *Audiol. Neurotol.* **2009**, *14* (Suppl. 1), 8–13. [CrossRef] [PubMed]
7. Gantz, B.J.; Turner, C.; Gfeller, K.E.; Lowder, M.W. Preservation of Hearing in Cochlear Implant Surgery: Advantages of Combined Electrical and Acoustical Speech Processing. *Laryngoscope* **2005**, *115*, 796–802. [CrossRef] [PubMed]
8. Gifford, R.H.; Dorman, M.F.; Skarzynski, H.; Lorens, A.; Polak, M.; Driscoll, C.L.W.; Roland, P.; Buchman, C.A. Cochlear Implantation with Hearing Preservation Yields Significant Benefit for Speech Recognition in Complex Listening Environments. *Ear Hear.* **2013**, *34*, 413–425. [CrossRef]

9. Irving, S.; Gillespie, L.; Richardson, R.; Rowe, D.; Fallon, J.B.; Wise, A.K. Electroacoustic Stimulation: Now and into the Future. *BioMed Res. Int.* **2014**, *2014*, 350504. [CrossRef]
10. Freni, F.; Gazia, F.; Slavutsky, V.; Scherdel, E.P.; Nicenboim, L.; Posada, R.; Portelli, D.; Galletti, B.; Galletti, F. Cochlear Implant Surgery: Endomeatal Approach versus Posterior Tympanotomy. *Int. J. Environ. Res. Public Health* **2020**, *17*, 4187. [CrossRef]
11. Helbig, S.; Settevendemie, C.; Mack, M.; Baumann, U.; Helbig, M.; Stöver, T. Evaluation of an Electrode Prototype for Atraumatic Cochlear Implantation in Hearing Preservation Candidates: Preliminary Results from a Temporal Bone Study. *Otol. Neurotol.* **2011**, *32*, 419–423. [CrossRef] [PubMed]
12. Kha, H.; Chen, B. Finite Element Analysis of Damage by Cochlear Implant Electrode Array's Proximal Section to the Basilar Membrane. *Otol. Neurotol.* **2012**, *33*, 1176–1180. [CrossRef] [PubMed]
13. Wardrop, P.; Whinney, D.; Rebscher, S.J.; Luxford, W.; Leake, P. A Temporal Bone Study of Insertion Trauma and Intracochlear Position of Cochlear Implant Electrodes. II: Comparison of Spiral Clarion and HiFocus II Electrodes. *Hear. Res.* **2005**, *203*, 68–79. [CrossRef] [PubMed]
14. Adunka, O.; Kiefer, J. Impact of Electrode Insertion Depth on Intracochlear Trauma. *Otolaryngol. Head Neck Surg.* **2006**, *135*, 374–382. [CrossRef] [PubMed]
15. Roland, P.S.; Wright, C.G. Surgical Aspects of Cochlear Implantation: Mechanisms of Insertional Trauma. *Adv. Otorhinolaryngol.* **2006**, *64*, 11–30. [CrossRef]
16. Cullen, R.D.; Higgins, C.; Buss, E.; Clark, M.; Pillsbury, H.C., 3rd; Buchman, C.A. Cochlear Implantation in Patients with Substantial Residual Hearing. *Laryngoscope* **2004**, *114*, 2218–2223. [CrossRef]
17. Gantz, B.J.; Turner, C.W. Combining Acoustic and Electrical Hearing. *Laryngoscope* **2003**, *113*, 1726–1730. [CrossRef]
18. Ishiyama, A.; Doherty, J.; Ishiyama, G.; Quesnel, A.M.; Lopez, I.; Linthicum, F.H. Post Hybrid Cochlear Implant Hearing Loss and Endolymphatic Hydrops. *Otol. Neurotol.* **2016**, *37*, 1516–1521. [CrossRef]
19. Ishiyama, A.; Ishiyama, G.; Lopez, I.A.; Linthicum, F.H., Jr. Temporal Bone Histopathology of First-Generation Cochlear Implant Electrode Translocation. *Otol. Neurotol.* **2019**, *40*, e581–e591. [CrossRef]
20. Lehnhardt, E. Intracochlear Placement of Cochlear Implant Electrodes in Soft Surgery Technique. *HNO* **1993**, *41*, 356–359.
21. Friedland, D.R.; Runge-Samuelson, C. Soft Cochlear Implantation: Rationale for the Surgical Approach. *Trends Amplif.* **2009**, *13*, 124–138. [CrossRef]
22. Briggs, R.J.S.; Tykocinski, M.; Xu, J.; Risi, F.; Svehla, M.; Cowan, R.; Stover, T.; Erfurt, P.; Lenarz, T. Comparison of Round Window and Cochleostomy Approaches with a Prototype Hearing Preservation Electrode. *Audiol. Neurotol.* **2006**, *11* (Suppl. 1), 42–48. [CrossRef] [PubMed]
23. Hochmair, I.; Hochmair, E.; Nopp, P.; Waller, M.; Jolly, C. Deep Electrode Insertion and Sound Coding in Cochlear Implants. *Hear. Res.* **2015**, *322*, 14–23. [CrossRef] [PubMed]
24. Helbig, S.; Adel, Y.; Rader, T.; Stöver, T.; Baumann, U. Long-Term Hearing Preservation Outcomes after Cochlear Implantation for Electric-Acoustic Stimulation. *Otol. Neurotol.* **2016**, *37*, e353–e359. [CrossRef] [PubMed]
25. Erixon, E.; Högstorp, H.; Wadin, K.; Rask-Andersen, H. Variational Anatomy of the Human Cochlea: Implications for Cochlear Implantation. *Otol. Neurotol.* **2009**, *30*, 14–22. [CrossRef]
26. Rask-Andersen, H.; Liu, W.; Erixon, E.; Kinnefors, A.; Pfaller, K.; Schrott-Fischer, A.; Glueckert, R. Human Cochlea: Anatomical Characteristics and Their Relevance for Cochlear Implantation. *Anat. Rec.* **2012**, *295*, 1791–1811. [CrossRef]
27. Avci, E.; Nauwelaers, T.; Lenarz, T.; Hamacher, V.; Kral, A. Variations in Microanatomy of the Human Cochlea: Variations in Microanatomy of the Human Cochlea. *J. Comp. Neurol.* **2014**, *522*, 3245–3261. [CrossRef] [PubMed]
28. Escudé, B.; James, C.; Deguine, O.; Cochard, N.; Eter, E.; Fraysse, B. The Size of the Cochlea and Predictions of Insertion Depth Angles for Cochlear Implant Electrodes. *Audiol. Neurootol.* **2006**, *11* (Suppl. 1), 27–33. [CrossRef]
29. Rebscher, S.J.; Hetherington, A.; Bonham, B.; Wardrop, P.; Whinney, D.; Leake, P.A. Considerations for Design of Future Cochlear Implant Electrode Arrays: Electrode Array Stiffness, Size, and Depth of Insertion. *J. Rehabil. Res. Dev.* **2008**, *45*, 731–747. [CrossRef]
30. Pietsch, M.; Aguirre Dávila, L.; Erfurt, P.; Avci, E.; Lenarz, T.; Kral, A. Spiral Form of the Human Cochlea Results from Spatial Constraints. *Sci. Rep.* **2017**, *7*, 7500. [CrossRef] [PubMed]
31. Margeta, J.; Hussain, R.; López Diez, P.; Morgenstern, A.; Demarcy, T.; Wang, Z.; Gnansia, D.; Martinez Manzanera, O.; Vandersteen, C.; Delingette, H.; et al. A Web-Based Automated Image Processing Research Platform for Cochlear Implantation-Related Studies. *J. Clin. Med.* **2022**, *11*, 6640. [CrossRef] [PubMed]
32. López Diez, P.; Sundgaard, J.V.; Patou, F.; Margeta, J.; Paulsen, R.R. Facial and Cochlear Nerves Characterization Using Deep Reinforcement Learning for Landmark Detection. In *Medical Image Computing and Computer Assisted Intervention—MICCAI 2021*; Springer International Publishing: Cham, Switzerland, 2021; pp. 519–528.
33. Leroy, G.; Rueckert, D.; Alansary, A. Communicative Reinforcement Learning Agents for Landmark Detection in Brain Images. In *Machine Learning in Clinical Neuroimaging and Radiogenomics in Neuro-Oncology*; Springer International Publishing: Cham, Switzerland, 2020; pp. 177–186.
34. Virtanen, P.; Gommers, R.; Oliphant, T.E.; Haberland, M.; Reddy, T.; Cournapeau, D.; Burovski, E.; Peterson, P.; Weckesser, W.; Bright, J.; et al. Author Correction: SciPy 1.0: Fundamental Algorithms for Scientific Computing in Python. *Nat. Methods* **2020**, *17*, 352. [CrossRef] [PubMed]

35. Pedregosa, F.; Varoquaux, G.; Gramfort, A.; Michel, V.; Thirion, B.; Grisel, O.; Blondel, M.; Müller, A.; Nothman, J.; Louppe, G.; et al. Scikit-Learn: Machine Learning in Python. *J. Mach. Learn. Res.* **2011**, *12*, 2825–2830. Available online: https://jmlr.org/papers/v12/pedregosa11a.html (accessed on 5 July 2022).
36. Yaniv, Z.; Lowekamp, B.C.; Johnson, H.J.; Beare, R. SimpleITK Image-Analysis Notebooks: A Collaborative Environment for Education and Reproducible Research. *J. Digit. Imaging* **2018**, *31*, 290–303. [CrossRef] [PubMed]
37. Hussain, R.; Lalande, A.; Marroquin, R.; Guigou, C.; Bozorg Grayeli, A. Video-Based Augmented Reality Combining CT-Scan and Instrument Position Data to Microscope View in Middle Ear Surgery. *Sci. Rep.* **2020**, *10*, 6767. [CrossRef]
38. Taha, A.A.; Hanbury, A. Metrics for Evaluating 3D Medical Image Segmentation: Analysis, Selection, and Tool. *BMC Med. Imaging* **2015**, *15*, 29. [CrossRef]
39. Mei, X.; Atturo, F.; Wadin, K.; Larsson, S.; Agrawal, S.; Ladak, H.M.; Li, H.; Rask-Andersen, H. Human Inner Ear Blood Supply Revisited: The Uppsala Collection of Temporal Bone-an International Resource of Education and Collaboration. *Upsala J. Med. Sci.* **2018**, *123*, 131–142. [CrossRef]
40. Schurzig, D.; Timm, M.E.; Batsoulis, C.; Salcher, R.; Sieber, D.; Jolly, C.; Lenarz, T.; Zoka-Assadi, M. A Novel Method for Clinical Cochlear Duct Length Estimation toward Patient-Specific Cochlear Implant Selection. *OTO Open* **2018**, *2*, 4. [CrossRef]
41. Goupell, M.J.; Stoelb, C.A.; Kan, A.; Litovsky, R.Y. The Effect of Simulated Interaural Frequency Mismatch on Speech Understanding and Spatial Release from Masking. *Ear Hear.* **2018**, *39*, 895–905. [CrossRef]
42. Thomas, J.; Klein, H.; Dazert, S.; Völter, C. Length Measurement of Cochlear Parameters Prior to Cochlear Implantation—Comparison of CT- vs. MRI-Based Results. In *Abstract- und Posterband—93. Jahresversammlung der Deutschen Gesellschaft für HNO-Heilkunde, Kopf- und Hals-Chirurgie e.V., Bonn Interface—Fokus Mensch im Zeitalter der Techniserten Medizin*; Georg Thieme: Leipzig, Germany, 2022.
43. Pirruccello, J.P.; Di Achille, P.; Nauffal, V.; Nekoui, M.; Friedman, S.F.; Klarqvist, M.D.R.; Chaffin, M.D.; Weng, L.-C.; Cunningham, J.W.; Khurshid, S.; et al. Genetic Analysis of Right Heart Structure and Function in 40,000 People. *Nat. Genet.* **2022**, *54*, 792–803. [CrossRef]
44. Alexiades, G.; Dhanasingh, A.; Jolly, C. Method to Estimate the Complete and Two-Turn Cochlear Duct Length. *Otol. Neurotol.* **2015**, *36*, 904–907. [CrossRef] [PubMed]
45. Reda, F.A.; McRackan, T.R.; Labadie, R.F.; Dawant, B.M.; Noble, J.H. Automatic Segmentation of Intra-Cochlear Anatomy in Post-Implantation CT of Unilateral Cochlear Implant Recipients. *Med. Image Anal.* **2014**, *18*, 605–615. [CrossRef] [PubMed]

Disclaimer/Publisher's Note: The statements, opinions and data contained in all publications are solely those of the individual author(s) and contributor(s) and not of MDPI and/or the editor(s). MDPI and/or the editor(s) disclaim responsibility for any injury to people or property resulting from any ideas, methods, instructions or products referred to in the content.

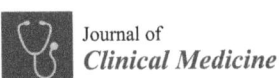

Article

A Web-Based Automated Image Processing Research Platform for Cochlear Implantation-Related Studies

Jan Margeta [1,*], Raabid Hussain [2], Paula López Diez [3], Anika Morgenstern [4], Thomas Demarcy [2], Zihao Wang [5], Dan Gnansia [2], Octavio Martinez Manzanera [2], Clair Vandersteen [6], Hervé Delingette [5], Andreas Buechner [4], Thomas Lenarz [4], François Patou [2] and Nicolas Guevara [6]

1 Research and Development, KardioMe, 01851 Nova Dubnica, Slovakia
2 Research and Technology Group, Oticon Medical, 2765 Smørum, Denmark
3 Department for Applied Mathematics and Computer Science, Technical University of Denmark, 2800 Kongens Lyngby, Denmark
4 Department of Otolaryngology, Medical University of Hannover, 30625 Hannover, Germany
5 Epione Team, Inria, Université Côte d'Azur, 06902 Sophia Antipolis, France
6 Institut Universitaire de la Face et du Cou, Centre Hospitalier Universitaire de Nice, Université Côte d'Azur, 06100 Nice, France
* Correspondence: jan@kardio.me

Abstract: The robust delineation of the cochlea and its inner structures combined with the detection of the electrode of a cochlear implant within these structures is essential for envisaging a safer, more individualized, routine image-guided cochlear implant therapy. We present Nautilus—a web-based research platform for automated pre- and post-implantation cochlear analysis. Nautilus delineates cochlear structures from pre-operative clinical CT images by combining deep learning and Bayesian inference approaches. It enables the extraction of electrode locations from a post-operative CT image using convolutional neural networks and geometrical inference. By fusing pre- and post-operative images, Nautilus is able to provide a set of personalized pre- and post-operative metrics that can serve the exploration of clinically relevant questions in cochlear implantation therapy. In addition, Nautilus embeds a self-assessment module providing a confidence rating on the outputs of its pipeline. We present a detailed accuracy and robustness analyses of the tool on a carefully designed dataset. The results of these analyses provide legitimate grounds for envisaging the implementation of image-guided cochlear implant practices into routine clinical workflows.

Keywords: cochlea; cochlear implant; image analysis; computed tomography; machine learning; deep learning; image segmentation; 3D model; tonotopic mapping; visualization

Citation: Margeta, J.; Hussain, R.; López Diez, P.; Morgenstern, A.; Demarcy, T.; Wang, Z.; Gnansia, D.; Martinez Manzanera, O.; Vandersteen, C.; Delingette, H.; et al. A Web-Based Automated Image Processing Research Platform for Cochlear Implantation-Related Studies. *J. Clin. Med.* **2022**, *11*, 6640. https://doi.org/10.3390/jcm11226640

Academic Editor: Giuseppe Magliulo

Received: 5 October 2022
Accepted: 28 October 2022
Published: 9 November 2022

Publisher's Note: MDPI stays neutral with regard to jurisdictional claims in published maps and institutional affiliations.

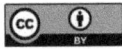

Copyright: © 2022 by the authors. Licensee MDPI, Basel, Switzerland. This article is an open access article distributed under the terms and conditions of the Creative Commons Attribution (CC BY) license (https://creativecommons.org/licenses/by/4.0/).

1. Introduction

Cochlear Implants (CI) are, to this day, the most successful neural interfaces ever engineered judging by their functional outcomes benefits, gains in quality of life, or widespread adoption in standard clinical practice [1]. More than 700,000 CI users worldwide have been eligible for and are undergoing CI therapy because of severe or profound deafness [2]. CI systems are neuroprosthetic devices generally composed of two parts. The first part is an external device called the sound processor and is usually worn behind the ear. It is responsible for real-time sensing, processing, and transmitting acoustic information (i.e., sound) to the other, internal, surgically implanted part of the system. This second part is in charge for transmitting the encoded acoustic information content to the auditory nerve by way of trains of electrical impulses delivered through an electrode array placed in the cochlea [2]. CI systems therefore bypass the cochlea altogether and replace the natural hearing mechanism with what is often referred to as "electrical hearing".

Despite its large overall success, CI therapy still presents significant shortcomings. In particular, documented clinical outcomes remain variable and generally not fully predictable. Additionally, perceptual adaptation to CI hearing, even when functionally successful in terms of speech recognition and communication abilities, often remain unsatisfactory when it comes to real-life scenarios, including complex, spatial, and musical soundscapes [1]. A large body of knowledge points to anatomical factors and our current limited ability to assess patient-specific cochlear anatomy (pre-implantation) and its relation to CI electrode placement (post-implantation) as impediments to the development of more adapted best practices in surgical and audiological CI therapy. The intrinsic inter-individual variability of inner ear anatomy, for instance, compounds the challenge to predict the insertion dynamics of a specific CI electrode, making it difficult to plan and predict how deep a surgeon may expect to insert the CI electrode, which may have consequences on the low-frequency percepts that the implant may be able to elicit—also known as a consequence for the preservation of residual hearing. Likewise, the challenge of assessing where exactly the electrode contacts lay within the cochlea post-operatively prevents a CI device fitting/programming that takes into account the natural tonotopicity of the spiral ganglions lining up the cochlea or the consideration of the fitting parameters set for the contra-lateral ear in bilateral CI users [3–5]. A common denominator to these aspects is, therefore, the need for an intimate assessment of individual anatomy and geometry of cochlear structures and CI electrode placement relative to these structures in individuals from various clinical population eligible for CI therapy. Importantly, if some of the mechanisms at play in limiting CI therapy performance outcomes (whichever ones we look at) are known, much obscurity remains as to how to harness individual anatomical information to optimize and personalize CI therapy in relevant clinical populations.

Nautilus is a web-based research-grade tool that allows the automated, accurate, robust, and uncertainty-transparent delineation of the cochlea, scala tympani (ST), scala vestibuli (SV), and of the electrode arrays with tonotopic mapping from conventional computed tomography (CT) and cone-beam computed tomography (CBCT) images (see Figure 1).

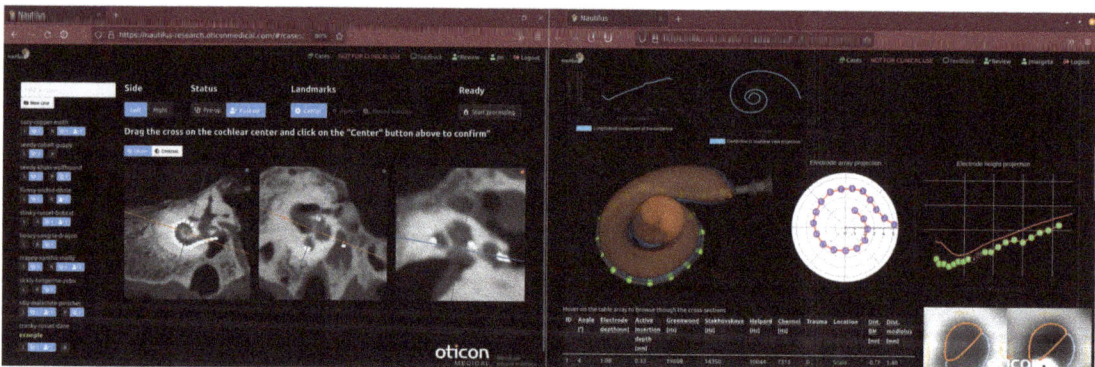

Figure 1. Nautilus offers a comprehensive set of research tools for pre- and post-operative cochlear image analysis for CI implantation and interactive visualization via a web browser. A number of metrics and additional outputs are generated by the pipeline and are made available for data export (e.g., spreadsheet of metrics for all cochleae in a user's collection or STL models of the cochlear meshes) for further data analysis and applications (e.g., simulation or 3D printing, novel electrode array development).

Background

The development of an automated imaging pipeline enabling the exploration of cochlear anatomy in clinical populations represents a significant challenge. The cochlear structures relevant to CI therapy, specifically the ST and SV, and the CI electrode array cannot always be easily delineated from clinical CT or CBCT images due to low image contrast and poor resolution. This prevents the manual delineation of ST and SV, which would anyway be a time-consuming, error-prone, and inconsistent process. More reasonably, semi- and fully automatic frameworks have been proposed to segment the cochlear bony labyrinth from pre-operative CT images. Earlier works focused on traditional segmentation techniques, such as level-set and interactive contour algorithms [6,7]. However, these required user input, were computationally time-consuming, and often led to incomplete segmentations. Recent works have focused on designing fully automatic convolutional neural networks capable of handling the intricate anatomy of the bony labyrinth [8–11]. The bony labyrinth is generally well identifiable in clinical CT or CBCT images, but its robust segmentation remains a challenge if one is to process images acquired with different scanners and image acquisition parameters, which may manifest in ranges of image resolution, contrast, and noise. Provided with a delineation of the bony labyrinth, various techniques permit the estimation of important metrics relevant to CI implantation, such as the cochlear duct length (CDL), which serves as an indicator of general cochlear size and what depth of insertion is reasonable to try to reach for that specific cochlea. The CDL and other metrics also enable the computation of normalized tonotopic frequencies according to Greenwood [12], Stakhovskaya [13], or Helpard et al. [14].

For all the information that can be gained from a segmentation of the bony labyrinth, many clinical questions call for the differentiation of ST from SV within the labyrinth. In this case, the automated image processing task becomes much more complex, since ST and SV are generally not visible in clinical CTs or CBCTs. Consequently, various atlases or shape models derived from temporal bone micro-CTs (µCTs) have been proposed to infer a ST/SV differentiation within the bony labyrinth when exploiting a clinical image [15–20]. The delineation of ST and SV is interesting in that CI implantation is preferentially done within ST as implantations or translocations in SV have been associated with observations of auditory pitch reversals and poorer speech intelligibility [21,22].

Post-operatively, CT imaging can provide information about the positioning of each electrode contact within or in the vicinity of the cochlea. However, the exploitation of post-operative CT/CBCT images is often compromised by metal artifacts emanating from the electrodes but generally affecting the region of interest around the electrodes enough so as to prevent the delineation of the bony labyrinth. Therefore, the post-implantation reconstruction of the CI electrode within cochlear structures often requires harnessing both the pre-operative and post-operative scans. Vanderbilt University's group first proposed to independently segment intra-cochlear structures from pre-operative images using active shape models, followed by detection of the electrode array midline from post-operative imaging before combining pre- and post-operative information through a rigid registration [23]. They also proposed to take advantage of the left/right symmetry of inner-ear anatomy by utilizing the pre-operative image of the normal contra-lateral ear for cochlear structure delineation for cases where pre-operative CT images were not available [24]. Granting the successful reconstruction of electrode placement within cochlear structures, the characteristic frequency (CF) at each contact can legitimately be computed at the estimated corresponding place on the organ of Corti (OC) [12] or at the nearest spiral ganglion (SG) [13,14,25]. The accurate inference of the relative position between an electrode and the basilar membrane (BM) lining up the ST can also enable the assessment of the potential translocation of the electrode in SV or inferential predictions of the degree of traumaticity of the insertion, e.g., if the electrode were to have either elevated or ripped through the BM and entered the SV. Although state-of-the-art research on cochlear imaging has resulted in imaging pipelines that do display accuracy levels that can warrant their use in specific settings, these pipelines have generally not been subject to a strict robustness evaluation: their ability to deal with images of heterogeneous quality as one may expect to have to deal with when working on datasets obtained across different clinical centers. Searching to facilitate the exploration of clinical questions related to the anatomical and geometrical considerations of CI therapy, Nautilus enables the automated, accurate, robust, and transparent-on-uncertainty segmentation of the cochlear bony labyrinth, ST, and SV from pre-operative CT/CBCTs. Post-operatively, Nautilus enables the automated identification and reconstruction of the electrode arrays within the cochlear structures extracted from the pre-operative image. This tool computes a range of metrics relevant to both surgical and audiological research in CI, including the characteristic frequencies at each electrode contact. Nautilus' predictions have been evaluated against several datasets annotated by experts and demonstrate state-of-the-art accuracy. Importantly, Nautilus was designed and stress-tested against images spanning a range of resolution, contrast, and noise, which results in its robust applicability, especially for a set of image input specifications that promote success, as we discuss later. Finally, the tool intends to transparently notify users of possible processing failures or complications using a set of caution flags to allow for the rejection of data points that may otherwise bias analysis.

2. Methods

Nautilus aims to be a gateway to advanced cochlear analysis. To maximize its availability, it has therefore been designed as a web application accessible via any modern web browser (e.g., Mozilla Firefox, Google Chrome, or Microsoft Edge) with no need for additional installation nor excessive requirements on the hardware. The data processing happens transparently on a cloud computing service. An overview of the processing pipeline can be seen in Figure 2, with Figure 3 illustrating the intermediary outputs of the process.

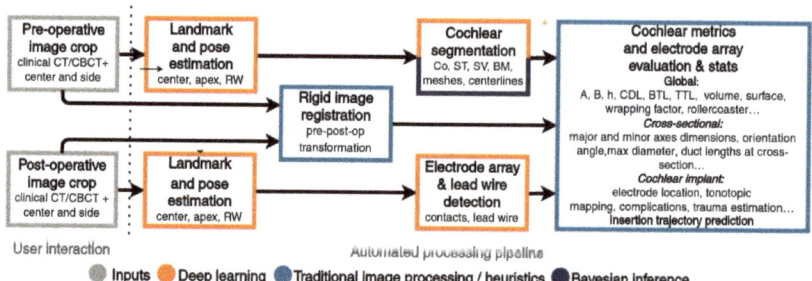

Figure 2. Nautilus pipeline overview. After the images are dropped onto a web browser window, the user moves a cross-hair roughly to the cochlea's center and selects the side (left/right) and whether it is a pre- or a post-operative scan. A crop (10 × 10 × 10 mm) centered on that landmark is then rid of personally identifiable information and uploaded for processing. First, relevant landmarks (the center, round window, and apex) are estimated and used for initial cochlear pose (reference coordinate system) computation. Segmentation of the cochlear bony labyrinth (CO) is obtained through a convolutional neural network, whereas subsequently, the scala tympani (ST) and scala vestibuli (SV) are obtained using Bayesian inference. From the post-operative image, electrode array contact coordinates and lead wire are extracted and fit to the Oticon Medical EVO electrode CAD model. An interactive visualization as well as pre- and post-operative metrics are available directly on the web browser. A number of additional outputs are generated by the pipeline and made available for data export for further processing and applications. The segmentations can be exported in STL format for 3D printing, for instance. An estimate of electrode trajectory is also provided from the pre-operative image to estimate the equivalent angular coverage for a given electrode insertion depth in millimeters.

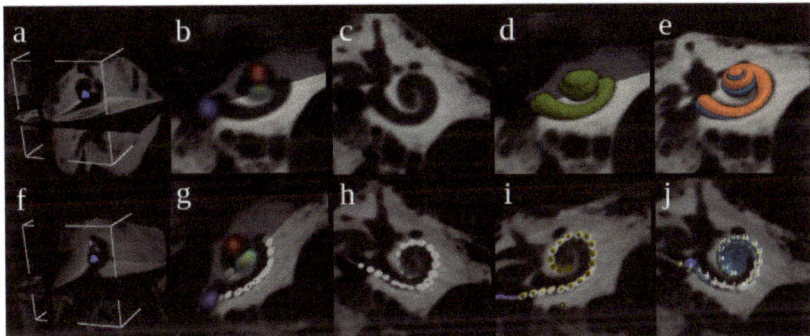

Figure 3. Steps of the image analysis pipeline in Nautilus. Regions of interest (10 × 10 × 10 mm) around a manually placed center (blue sphere) are cropped from both pre-operative (**a**) and post-operative (**f**) images. Landmark heatmaps are estimated (**b**,**g**) for the center (green), round window (blue), and apex (red). Images are aligned with rigid registration (**c**,**h**) as shown in cochlear view. Segmentation of the cochlear bony labyrinth (CO) (**d**) is subsequently split into the scala tympani (ST) and scala vestibuli (SV) (**e**). From the post-operative image, electrode array contact coordinates and lead wire are extracted (**i**), and an Oticon Medical EVO electrode CAD model is fit (**j**).

2.1. Data Upload and Pseudonymization via a Web-Based Frontend

Each user can create their private collection of images and associate each image to a specific case/individual. For each case, a unique anonymous identifier is generated upon creation. Once the image (most of the standard medical imaging formats are admissible (e.g., DICOM, NIFTI, MHA), as they can be loaded by ITK [26]) is loaded on the local browser, the image metadata (if any) are cleared of all personal identifiable information (PII). The user must then inform the laterality of the cochlea (left or right), whether it is a pre- or post-operative scan, and roughly place a cross on the targeted cochlea so as to allow the cropping and upload of a region of interest (ROI) from the original (albeit anonymized) image. After the data are uploaded, a processing job is queued and handled by the backend as soon as required computing resources become available.

2.2. Cochlear Landmarks and Canonical Pose Estimation

Cochlear pose estimation is essential to determine an initial orientation of the cochlea within the image and serves for image visualization in the standardized views [27]. The estimation of cochlear pose is also used for inferring the characteristic equation of the modiolar axis of the cochlea, which, in turn, is used to derive a number of metrics. We estimate the cochlear pose from a set of three automatically estimated landmarks—the center of the basal turn of the cochlea (C), the round window (RW—defined at its center), and the apex (Ap—defined at the helicotrema), as prescribed in [16]. Ap and C form the modiolar axis, which coincides with the z-axis. The basal plane passes through the RW, which defines the direction of the x-axis. The origin of the canonical reference coordinated is the intersection of the basal plane and the modiolar axis. Finally, the remaining axis is chosen such that the angle increases as we follow the cochlear duct starting from 0 deg at the RW. The canonical reference frame allows Nautilus' users to consistently compare cochleae of different sizes and allows equal treatment for both left and right cochleae.

A number of approaches have been proposed to estimate the landmarks or the pose, including registration and one-shot learning [28] or using regression forests to vote for the location of the landmarks [29]. More recently, reinforcement learning methods [30–32] have also been used to efficiently locate landmarks or to generate clinically meaningful image views [33] and, relevantly for our domain of application, to locate cochlear nerve landmarks [34]. Heatmap-based approaches consistently demonstrate robustness, explainability, and computational efficiency and offer an elegant form of uncertainty modelling and failure detection [35]. They do, however, sometimes have difficulties locating landmarks present around the image borders. We employ a conventional U-Net convolutional neural network architecture [36] as implemented in [37] with three output channels, one for each landmark. We modeled each landmark with a Gaussian heatmap and trained the network to map the input image to the three target heatmaps simultaneously. Our network architecture (detailed in the Supplementary Material) has 3 encoding blocks, 8 channels after the first layer and 16 output channels for the final feature map before the final projection onto the 3 heatmap channels (see Figure S1).

Our training set consists of an assortment of 279 pre- and post-operative clinical CT and CBCT images obtained from diverse sources. Our landmark detection block must be capable of handling (and was therefore trained on) both pre- and post-operative images. It is, however, significantly more difficult to accurately annotate C, RW, and Ap on the post-operative images due to the metallic artifacts. As a workaround, the pre-operative images were registered with the post-operative images, and the landmarks from pre-operative images were transported onto the post-operative images.

For training and inference, we resampled the input images to isotropic 0.3 mm spacing and normalized the intensities between the 5–95% percentile to 0–1 with no clipping. To increase the variability of our training set, we randomly sampled from a combination of data augmentations, such as random noise, flipping in all three dimensions, Gaussian blurring, random anisotropy [38], rigid transformations, and small elastic deformations as implemented by the TorchIO library [39]. Similarly to [40], we have observed that focal loss worked particularly well for sufficiently accurate landmark detection. During the inference, we transformed the predictions with the sigmoid activation to normalize them between 0 and 1, and for each output, we pick the mode of the output distribution (the hottest voxel of the heatmap) as the corresponding landmark.

2.3. Segmentation of Cochlear Structures

Nautilus is built with cochlear surgery planning, evaluation, and audiological fitting in mind. Therefore, in the current version, we focus on segmenting the two main cochlear ducts—ST and SV—and compute relevant measurements from these structures as others before us [41]. At a later stage, the delineation of ST and SV serves to relate the placement electrode array placement within the cochlea and infer information such as the characteristic frequency of each electrode contact [23]. An accurate and robust segmentation of ST and SV is therefore critical. Recent approaches based on convolutional neural networks have shown the most promise. Nikan et al., for instance [9], segmented various temporal bone structures including the labyrinth, ossicles, and facial nerve. Most of the cochlear segmentation approaches perform remarkably well on the cochlea and neighboring structures. They do not, however, separate the scalae [8,42], nor do they estimate the position of the BM, the delicate structure responsible for the transduction of mechanical waves within the cochlea into trains of electrical impulses, an essential structure to preserve in anticipation of restorative therapeutic advances. The separation of the scalae on clinical CTs is challenging as ST and SV are not discernible on clinical scans, mainly due to limited image resolution and contrast. To circumvent this issue, a shape model is often used to serve as a priori information on ST/SV distinction within the cochlear labyrinth. Recently, atlases [43] and a hybrid active shape model combined with deep learning [44] have been used with success for the separation of the scalae.

We used a pre-operative image of the implanted cochlea as the reference image for segmentation. Nautilus uses an approach similar to [44], which merges deep learning for appearance modelling with a strong shape prior constraining the final segmentation [45]. Instead of an active shape model, we build on top of a well-validated Bayesian joint appearance and shape inference model [20,46]. The parameters of this shape model were tuned and validated on µCT data. The model can then serve as a strong prior constraining the final output for the lower-resolution clinical CT images. This approach provides a probabilistic separation of ST and SV even in images of poor resolution. We provide an estimate of the BM location from the intersection of ST and SV's probability maps.

Demarcy et al.'s original Bayesian framework proposed to model the foreground and background appearance (i.e., intensity) as mixtures of Student distributions. We observed that this initialization is fairly sensitive to the type of scanner used for image acquisition and to image quality despite using normative Hounsfield units. To achieve better generalization, we therefore replaced the original appearance model with a trained convolutional neural network [36].

Similarly to our landmark detection approach, we used a reference 3D U-Net implementation of MONAI [37] with 6 encoding blocks, 8 output channels after the first layer (see Figure S2), and PReLU as the activation function and trained it on 130 images. We normalized the data by resampling the images to 0.125 mm spacing and rescaled the intensities such that the 5th and 95th percentile of the intensity distribution of each image were mapped to 0 and 1. In addition to augmentations used for landmark detection, we used random patch swapping [47] to increase the robustness to artifacts and force the network to learn a stronger shape prior. The model was trained on 128 × 128 × 128 patches with the AdamW [48] optimizer minimizing the Dice focal loss [37,49].

A large number of the metrics we extract from both pre- and post-operative processes depend on reliable estimation of the cochlear ducts' centerline. Because our segmentation of ST and SV is based on a parametric shape model [46], extracting an approximate centerline is straightforward. We then refine this curve and estimate ST and SV centerlines from cross-sections of the segmentations along this curve. At each cross-section, we estimate the coordinates of the lateral wall landmark as the furthest point on the ST from the modiolar axis, OC at 80% of the distance to the LW [13], and the SG offset by −0.35 mm both radially and longitudinally from the modiolar wall landmarks (i.e., the point on the ST closest to the modiolus) as an approximation of Rosenthal's canal.

2.4. Electrode Depth-to-Angular Coverage Prediction

The centerline can be discretized based on angles (in cylindrical coordinates), which can be used to predict a priori the angular coverage an electrode array is expected to reach as a function of the number of electrodes inserted beyond the RW. Shurzig et al. [50,51] proposed an ideal trajectory for the electrode, to be computed by subtracting the radius of the electrode from the radius of the cochlear spiral. A retrospective analysis of our predictions carried out on 98 images from our clinical dataset hinted that, on average, the CI electrode only follows an ideal trajectory after hitting the lateral wall around 150 deg. This observation leads us to propose the following statistical predictive model:

$$\delta_i = \rho - \begin{cases} 1.3 - 0.007\theta_i, & \text{if } i \leq 150° \\ r_i, & \text{otherwise} \end{cases} \quad (1)$$

where ρ is the radius of the centerline in cylindrical coordinates, and r and θ represent the radius of the ith electrode. Figure 4 depicts the angular errors based on Equation (1). Our predictions fall, on average, within 20° of the observed insertion angular coverage (n = 58).

2.5. Registration of the Pre- and Post-Operative Images

To evaluate the electrode array placement within the cochlea, we need to be able to fuse the segmentation of the pre-operative scan and the electrode contacts of the post-operative scan to the same reference coordinate system. Although the post-operative scan is deteriorated by the metallic artifacts generated by the electrode contact, it still represents the bony structures somewhat similarly to what is seen in the pre-operative image. Rigid transformation is therefore possible for aligning pre- and post-operative images. We first pre-align the pre- and post-op image pair into their canonical poses with the previously estimated landmarks and fine-tune the final transform using the Elastix package [52,53]. We have observed that even for CT or CBCT images in Hounsfield units, the Advanced Mattes mutual information [54] with 64 histogram bins performs adequately. Invalid voxels (usually found at the boundaries of the image) and metallic artifacts in all voxels with $HU > 2500$ are masked out and not used for computing the similarity.

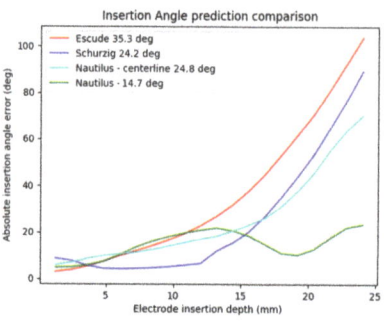 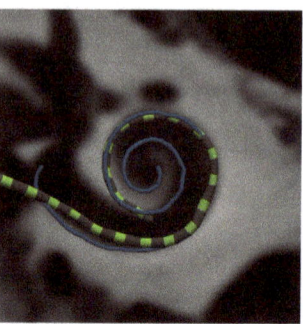

Figure 4. Angular insertion depth estimation based on the number of electrodes inserted inside the cochlea. The comparison graph shows (**left**), contrarily to our approach, how the performance of state-of-the-art approaches decreases exponentially with insertion depth. On the (**right**) is an example of a predicted trajectory (blue) and inserted electrode.

2.6. Electrode Array Detection

The electrode array detection starts with the estimation of the 3D coordinates for each of the 20 electrode contacts before the subsequent evaluation of their placement, e.g., with relative distances from relevant cochlear structures such as SG, MW, LW, BM (distances which could presumably be used to infer an indicator of traumaticity [55]). The reconstruction of the electrode array can also help with the visual inspection and assessment of complications such as kinking, tip fold-over, or buckling [56]. Most of these patterns are difficult to identify on 2D images [57], and the 3D processing approaches provide significant advantages. Various approaches can be used to locate electrode contacts. Measuring peaks of an image intensity profile is a straightforward method [58]. When these peaks are less discriminative, modelling intensity and shape with Markov random fields can help [59], and so can morphological or filtering approaches with handcrafted rules [23,60,61] or graph-based approaches [62]. Many of these approaches work well when the image resolution is fine and the contacts are well resolved, with sufficient contrast and limited metallic artifacts, no significant kinking or tip fold-over; they often can be well tuned to a particular set of scanners. With our heterogeneous dataset, the evaluated methods suffer under uneven image quality and artifacts of various appearances. We used machine learning to enhance and detect the electrode contacts of the array and to generalize over differences in appearance and image quality between the different imaging vendors. We have designed a pipeline similar to our landmark estimation similar to [63] and trained a U-Net [36,37] to estimate the likelihood of a voxel being a center of a contact. However, in addition to the contact probability estimation, our network performs two additional tasks, which share a common feature extraction backbone (see Figure S3). For training, we annotated a dataset of 106 post-operative images with ITK-SNAP [64] containing all the individual electrodes (1–20) and lead wires (where visible). From the annotations, we generated 3 different target labels: electrode location heatmap common for all electrodes (with value 1 at the centers of the electrodes and 0 away from them). By connecting electrode coordinates, we constructed a curve, which we turned into a probability map for the electrode array, and lastly, we created a discrete label map with 5 classes (background, proximal electrode, mid-electrode, distal-electrode, and lead wire) used for semantic segmentation of the post-op images.

During the inference, we first estimated the contact probabilities and considered all peaks to be contact candidates. To create an electrode array out of this unsorted set of candidates, we started with the two most central points. We then iteratively fit a cubic

B-spline to the already existing set and extrapolated at the two ends to search for the next probable point until no further expansion was plausible. This gave us a sorted array of contacts. To determine the final order, we assumed that the electrode array enters the cochlear around the round window and ascends along the cochlear duct towards the apex, i.e., the signed distance to the basal plane of the first contact should be smaller than that of the last most distal contact. We have observed that this strategy performs well even in the presence of mild to moderate aforementioned electrode array insertion complications. The lead wire is then estimated from the semantic segmentation by fitting a curve to the skeleton of the closest wire-like object near the first contact. This can serve to provide a more reliable estimation of the insertion angle [65].

This electrode array detection block is designed to operate on clinical CT and CBCT images, with, for the best performance, images of resolution of 0.3 mm or finer with little anisotropy. The electrode array detector has currently been tuned for and tested with the CLA and EVO electrode array from Oticon Medical (24 mm long with 20 electrodes with 1.2 mm pitch and diameter ranging from 0.5 mm proximally to 0.4 mm distally) [66]. There is, however, no significant limitation to using it for models from other vendors (see Figure 5).

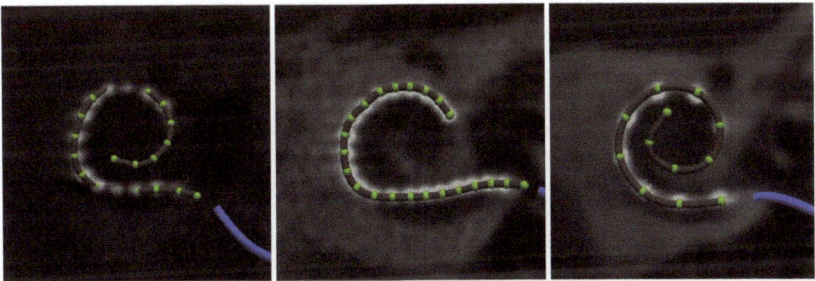

Figure 5. Electrode array detection in Nautilus has been developed and validated with Oticon Medical EVO electrode arrays (**left**) in mind. However, the same approach can be used with other electrode arrays. Example detection outputs for Cochlear Nucleus CI622 (**middle**), and MED-EL FLEX24 (**right**) cochlear implants

2.7. Extracted Measurements

Both pre- and post-operative processing pipelines output several clinically relevant metrics, some of which are depicted in Figure 6.

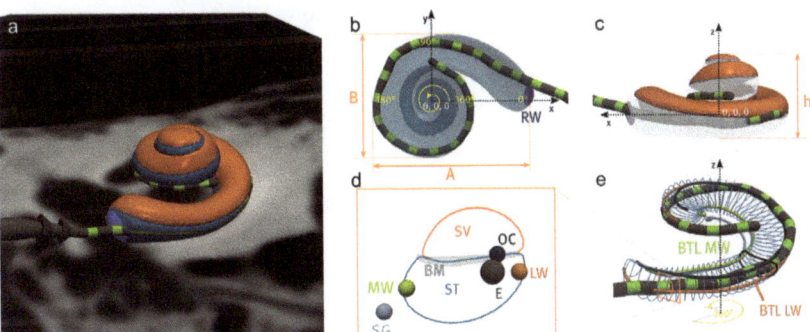

Figure 6. Cochlea and cochlear implant in the reference coordinate frame (**a**) and representation of different global (**b,c**) or cross-sectional metrics (**d,e**) that can be obtained using Nautilus. Examples include A, B, and the basal turn length (BTL) along various paths within the bony labyrinth (here, BTL LW and BTL MW are the 360-degree lengths covered while following the lateral wall (LW) or the modiolar wall (MW), respectively).

2.7.1. Global Pre-Operative Metrics

Global metrics characterize the overall shape and size of the cochlea. These include the volume and surface area of the cochlea along with cochlear dimensions A and B originally proposed by Escude et al. [67], which are defined by the length of the straight line between the round window, passing through the modiolar axis, and reaching the furthest point around the 180° cochlear angle and its perpendicular line, respectively (Figure 6b). Cochlear height h is computed along the modiolar axis. These measurements can be computed for the labyrinth or specifically for ST or SV. Cochlear shape is also defined by its potential "*rollercoaster*", which represents the largest deviation in height from a linear fit of the spiral height—or the vertical "dip" of the basal turn before the cochlear spirals upwards around the modiolar axis [68]. Nautilus also supports automatic computations of cochlear, basal and two-turn duct lengths of the labyrinth, ST, and SV along various trajectories within these structures: along the estimated paths of the lateral wall (LW), modiolar wall (MW), organ of Corti (OC) and spiral ganglion (SG) [68] (Figure 6d). The extraction of these metrics allows the computation of the cochlear wrapping factor, which represents the logarithmic spiral angle of the cochlea, and the wrapping ratio, which represents the ratio of the maximum cochlear angle (at the helicotrema) and the lateral wall duct length.

2.7.2. Local Pre- and Post-Operative Metrics

Local metrics characterize cochlear structures at particular places along the cochlear spiral. From pre-operative image processing, cochlear duct cross-sections are extracted at fixed angular displacements based on the labyrinth centerline. Cross-sectional area, radius, height, angle, minor and major axis lengths can then be computed by fitting an ellipse within each specific cross-section [69,70].

Post-operatively, registration parameters and the estimated locations of each electrode allow the computation of other important metrics. Electrode intracochlear positioning is characterized both by distance and angular measures at each electrode contact (where RW relates to 0° and Ap corresponds to the maximum cochlear angle, which is typically around 900°) cochlear coverage). From these, the characteristic frequencies associated with each electrode are proposed in relation to OC [12] or SG [13,14]. In addition, the distance of each electrode contact to the MW and the estimated BM position are also computed.

2.8. Failure Flagging Mechanisms

Any automated system can occasionally fail. Transparency to the user (e.g., in the form of notifications or flags) in case of such failures is particularly important in order to identify which data point to exclude in any further observation or statistical analysis realized on Nautilus' outputs. Therefore, Nautilus embeds a self-check flagging module that looks for signs of failures (e.g., detects suspicious segmentation or unexpected electrode array parameters) and explicitly notifies the user that images might not have been successfully processed and that the results should therefore be checked and/or used with caution. Whenever a flag is raised, a corresponding message is shown to the user (see Figure S4 for an example). Specific flags have been implemented at each processing stage. They are presented in Table 1. Figure S5 depicts the receiver operating curve (ROC) for the combined flags, based on which the cutoff values for notifying the user of a potentially faulty processing were chosen.

2.9. Data Export

The user can generate an export bundle containing all the outputs of the analysis in diverse export formats (Parquet, Excel, JSON) allowing further data analysis in their tool of choice. These analysis results are tagged with the unique version identifier for the specific processing pipeline version that was used for processing. Users may generate an export file for each case individually or a group of cases filtered on date. Figure S6 presents distributions of cochlear metrics computed by our pipeline using the export.

Table 1. Description of different flags from the self-check module as implemented in Nautilus. The failure flags trigger a decreased level of confidence in the processed results when extra attention is needed.

Category	Flags Implemented
Image	poor image quality (resolution)
Segmentation	low cochlear volume low segmentation reliability irregular cochlear centerline irregular voxel intensities within segmented region
Registration	low correlation between pre-op and post-op large difference between registered landmarks too many electrode detected outside cochlea too many electrodes detected outside scala tympani non-basal electrodes detected outside cochlea
Electrode detection	incorrect number of electrodes detected irregular electrode ordering incorrect intensity at electrode locations irregular electrode pitch detected electrodes clustered together incorrect distance to modiolar axis electrodes detected near image boundaries

3. Results

3.1. Evaluation Datasets

A well-curated multi-centric dataset, comprising both clinical and cadaver bones, was chosen for tye evaluation of Nautilus. CT images acquired from various scanners, using various acquisition parameters, and presenting heterogeneous resolutions, contrasts, and signal-to-noise ratios were included both for training and evaluation (see Figures S7 and S8 in the Supplementary Material). Groundtruth annotations, comprising the C, Ap and RW landmarks, cochlear structures and the electrode center points, were delineated by an expert radiologist using ITK-SNAP [64]. Limited by the poor resolution and imaging conditions of clinical images, only the cochlea could be manually delineated for clinical scans. On the other hand, ST and SV were successfully delineated in cadaver head CT scans since better contrast and resolutions could be achieved. The number of images used for training and evaluation for each process are mentioned in their respective sections. Each part of the pipeline was independently evaluated, as detailed below. A summary of the results is presented in Table 2.

3.2. Accuracy

3.2.1. Landmark Detection

The landmark detection pipeline, utilized both pre- and post-operatively, was evaluated on a dataset of 60 images. The images were passed through the landmark detector, and the distance between the predicted and groundtruth annotation landmarks was computed. Mean detection errors of 0.71 ± 1.0 mm, 0.75 ± 1.14 mm, and 1.30 ± 1.73 mm were observed for C, Ap and RW, respectively. All the individual errors were within a distance of two voxels, with the RW landmark yielding the worst performance.

Table 2. Accuracy and robustness analysis for each pipeline process. ASSD: average symmetric surface distance, RAVD: relative absolute volume difference, HD95: 95% Hausdorff distance.

	Landmark Detection		
Dataset	Apex (mm)	Center (mm)	Round Window (mm)
Clinical (n = 60)	0.71	0.75	1.30

Segmentation												
Dataset	Dice (%)			ASSD (mm)			RAVD			HD95 (mm)		
Structure	CO	ST	SV	CO	ST	SV	CO	ST	SV	CO	ST	SV
TB set 1 (n = 9)	83	67	64	0.17	0.21	0.18	−0.10	−0.02	−0.20	0.43	0.61	0.43
TB set 2 (n = 9)	77	64	58	0.21	0.23	0.24	−0.10	0.23	−0.38	0.76	0.77	0.99
TB set 3 (n = 5)	79	64	56	0.19	0.22	0.20	−0.21	−0.04	−0.40	0.62	0.71	0.64
Clinical (n = 58)	86			0.14			−0.13			0.35		
Mean	84	65	60	0.15	0.22	0.20	−0.14	0.02	−0.32	0.41	0.68	0.63

	Electrode Detection
Dataset	Electrode Distance (mm)
Clinical (n = 60)	0.09

	Registration	
Dataset	Mutual Information	Mean Registration Error (mm)
Clinical (n = 15)	0.15	0.88

	Robustness Analysis	
Dataset	Reviewer 1 (%)	Reviewer 2 (%)
Pre-operative (n = 156)	98.7	98.1
Post-operative (n = 156)	88.3 (76.2)	85.2 (78.4)

	Failure Detection		
Dataset	Sensitivity (%)	Specificity (%)	Accuracy (%)
Pre-operative (n = 156)	100	97.4	97.4
Post-operative (n = 156)	97.3	57.7	68.6

Computational Time	
Process	Approximate Time (s)
Landmark estimation	5.9
Cochlear view generation	12.5
Segmentation and pre-operative analysis	468.9
Electrode detection and post-operative analysis	148.2
Registration	49.8

3.2.2. Segmentation

Nautilus' segmentation pipeline was evaluated on four different clinical and cadaver datasets. The clinical dataset consisted of 58 pre-operative images with voxel resolutions ranging from 0.1 to 0.4 mm in the x-y plane and slice thickness ranging from 0.1 to 1 mm. The images were uploaded on Nautilus, and the union of ST and SV segmentation masks were obtained and compared with the manually labelled cochlea annotations. All the images were successfully processed, and a mean dice similarity coefficient and average surface error [71] of 86 ± 3% and 0.14 ± 0.03 mm were, respectively, observed for the clinical dataset. The cadaver datasets comprised 23 temporal bone (TB) µCT images in total. For computational limitations, the CT scans were resampled to an isotropic resolution of 0.1 mm. The images were uploaded on Nautilus, and the segmentation masks were obtained and compared with the manually labelled ST and SV annotations. All the images were successfully processed, and a mean dice similarity coefficient and average surface error of 80 ± 3% and 0.19 ± 0.04 mm were, respectively, observed for this cadaveric image dataset.

Figure 7 depicts segmentation results for each dataset. For a more thorough analysis, the cochlea was sectioned along its centerline at an 18° angular interval. Dice similarity coefficients were computed for each segment (see Figure S9), where it appears that Dice scores decrease towards the apical area.

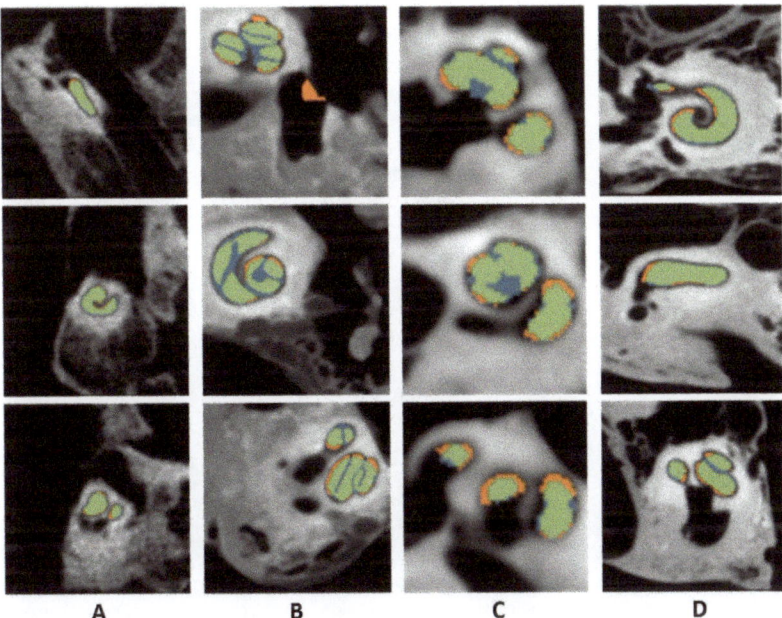

Figure 7. Segmentation output for different patients. (**A**) Clinical dataset, (**B**) cadaver dataset 1, (**C**) cadaver dataset 2, (**D**) cadaver dataset 3, blue: Nautilus estimation, orange: ground truth, green: overlap between the two.

3.2.3. Registration

The registration pipeline was evaluated on a dataset containing 15 sets of pre- and post-operative images with resolutions ranging from 0.1 to 0.3 mm. These image pairs did not necessarily have the same resolution. Each post-operative image of each pair was registered together with its pre-operative counterpart, and the average distances between the pre- and post-operative *RW*, *Ap*, and *C* landmarks within the registered coordinate system were computed to quantify the registration error. A mean target registration error of 0.88 ± 0.39 mm was obtained.

3.2.4. Electrode Detection

The electrode detection pipeline was evaluated on a dataset of 60 post-operative images. The electrode coordinates for each image were determined using Nautilus and compared with their corresponding groundtruth coordinates. An average electrode detection distance error of 0.09 ± 0.16 mm was achieved for successfully processed images (those that did not were rated as failures as part of our failure detection analysis—see Section 2.8).

3.3. Robustness

A retrospective robustness analysis was carried out, in which two experts from the Hannover Medical School, Hannover, Germany, and the Institut de la Face et du Cou, Nice, France, independently verified the subjective quality of both pre- and post-operative analysis outputs. A dataset of 156 ears (81 left, 75 right) was used for this study. The reviewers were presented with an assessment sheet in which they reported their subjective evaluations of the quality of the input image (both pre- and post-operative), the quality of the segmentation, and the quality of the reconstruction of the electrode array. Reviewer 1 marked 87 pre- and 59 and post-operative images as being of "good quality". The remaining pre-operative images were either classified as having poor resolution, being very noisy or already containing an electrode array. A total of 2 out of 156 cases were marked as failures, yielding a pre-operative processing success rate of 98.7%. For the post-operative assessment, 37 cases were marked as failures, yielding a success rate of 76.2%. However, a success rate of 88.3% was realized if out-of-specification images (images that the reviewers judged as being of poor quality) were excluded from the cohort. Reviewer 2 marked 126 pre- and 60 post-operative images as being of good quality. A total of 5 out of 156 cases were marked as failures, yielding a pre-operative success rate of 98.1%. For the post-operative assessment, 33 cases were marked as failures, yielding a success rate of 78.4% or 85.2% if images judged of poor quality by the reviewer herself were excluded from the cohort.

3.4. Failure Detection

The outputs of Nautilus' flagging system were compared with the qualitative assessment of the two reviewers, as detailed in the previous section. Figure S10 presents a performance summary of each flagging mechanism. An overall pre-operative failure detection sensitivity and specificity 100% and 97.4%, respectively, was achieved, with a corresponding post-operative failure detection sensitivity and specificity of 97.3% and 59.7%, respectively.

3.5. Computational Performances

Average computation times for each process are listed in Table 2. Computation times were obtained for a processing run on a standard Azure cloud VMs (Standard DS3 v2). On average, a complete pre- and post-operative analysis took around 10–12 min, with data storage and shape model adaptation for the segmentation taking the most time. All the other processes take less than two minutes combined. Nautilus is orchestrated with Azure Kubernetes with scalability in mind, and the throughput can be trivially scaled up by increasing the number of worker nodes.

4. Discussion

We present a web-based imaging research platform enabling the segmentation of cochlear structures and reconstruction of a cochlear implant electrode from conventional pre- and post-operative CT scans, respectively. Detailed analyses of accuracy, robustness, and failure detection provide legitimate grounds for using Nautilus for the exploration of clinically relevant questions on cochlear implantation and envisage further developments towards image-guided CI therapy.

Nautilus demonstrates segmentation performances in the range of previously presented academic results. More recent works have reported average cochlear Dice scores and average surface errors in the range of 72–91% and 0.11–0.27 mm, respectively [8–10,20,72]. Some of these groups have achieved higher Dice scores on limited datasets with high-resolution CT and μCT images [8,72]. A direct comparison between the works is not possible since our dataset and analysis focused on clinical and downsampled μCT images. Moreover, there is no publicly available benchmark analysis available for a fair comparison between different approaches. Nevertheless, our results on a varied dataset supports our claim of high accuracy and usability with conventional clinical CTs.

Many prior works have focused on inferring cochlea shape from μCT or high-resolution CTs as they offer good contrast and resolution compared to routine clinical CTs [8,72]. Our segmentation approach relies on JASMIN-inspired shape analysis [20], which offers the advantage of more interpretability of the estimated model parameters allowing further statistical studies. However, the same process is the bottleneck of our pipeline in terms of computational efficiency. This process could be adapted to benefit from learned shape models and anatomically inspired post-processing [73,74]. Our analysis also suggests that Nautilus performs better on clinical CT scans compared to cadaver head scans, which might be inherent to the cadaver head preparation process that often results in random air pockets, leading to a different intensity profile [75]. Additionally, our training dataset is comprised of mainly clinical scans. In future, a cadaver-specific pipeline may be developed to support cadaver-based research. Regardless, this is not a limiting factor in the applicability of Nautilus, as the main foreseen applications are in clinical research. Furthermore, our discretized analysis of the segmentation revealed that the performance decreases beyond two turns of the cochlea because of the small diameter of the cochlear ducts relative to image resolutions. This, however, is also not a limiting factor as most of the CI electrode arrays only reach around 450–600° of insertion coverage.

Post-operatively, our electrode detection process outperforms previously reported works, which have reported localization errors in the range of 0.1–0.35 mm [58,61,62]. The electrode contact-BM distances could serve for inferring insertion trauma according to the Eshraghi trauma scales [55]. This would require distance-trauma evaluation against either cadaveric histology samples or high-resolution μCT scans where the various grades of BM trauma would be resolvable. We must note that metallic artifacts emanating from the electrodes do not permit direct segmentation of cochlear structures. This warrants the necessity of a pre-operative CT-scan to infer information about the cochlear structures. The post-operative images can be converted into pseudo-pre-operative images suitable for segmentation using artifact reduction techniques [76], or an atlas can be adapted on the post-operative to segment it directly [77]. The metallic artifacts might have an impact on pre-post registration as well. However, the challenge of post- to pre-operative image conversion can be circumvented by simply using a mirrored version of the contralateral cochlea in the post-operative scan if that contralateral ear is not implanted [24].

Although accuracy is an elementary performance metric for any segmentation pipeline, robustness is key for the usefulness of a tool such as Nautilus, especially given the heterogeneity of image quality expected to be input to the tool. Our subjective quality assessment provides an indication that Nautilus can be used with confidence when dealing with images of various resolutions, contrast, and signal-to-noise ratios. To the best of our knowledge, no other work in this domain has focused on robustness analysis from a comprehensive multi-centric dataset with varying image qualities. Recently, Fan et al. achieved 85% robustness for cochlea segmentation on their 177-image dataset [44]. Contrarily, our qualitative analysis depicts a robustness of around 97% with clinically reasonable performance. Our analysis enabled us to identify a resolution cutoff beyond which robustness seems to drop. The processing of images presenting voxel sizes superior to 0.3 mm does result in a significantly greater number of failures or inadequate outputs. This assessment, therefore, sets input specifications for recommended input image resolutions.

Because the probability of failure of our pipelines is non-zero, especially if out-of-specification images are input to the tool, Nautilus does provide cautionary flagging mechanisms that embody our guiding design principle of transparency. Our current set of flags has been 100 percent sensitive and about 60 percent specific, meaning that processing failures are very unlikely to go unaccounted for and that the system will result in false positives (notified non-failures) in less than half of the time, which we deemed an acceptable threshold for usability, especially as Nautilus is robust. A further observation for failures related to electrode detection in particular is that any failures are hard failures and easily noticed by the user. All in all, our flagging mechanisms should be useful to call for manual verification and potentially discard faulty analyses.

The set of features proposed by Nautilus provides legitimate grounds for exploring many relevant clinical and basic questions related to cochlear anatomy. Nautilus' statistical model of the electrode insertion trajectory from pre-operative images, for instance, could be used prospectively to aim at a specific insertion angular coverage. The accuracy of these predictions could be validated using Nautilus with the post-operative images. Post-operatively,

Nautilus makes possible the exploration of anatomo-physiologically-tuned fitting [78,79] or the exploration of the relationship between electrode geometrical configuration within the cochlea and clinical outcomes, including perhaps residual hearing. For all its utility, Nautilus could in the future be extended with additional features to address a broader spectrum of investigations, such as these related to the prediction of insertion difficulties during surgical planning, including for abnormal anatomies [80,81]. The delineation of other structures, including the facial nerve, chorda tympani, or RW would then be required. Other imaging modalities (e.g., MRI) and electrode arrays could be the subject of future developments. Bridging pre- and post-operative use-cases, an augmented reality setup inspired by [82] could be envisaged for intraoperative guidance.

Supplementary Materials: The following supporting information can be downloaded at: https://www.mdpi.com/article/10.3390/jcm11226640/s1, Figure S1: Landmark prediction model architecture; Figure S2: Pre-operative U-Net used for cochlear segmentation; Figure S3: Post-operative U-Net for cochlear implant detection; Figure S4: An example of a failure flag being triggered and shown to caution the user about possible processing failure; Figure S5: ROC curve for failure detection process; Figure S6: Pre-operative statistics from the qualitative assessment cohort automatically computed from the segmentations; Figure S7: Qualitative segmentation performance with respect to image quality criteria; Figure S8: Qualitative registration performance with respect to image quality criteria; Figure S9: Dice scores per cochlear angle for the cadaver bone dataset (n = 23); Figure S10: Quantitative evaluation of the failure detection pipeline with respect to reviewer's grading.

Author Contributions: Conceptualization, J.M., T.D., D.G. and F.P.; methodology, J.M., R.H., P.L.D., T.D., Z.W. and H.D.; software, J.M., R.H., P.L.D., T.D., Z.W., O.M.M. and H.D.; validation, R.H., A.M., C.V. and N.G.; formal analysis, J.M., R.H., T.D., Z.W. and D.G.; investigation, J.M., R.H., P.L.D., A.M., T.D. and Z.W.; resources, R.H., A.M., T.D., A.B., T.L., F.P. and N.G.; data curation, J.M., R.H., P.L.D., A.M., T.D., C.V., A.B. and N.G.; writing—original draft preparation, J.M., R.H., P.L.D. and F.P.; writing—review and editing, J.M., R.H., P.L.D., A.M., T.D., Z.W., D.G., O.M.M., C.V., H.D., A.B., T.L., F.P. and N.G; visualization, J.M., R.H. and P.L.D.; supervision, J.M., R.H., D.G., H.D., A.B., T.L., F.P. and N.G.; project administration, F.P.; funding acquisition, D.G. and F.P. All authors have read and agreed to the published version of the manuscript.

Funding: This research received no external funding.

Institutional Review Board Statement: All clinical CT images used for the development of Nautilus were anonymized. These clinical scans are part of the clinical routine at the Hannover Medical School to pre-operatively evaluate the condition of the cochlea and post-operatively confirm correct intracochlear array placement. The institutional ethics committee at Hannover Medical School approved the use of anonymized imaging data obtained within the clinical routine.

Informed Consent Statement: Informed consent was obtained from all patients, and all experiments were performed in accordance with relevant guidelines and regulations and in accordance with the Declaration of Helsinki.

Data Availability Statement: The datasets analysed within the scope of the current study cannot be made publicly available as they have been made available to the authors under the specific authorization of the Hannover Medical School. The Hannover Medical School has collected the authorization of their patients to share their data anonymously for third-party analyses in the context of clinical research. This authorization does not extend to the public publication and distribution of the data. Access to the tool is, however, available upon reasonable request at nautilus_info@oticonmedical.com.

Acknowledgments: We would like to thank all beta-testers and early users for critical feedback on the platform. We are also grateful to the developers of the many software tools and packages used for this project, including, but not limited to, PyTorch [83], MONAI [37], TorchIO [39], ITK [26], ITK-SNAP [64], Elastix [53], VTK [84], NumPy [85], SciPy [86], scikit-learn [87], Django, Django REST framework, Celery, Kubernetes, Docker, PostgreSQL, Redis, React, react-vtkjs-viewport [88], React, Chart.js, Plotly.js, Bulma, and PyVista [89].

Conflicts of Interest: J.M. is a consultant for, and at the time of this study, R.H., T.D., O.M.M., D.G. and F.P. worked in the Research & Technology Department at Oticon Medical, manufacturer of the Neuro Zti cochlear implant system. The remaining authors declare no conflict of interest.

Abbreviations

The following abbreviations are used in this manuscript:

ASSD	Average symmetric surface distance
BM	Basilar membrane
BTL	Basal turn length
CBCT	Cone-beam computed tomography
CDL	Cochlear duct length
HD95	Hausdorff distance at the 95th percentile
MRI	Magnetic resonance imaging
MW	Modiolar wall
μCT	Micro computed tomography
LW	Lateral wall
OC	Organ of Corti
RAVD	Relative absolute volume difference
ROC	Receiver operating characteristic curve
RW	Round window
SG	Spiral ganglion
ST	Scala tympani
SV	Scala vestibuli
TB	Temporal bone

References

1. Carlson, M.L. Cochlear Implantation in Adults. *N. Engl. J. Med.* **2020**, *382*, 1531–1542. [CrossRef] [PubMed]
2. NIDCD. Cochlear Implants—Who Gets Cochlear Implants? 2021. Available online: https://www.nidcd.nih.gov/health/cochlear-implants (accessed on 22 July 2022).
3. Kan, A.; Stoelb, C.; Litovsky, R.Y.; Goupell, M.J. Effect of Mismatched Place-of-Stimulation on Binaural Fusion and Lateralization in Bilateral Cochlear-Implant Usersa. *J. Acoust. Soc. Am.* **2013**, *134*, 2923. [CrossRef] [PubMed]
4. Goupell, M.J.; Stakhovskaya, O.A.; Bernstein, J.G.W. Contralateral Interference Caused by Binaurally Presented Competing Speech in Adult Bilateral Cochlear-Implant Users. *Ear Hear.* **2018**, *39*, 110–123. [CrossRef] [PubMed]
5. Peng, Z.E.; Litovsky, R.Y. Novel Approaches to Measure Spatial Release From Masking in Children with Bilateral Cochlear Implants. *Ear Hear.* **2022**, *43*, 101–114. [CrossRef] [PubMed]
6. Yoo, K.S.; Wang, G.; Rubinstein, J.T.; Vannier, M.W. Semiautomatic Segmentation of the Cochlea Using Real-Time Volume Rendering and Regional Adaptive Snake Modeling. *J. Digit. Imaging* **2001**, *14*, 173–181. [CrossRef]
7. Xianfen, D.; Siping, C.; Changhong, L.; Yuanmei, W. 3D Semi-automatic Segmentation of the Cochlea and Inner Ear. In Proceedings of the 2005 27th Annual Conference of the IEEE Engineering in Medicine and Biology, Shanghai, China, 31 August–3 September 2005; pp. 6285–6288. [CrossRef]
8. Hussain, R.; Lalande, A.; Girum, K.B.; Guigou, C.; Bozorg Grayeli, A. Automatic Segmentation of Inner Ear on CT-scan Using Auto-Context Convolutional Neural Network. *Sci. Rep.* **2021**, *11*, 4406. [CrossRef]
9. Nikan, S.; Van Osch, K.; Bartling, M.; Allen, D.G.; Rohani, S.A.; Connors, B.; Agrawal, S.K.; Ladak, H.M. PWD-3DNet: A Deep Learning-Based Fully-Automated Segmentation of Multiple Structures on Temporal Bone CT Scans. *IEEE Trans. Image Process.* **2021**, *30*, 739–753. [CrossRef]
10. Lv, Y.; Ke, J.; Xu, Y.; Shen, Y.; Wang, J.; Wang, J. Automatic Segmentation of Temporal Bone Structures from Clinical Conventional CT Using a CNN Approach. *Int. J. Med Robot. Comput. Assist. Surg.* **2021**, *17*, e2229. [CrossRef]
11. Heutink, F.; Koch, V.; Verbist, B.; van der Woude, W.J.; Mylanus, E.; Huinck, W.; Sechopoulos, I.; Caballo, M. Multi-Scale Deep Learning Framework for Cochlea Localization, Segmentation and Analysis on Clinical Ultra-High-Resolution CT Images. *Comput. Methods Programs Biomed.* **2020**, *191*, 105387. [CrossRef]
12. Greenwood, D.P. Bandwidth Specification for Adaptive Optics Systems*. *JOSA* **1977**, *67*, 390–393. [CrossRef]
13. Stakhovskaya, O.; Sridhar, D.; Bonham, B.H.; Leake, P.A. Frequency Map for the Human Cochlear Spiral Ganglion: Implications for Cochlear Implants. *J. Assoc. Res. Otolaryngol.* **2007**, *8*, 220. [CrossRef] [PubMed]
14. Helpard, L.; Li, H.; Rohani, S.A.; Zhu, N.; Rask-Andersen, H.; Agrawal, S.; Ladak, H.M. An Approach for Individualized Cochlear Frequency Mapping Determined From 3D Synchrotron Radiation Phase-Contrast Imaging. *IEEE Trans. Biomed. Eng.* **2021**, *68*, 3602–3611. [CrossRef] [PubMed]
15. Gerber, N.; Reyes, M.; Barazzetti, L.; Kjer, H.M.; Vera, S.; Stauber, M.; Mistrik, P.; Ceresa, M.; Mangado, N.; Wimmer, W.; et al. A Multiscale Imaging and Modelling Dataset of the Human Inner Ear. *Sci. Data* **2017**, *4*, 170132. [CrossRef] [PubMed]
16. Wimmer, W.; Anschuetz, L.; Weder, S.; Wagner, F.; Delingette, H.; Caversaccio, M. Human Bony Labyrinth Dataset: Co-registered CT and Micro-CT Images, Surface Models and Anatomical Landmarks. *Data Brief* **2019**, *27*, 104782. [CrossRef] [PubMed]
17. Sieber, D.; Erfurt, P.; John, S.; Santos, G.R.D.; Schurzig, D.; Sørensen, M.S.; Lenarz, T. The OpenEar Library of 3D Models of the Human Temporal Bone Based on Computed Tomography and Micro-Slicing. *Sci. Data* **2019**, *6*, 180297. [CrossRef]

18. Noble, J.H.; Gifford, R.H.; Labadie, R.F.; Dawant, B.M. Statistical Shape Model Segmentation and Frequency Mapping of Cochlear Implant Stimulation Targets in CT. In Proceedings of the Medical Image Computing and Computer-Assisted Intervention—MICCAI, Nice, France, 1–5 October 2012; Ayache, N., Delingette, H., Golland, P., Mori, K., Eds.; Springer: Berlin/Heidelberg, Germany, 2012; pp. 421–428. [CrossRef]
19. Noble, J.H.; Labadie, R.F.; Majdani, O.; Dawant, B.M. Automatic Segmentation of Intra-Cochlear Anatomy in Conventional CT. *IEEE Trans. BioMed Eng.* **2011**, *58*, 2625–2632. [CrossRef]
20. Wang, Z.; Demarcy, T.; Vandersteen, C.; Gnansia, D.; Raffaelli, C.; Guevara, N.; Delingette, H. Bayesian Logistic Shape Model Inference: Application to Cochlear Image Segmentation. *Med. Image Anal.* **2022**, *75*, 102268. [CrossRef]
21. Finley, C.C.; Holden, T.A.; Holden, L.K.; Whiting, B.R.; Chole, R.A.; Neely, G.J.; Hullar, T.E.; Skinner, M.W. Role of Electrode Placement as a Contributor to Variability in Cochlear Implant Outcomes. *Otol. Neurotol.* **2008**, *29*, 920–928. [CrossRef]
22. Macherey, O.; Carlyon, R.P. Place-Pitch Manipulations with Cochlear Implants. *J. Acoust. Soc. Am.* **2012**, *131*, 2225–2236. [CrossRef]
23. Schuman, T.A.; Noble, J.H.; Wright, C.G.; Wanna, G.B.; Dawant, B.; Labadie, R.F. Anatomic Verification of a Novel Method for Precise Intrascalar Localization of Cochlear Implant Electrodes in Adult Temporal Bones Using Clinically Available Computed Tomography. *Laryngoscope* **2010**, *120*, 2277–2283. [CrossRef]
24. Reda, F.A.; McRackan, T.R.; Labadie, R.F.; Dawant, B.M.; Noble, J.H. Automatic Segmentation of Intra-Cochlear Anatomy in Post-Implantation CT of Unilateral Cochlear Implant Recipients. *Med. Image Anal.* **2014**, *18*, 605–615. [CrossRef]
25. Dillon, M.T.; Canfarotta, M.W.; Buss, E.; O'Connell, B.P. Comparison of Speech Recognition with an Organ of Corti versus Spiral Ganglion Frequency-to-Place Function in Place-Based Mapping of Cochlear Implant and Electric-Acoustic Stimulation Devices. *Otol. Neurotol. Off. Publ. Am. Otol. Soc. Am. Neurotol. Soc. Eur. Acad. Otol. Neurotol.* **2021**, *42*, 721–725. [CrossRef] [PubMed]
26. Johnson, H.J.; McCormick, M.; Ibáñez, L.; Consortium, T.I.S. *The ITK Software Guide*, 3rd ed.; Kitware, Inc.: Clifton Park, NY, USA, 2013.
27. Verbist, B.M.; Joemai, R.M.S.; Briaire, J.J.; Teeuwisse, W.M.; Veldkamp, W.J.H.; Frijns, J.H.M. Cochlear Coordinates in Regard to Cochlear Implantation: A Clinically Individually Applicable 3 Dimensional CT-Based Method. *Otol. Neurotol.* **2010**, *31*, 738–744. [CrossRef] [PubMed]
28. Wang, Z.; Vandersteen, C.; Raffaelli, C.; Guevara, N.; Patou, F.; Delingette, H. One-Shot Learning for Landmarks Detection. In *Deep Generative Models, and Data Augmentation, Labelling, and Imperfections*; Engelhardt, S., Oksuz, I., Zhu, D., Yuan, Y., Mukhopadhyay, A., Heller, N., Huang, S.X., Nguyen, H., Sznitman, R., Xue, Y., Eds.; Lecture Notes in Computer Science; Springer International Publishing: Cham, Switzerland, 2021; pp. 163–172. [CrossRef]
29. Criminisi, A.; Shotton, J.; Robertson, D.; Konukoglu, E. Regression Forests for Efficient Anatomy Detection and Localization in CT Studies. In *Medical Computer Vision. Recognition Techniques and Applications in Medical Imaging*; Menze, B., Langs, G., Tu, Z., Criminisi, A., Eds.; Springer: Berlin/Heidelberg, Germany, 2011; Volume 6533, pp. 106–117. [CrossRef]
30. Ghesu, F.C.; Georgescu, B.; Mansi, T.; Neumann, D.; Hornegger, J.; Comaniciu, D. An Artificial Agent for Anatomical Landmark Detection in Medical Images. In *Medical Image Computing and Computer-Assisted Intervention—MICCAI 2016*; Ourselin, S., Joskowicz, L., Sabuncu, M.R., Unal, G., Wells, W., Eds.; Springer International Publishing: Cham, Switzerland, 2016; Volume 9902, pp. 229–237. [CrossRef]
31. Alansary, A.; Oktay, O.; Li, Y.; Folgoc, L.L.; Hou, B.; Vaillant, G.; Kamnitsas, K.; Vlontzos, A.; Glocker, B.; Kainz, B.; et al. Evaluating Reinforcement Learning Agents for Anatomical Landmark Detection. *Med. Image Anal.* **2019**, *53*, 156–164. [CrossRef] [PubMed]
32. Leroy, G.; Rueckert, D.; Alansary, A. Communicative Reinforcement Learning Agents for Landmark Detection in Brain Images. In *Machine Learning in Clinical Neuroimaging and Radiogenomics in Neuro-Oncology*; Kia, S.M., Mohy-ud-Din, H., Abdulkadir, A., Bass, C., Habes, M., Rondina, J.M., Tax, C., Wang, H., Wolfers, T., Rathore, S., et al., Eds.; Springer International Publishing: Cham, Switzerland, 2020; pp. 177–186. [CrossRef]
33. Alansary, A.; Folgoc, L.L.; Vaillant, G.; Oktay, O.; Li, Y.; Bai, W.; Passerat-Palmbach, J.; Guerrero, R.; Kamnitsas, K.; Hou, B.; et al. Automatic View Planning with Multi-Scale Deep Reinforcement Learning Agents. In *Medical Image Computing and Computer Assisted Intervention—MICCAI 2018*; Frangi, A.F., Schnabel, J.A., Davatzikos, C., Alberola-López, C., Fichtinger, G., Eds.; Springer International Publishing: Cham, Switzerland, 2018; pp. 277–285. [CrossRef]
34. López Diez, P.; Sundgaard, J.V.; Patou, F.; Margeta, J.; Paulsen, R.R. Facial and Cochlear Nerves Characterization Using Deep Reinforcement Learning for Landmark Detection. In *Medical Image Computing and Computer Assisted Intervention—MICCAI 2021*; de Bruijne, M., Cattin, P.C., Cotin, S., Padoy, N., Speidel, S., Zheng, Y., Essert, C., Eds.; Springer International Publishing: Cham, Switzerland, 2021; Volume 12904, pp. 519–528. [CrossRef]
35. McCouat, J.; Voiculescu, I. Contour-Hugging Heatmaps for Landmark Detection. In Proceedings of the IEEE/CVF Conference on Computer Vision and Pattern Recognition (CVPR), New Orleans, LA, USA, 19–20 June 2022; pp. 20597–20605.
36. Ronneberger, O.; Fischer, P.; Brox, T. U-Net: Convolutional Networks for Biomedical Image Segmentation. In *Medical Image Computing and Computer-Assisted Intervention—MICCAI 2015*; Navab, N., Hornegger, J., Wells, W.M., Frangi, A.F., Eds.; Springer International Publishing: Cham, Switzerland, 2015; pp. 234–241. [CrossRef]
37. MONAI Consortium. MONAI: Medical Open Network for AI (1.0.0). Zenodo. 2022. Available online: https://zenodo.org/record/7086266 (accessed on 22 September 2022). [CrossRef]

38. Billot, B.; Robinson, E.; Dalca, A.V.; Iglesias, J.E. Partial Volume Segmentation of Brain MRI Scans of Any Resolution and Contrast. In *Medical Image Computing and Computer Assisted Intervention—MICCAI 2020*; Martel, A.L., Abolmaesumi, P., Stoyanov, D., Mateus, D., Zuluaga, M.A., Zhou, S.K., Racoceanu, D., Joskowicz, L., Eds.; Lecture Notes in Computer Science; Springer International Publishing: Cham, Switzerland, 2020; pp. 177–187. [CrossRef]
39. Pérez-García, F.; Sparks, R.; Ourselin, S. TorchIO: A Python Library for Efficient Loading, Preprocessing, Augmentation and Patch-Based Sampling of Medical Images in Deep Learning. *Comput. Methods Programs Biomed.* **2021**, *208*, 106236. [CrossRef]
40. Lin, T.Y.; Goyal, P.; Girshick, R.; He, K.; Dollár, P. Focal Loss for Dense Object Detection. In Proceedings of the 2017 IEEE International Conference on Computer Vision (ICCV), Venice, Italy, 22–29 October 2017; pp. 2999–3007. [CrossRef]
41. Schurzig, D.; Timm, M.E.; Majdani, O.; Lenarz, T.; Rau, T.S. The Use of Clinically Measurable Cochlear Parameters in Cochlear Implant Surgery as Indicators for Size, Shape, and Orientation of the Scala Tympani. *Ear Hear.* **2021**, *42*, 1034–1041. [CrossRef]
42. Fauser, J.; Stenin, I.; Bauer, M.; Hsu, W.H.; Kristin, J.; Klenzner, T.; Schipper, J.; Mukhopadhyay, A. Toward an Automatic Preoperative Pipeline for Image-Guided Temporal Bone Surgery. *Int. J. Comput. Assist. Radiol. Surg.* **2019**, *14*, 967–976. [CrossRef]
43. Powell, K.A.; Wiet, G.J.; Hittle, B.; Oswald, G.I.; Keith, J.P.; Stredney, D.; Andersen, S.A.W. Atlas-Based Segmentation of Cochlear Microstructures in Cone Beam CT. *Int. J. Comput. Assist. Radiol. Surg.* **2021**, *16*, 363–373. [CrossRef]
44. Fan, Y.; Zhang, D.; Banalagay, R.; Wang, J.; Noble, J.H.; Dawant, B.M. Hybrid Active Shape and Deep Learning Method for the Accurate and Robust Segmentation of the Intracochlear Anatomy in Clinical Head CT and CBCT Images. *J. Med. Imaging* **2021**, *8*, 064002. [CrossRef]
45. Margeta, J.; Demarcy, T.; Lopez Diez, P.; Hussain, R.; Vandersteen, C.; Guevarra, N.; Delingette, H.; Gnansia, D.; Kamaric Riis, S.; Patou, F. Nautilus: A Clinical Tool for the Segmentation of Intra-Cochlear Structures and Related Applications. In Proceedings of the Conference on Implantable Auditory Prostheses (CIAP), Lake Tahoe, CA, USA, 12–16 July 2021.
46. Demarcy, T. Segmentation and Study of Anatomical Variability of the Cochlea from Medical Images. Ph.D. Thesis, Université Côte d'Azur, Nice, France, 2017.
47. Chen, L.; Bentley, P.; Mori, K.; Misawa, K.; Fujiwara, M.; Rueckert, D. Self-Supervised Learning for Medical Image Analysis Using Image Context Restoration. *Med. Image Anal.* **2019**, *58*, 101539. [CrossRef]
48. Loshchilov, I.; Hutter, F. Decoupled Weight Decay Regularization. *arXiv* **2019**, arXiv:1711.05101.
49. Yeung, M.; Sala, E.; Schönlieb, C.B.; Rundo, L. Unified Focal Loss: Generalising Dice and Cross Entropy-Based Losses to Handle Class Imbalanced Medical Image Segmentation. *Comput. Med. Imaging Graph.* **2022**, *95*, 102026. [CrossRef] [PubMed]
50. Schurzig, D.; Timm, M.E.; Batsoulis, C.; Salcher, R.; Sieber, D.; Jolly, C.; Lenarz, T.; Zoka-Assadi, M. A Novel Method for Clinical Cochlear Duct Length Estimation toward Patient-Specific Cochlear Implant Selection. *OTO Open* **2018**, *2*, 2473974X18800238. [CrossRef] [PubMed]
51. Mertens, G.; Van Rompaey, V.; Van de Heyning, P.; Gorris, E.; Topsakal, V. Prediction of the Cochlear Implant Electrode Insertion Depth: Clinical Applicability of Two Analytical Cochlear Models. *Sci. Rep.* **2020**, *10*, 3340. [CrossRef] [PubMed]
52. Shamonin, D. Fast Parallel Image Registration on CPU and GPU for Diagnostic Classification of Alzheimer's Disease. *Front. Neuroinform.* **2013**, *7*, 50. [CrossRef]
53. Klein, S.; Staring, M.; Murphy, K.; Viergever, M.; Pluim, J. Elastix: A Toolbox for Intensity-Based Medical Image Registration. *IEEE Trans. Med. Imaging* **2010**, *29*, 196–205. [CrossRef]
54. Mattes, D.; Haynor, D.; Vesselle, H.; Lewellen, T.; Eubank, W. PET-CT Image Registration in the Chest Using Free-Form Deformations. *IEEE Trans. Med. Imaging* **2003**, *22*, 120–128. [CrossRef]
55. Eshraghi, A.A.; Van De Water, T.R. Cochlear Implantation Trauma and Noise-Induced Hearing Loss: Apoptosis and Therapeutic Strategies. *Anat. Rec. Part A Discov. Mol. Cell. Evol. Biol.* **2006**, *288A*, 473–481. [CrossRef]
56. Ishiyama, A.; Risi, F.; Boyd, P. Potential Insertion Complications with Cochlear Implant Electrodes. *Cochlear Implant. Int.* **2020**, *21*, 206–219. [CrossRef]
57. McClenaghan, F.; Nash, R. The Modified Stenver's View for Cochlear Implants—What Do the Surgeons Want to Know? *J. Belg. Soc. Radiol.* **2020**, *104*, 37. [CrossRef]
58. Bennink, E.; Peters, J.P.; Wendrich, A.W.; Vonken, E.j.; van Zanten, G.A.; Viergever, M.A. Automatic Localization of Cochlear Implant Electrode Contacts in CT. *Ear Hear.* **2017**, *38*, e376–e384. [CrossRef] [PubMed]
59. Hachmann, H.; Krüger, B.; Rosenhahn, B.; Nogueira, W. Localization Of Cochlear Implant Electrodes From Cone Beam Computed Tomography Using Particle Belief Propagation. In Proceedings of the 2021 IEEE 18th International Symposium on Biomedical Imaging (ISBI), Nice, France, 13–16 April 2021; pp. 593–597. [CrossRef]
60. Zhao, Y.; Dawant, B.M.; Labadie, R.F.; Noble, J.H. Automatic Localization of Closely Spaced Cochlear Implant Electrode Arrays in Clinical CTs. *Med. Phys.* **2018**, *45*, 5030–5040. [CrossRef] [PubMed]
61. Zhao, Y.; Dawant, B.M.; Labadie, R.F.; Noble, J.H. Automatic Localization of Cochlear Implant Electrodes in CT. In *Medical Image Computing and Computer-Assisted Intervention—MICCAI 2014*; Golland, P., Hata, N., Barillot, C., Hornegger, J., Howe, R., Eds.; Springer International Publishing: Cham, Switzerland, 2014; Volume 8673, pp. 331–338. [CrossRef]
62. Zhao, Y.; Chakravorti, S.; Labadie, R.F.; Dawant, B.M.; Noble, J.H. Automatic Graph-Based Method for Localization of Cochlear Implant Electrode Arrays in Clinical CT with Sub-Voxel Accuracy. *Med. Image Anal.* **2019**, *52*, 1–12. [CrossRef]
63. Chi, Y.; Wang, J.; Zhao, Y.; Noble, J.H.; Dawant, B.M. A Deep-Learning-Based Method for the Localization of Cochlear Implant Electrodes in CT Images. In Proceedings of the 2019 IEEE 16th International Symposium on Biomedical Imaging (ISBI 2019), Venice, Italy, 8–11 April 2019; IEEE: Venice, Italy, 2019; pp. 1141–1145. [CrossRef]

64. Yushkevich, P.A.; Piven, J.; Hazlett, H.C.; Smith, R.G.; Ho, S.; Gee, J.C.; Gerig, G. User-Guided 3D Active Contour Segmentation of Anatomical Structures: Significantly Improved Efficiency and Reliability. *NeuroImage* **2006**, *31*, 1116–1128. [CrossRef] [PubMed]
65. Torres, R.; Jia, H.; Drouillard, M.; Bensimon, J.L.; Sterkers, O.; Ferrary, E.; Nguyen, Y. An Optimized Robot-Based Technique for Cochlear Implantation to Reduce Array Insertion Trauma. *Otolaryngol. Head Neck Surg.* **2018**, *159*, 019459981879223. [CrossRef]
66. Bento, R.; Danieli, F.; Magalhães, A.; Gnansia, D.; Hoen, M. Residual Hearing Preservation with the Evo® Cochlear Implant Electrode Array: Preliminary Results. *Int. Arch. Otorhinolaryngol.* **2016**, *20*, 353–358. [CrossRef]
67. Escudé, B.; James, C.; Deguine, O.; Cochard, N.; Eter, E.; Fraysse, B. The Size of the Cochlea and Predictions of Insertion Depth Angles for Cochlear Implant Electrodes. *Audiol. Neurotol.* **2006**, *11*, 27–33. [CrossRef]
68. Pietsch, M.; Aguirre Dávila, L.; Erfurt, P.; Avci, E.; Lenarz, T.; Kral, A. Spiral Form of the Human Cochlea Results from Spatial Constraints. *Sci. Rep.* **2017**, *7*, 7500. [CrossRef]
69. Fitzgibbon, A.; Pilu, M.; Fisher, R. Direct Least Square Fitting of Ellipses. *IEEE Trans. Pattern Anal. Mach. Intell.* **1999**, *21*, 476–480. [CrossRef]
70. Burger, W.; Burge, M.J. *Principles of Digital Image Processing: Core Algorithms*; Springer Science & Business Media: New York, NY, USA, 2010.
71. Maier-Hein, L.; Reinke, A.; Christodoulou, E.; Glocker, B.; Godau, P.; Isensee, F.; Kleesiek, J.; Kozubek, M.; Reyes, M.; Riegler, M.A.; et al. Metrics Reloaded: Pitfalls and Recommendations for Image Analysis Validation. *arXiv* **2022**, arXiv:2206.01653.
72. Ruiz Pujadas, E.; Kjer, H.M.; Piella, G.; Ceresa, M.; González Ballester, M.A. Random Walks with Shape Prior for Cochlea Segmentation in Ex Vivo μCT. *Int. J. Comput. Assist. Radiol. Surg.* **2016**, *11*, 1647–1659. [CrossRef] [PubMed]
73. Girum, K.B.; Lalande, A.; Hussain, R.; Créhange, G. A Deep Learning Method for Real-Time Intraoperative US Image Segmentation in Prostate Brachytherapy. *Int. J. Comput. Assist. Radiol. Surg.* **2020**, *15*, 1467–1476. [CrossRef] [PubMed]
74. Painchaud, N.; Skandarani, Y.; Judge, T.; Bernard, O.; Lalande, A.; Jodoin, P.M. Cardiac Segmentation With Strong Anatomical Guarantees. *IEEE Trans. Med. Imaging* **2020**, *39*, 3703–3713. [CrossRef] [PubMed]
75. Soldati, E.; Pithioux, M.; Guenoun, D.; Bendahan, D.; Vicente, J. Assessment of Bone Microarchitecture in Fresh Cadaveric Human Femurs: What Could Be the Clinical Relevance of Ultra-High Field MRI. *Diagnostics* **2022**, *12*, 439. [CrossRef]
76. Wang, Z.; Vandersteen, C.; Demarcy, T.; Gnansia, D.; Raffaelli, C.; Guevara, N.; Delingette, H. Inner-Ear Augmented Metal Artifact Reduction with Simulation-Based 3D Generative Adversarial Networks. *Comput. Med. Imaging Graph.* **2021**, *93*, 101990. [CrossRef]
77. Wang, J.; Su, D.; Fan, Y.; Chakravorti, S.; Noble, J.H.; Dawant, B.M. Atlas-Based Segmentation of Intracochlear Anatomy in Metal Artifact Affected CT Images of the Ear with Co-trained Deep Neural Networks. In *Medical Image Computing and Computer Assisted Intervention—MICCAI 2021*; de Bruijne, M., Cattin, P.C., Cotin, S., Padoy, N., Speidel, S., Zheng, Y., Essert, C., Eds.; Springer International Publishing: Cham, Switzerland, 2021; Volume 12904, pp. 14–23. [CrossRef]
78. Mertens, G.; Van de Heyning, P.; Vanderveken, O.; Topsakal, V.; Van Rompaey, V. The Smaller the Frequency-to-Place Mismatch the Better the Hearing Outcomes in Cochlear Implant Recipients? *Eur. Arch. Oto-Rhino* **2022**, *279*, 1875–1883. [CrossRef]
79. Canfarotta, M.W.; Dillon, M.T.; Buss, E.; Pillsbury, H.C.; Brown, K.D.; O'Connell, B.P. Frequency-to-Place Mismatch: Characterizing Variability and the Influence on Speech Perception Outcomes in Cochlear Implant Recipients. *Ear Hear.* **2020**, *41*, 1349–1361. [CrossRef] [CrossRef]
80. López Diez, P.; Sørensen, K.; Sundgaard, J.V.; Diab, K.; Margeta, J.; Patou, F.; Paulsen, R.R. Deep Reinforcement Learning for Detection of Inner Ear Abnormal Anatomy in Computed Tomography. In Proceedings of the Medical Image Computing and Computer Assisted Intervention—MICCAI 2022, Singapore, 18–22 September 2022; Wang, L., Dou, Q., Fletcher, P.T., Speidel, S., Li, S., Eds.; Springer Nature Switzerland: Cham, Switzerland, 2022; Lecture Notes in Computer Science, pp. 697–706. [CrossRef]
81. López Diez, P.; Juhl, K.A.; Sundgaard, J.V.; Diab, H.; Margeta, J.; Patou, F.; Paulsen, R.R. Deep Reinforcement Learning for Detection of Abnormal Anatomies. In Proceedings of the Northern Lights Deep Learning Workshop, North Pole, Norway, 10–12 January 2022; Volume 3. [CrossRef]
82. Hussain, R.; Lalande, A.; Guigou, C.; Bozorg-Grayeli, A. Contribution of Augmented Reality to Minimally Invasive Computer-Assisted Cranial Base Surgery. *IEEE J. Biomed. Health Inform.* **2020**, *24*, 2093–2106. [CrossRef]
83. Paszke, A.; Gross, S.; Massa, F.; Lerer, A.; Bradbury, J.; Chanan, G.; Killeen, T.; Lin, Z.; Gimelshein, N.; Antiga, L.; et al. PyTorch: An Imperative Style, High-Performance Deep Learning Library. In Proceedings of the 33rd International Conference on Neural Information Processing Systems, Vancouver, BC, Canada, 8–14 December 2019; Number 721; Curran Associates Inc.: Red Hook, NY, USA, 2019; pp. 8026–8037.
84. Schroeder, W.; Martin, K.; Lorensen, B. *The Visualization Toolkit—An Object-Oriented Approach to 3D Graphics*, 4th ed.; Kitware, Inc.: Clifton Park, NY, USA, 2006.
85. Harris, C.R.; Millman, K.J.; van der Walt, S.J.; Gommers, R.; Virtanen, P.; Cournapeau, D.; Wieser, E.; Taylor, J.; Berg, S.; Smith, N.J.; et al. Array Programming with NumPy. *Nature* **2020**, *585*, 357–362. [CrossRef]
86. Virtanen, P.; Gommers, R.; Oliphant, T.E.; Haberland, M.; Reddy, T.; Cournapeau, D.; Burovski, E.; Peterson, P.; Weckesser, W.; Bright, J.; et al. SciPy 1.0: Fundamental Algorithms for Scientific Computing in Python. *Nat. Methods* **2020**, *17*, 261–272. [CrossRef]
87. Pedregosa, F.; Varoquaux, G.; Gramfort, A.; Michel, V.; Thirion, B.; Grisel, O.; Blondel, M.; Prettenhofer, P.; Weiss, R.; Dubourg, V.; et al. Scikit-Learn: Machine Learning in Python. *J. Mach. Learn. Res.* **2011**, *12*, 2825–2830.

88. Ziegler, E.; Urban, T.; Brown, D.; Petts, J.; Pieper, S.D.; Lewis, R.; Hafey, C.; Harris, G.J. Open Health Imaging Foundation Viewer: An Extensible Open-Source Framework for Building Web-Based Imaging Applications to Support Cancer Research. *JCO Clin. Cancer Inform.* **2020**, *4*, 336–345. [CrossRef] [PubMed]
89. Sullivan, C.B.; Kaszynski, A. PyVista: 3D Plotting and Mesh Analysis through a Streamlined Interface for the Visualization Toolkit (VTK). *J. Open Source Softw.* **2019**, *4*, 1450. [CrossRef]

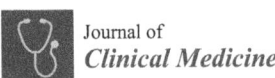

Systematic Review

Short- and Long-Term Effect of Cochlear Implantation on Disabling Tinnitus in Single-Sided Deafness Patients: A Systematic Review

Samar A. Idriss [1,2], Pierre Reynard [1,3,4], Mathieu Marx [5,6], Albane Mainguy [7], Charles-Alexandre Joly [1,3,4], Eugen Constant Ionescu [1,3], Kelly K. S. Assouly [8,9,10] and Hung Thai-Van [1,3,4,7,*]

1. Department of Audiology and Otoneurological Evaluation, Edouard Herriot Hospital, Hospices Civils de Lyon, 69002 Lyon, France
2. Department of Otorhinolaryngology and Head and Neck Surgery, Eye and Ear University Hospital, Holy Spirit University of Kaslik, Beirut 1202, Lebanon
3. Institut de l'Audition, Institut Pasteur, University of Paris, INSERM, 75012 Paris, France
4. Faculty of Medicine, University Claude Bernard Lyon 1, 69100 Villeurbanne, France
5. Department of Otology, Otoneurology and Pediatric Otolaryngology, Pierre-Paul Riquet Hospital, Toulouse Purpan University Hospital, 31300 Toulouse, France
6. Brain and Cognition Laboratory, UMR 5549, Toulouse III University, 31062 Toulouse, France
7. National Commission for the Evaluation of Medical Devices and Health Technologies, Haute Autorité de Santé, 93210 La Plaine St Denis, France
8. Department of Otorhinolaryngology and Head & Neck Surgery, University Medical Center Utrecht, 3584 CX Utrecht, The Netherlands
9. UMC Utrecht Brain Center, University Medical Center Utrecht, 3584 CX Utrecht, The Netherlands
10. Cochlear Technology Centre, 2800 Mechelen, Belgium
* Correspondence: hung.thai-van@chu-lyon.fr

Abstract: Patients with single-sided deafness can experience an ipsilateral disabling tinnitus that has a major impact on individuals' social communication and quality of life. Cochlear implants appear to be superior to conventional treatments to alleviate tinnitus in single-sided deafness. We conducted a systematic review to evaluate the effectiveness of cochlear implants in single-sided deafness with disabling tinnitus when conventional treatments fail to alleviate tinnitus (PROSPERO ID: CRD42022353292). All published studies in PubMed/MEDLINE and SCOPUS databases until December 2021 were included. A total of 474 records were retrieved, 31 studies were included and were divided into two categories according to whether tinnitus was assessed as a primary complaint or not. In all studies, cochlear implantation, evaluated using subjective validated tools, succeeded in reducing tinnitus significantly. Objective evaluation tools were less likely to be used but showed similar results. A short-(3 months) and long-(up to 72 months) term tinnitus suppression was reported. When the cochlear implant is disactivated, complete residual tinnitus inhibition was reported to persist up to 24 h. The results followed a similar pattern in studies where tinnitus was assesed as a primary complaint or not. In conclusion, the present review confirmed the effectiveness of cochlear implantation in sustainably reducing disabling tinnitus in single-sided deafness patients.

Keywords: single-sided deafness; cochlear implant; disabling tinnitus; systematic review; speech perception; sound localization; hyperacusis; quality of life

1. Introduction

Single-sided deafness (SSD), also known as unilateral profound hearing loss [1], is associated with a hearing impairment with higher perception of hearing handicap and visual annalog scores [2]. Despite normal or near-normal contralateral hearing status, monaural stimulation can lead to a wide range of audiological disabilities such as poor speech perception in noise and sound localization [3,4]. In addition, patients with SSD can experience an ipsilateral severe tinnitus [5–7]. These issues can have a crucial impact on individuals' social communication and interaction, in addition to significant effects on their quality of life (QoL) [8]; it can also lead to a psychological distress [9].

Tinnitus severity is graded using various validated subjective tools such as Tinnitus Questionnaire (TQ) [10,11], Tinnitus Handicap Index (THI) [12], Tinnitus Reaction Questionnaire (TRQ) [13], Visual Analog Score (VAS) [14], Tinnitus Rating Score (TRS) [15], Subjective Tinnitus Severity Scale (STSS) [16], and Numeric Rating Scale (NRS) [17], among others. Severe disabling tinnitus is defined by a TFI > 32/100, THI > 58/100, TQ > 42/84, or VAS loudness or annoyance >6/10 [18]. It is a difficult-to-treat disabling condition, and is frequently associated with by hearing loss [19]. One of its main pathophysiological mechanisms involves a paradoxical enhanced central activity associated with loss of peripheral input [20]. Persistent bothersome tinnitus can be very harmful to psychological health [9,21] and co-occurs with several comorbidities [22]. Notably, it can be associated with sleeping disturbances, cardiovascular diseases, and metabolic disorders [23]. The American Academy of Otolaryngology and the European societies have published guidelines for the management of tinnitus [24,25]. Drugs, including antidepressants [26] anticonvulsants [27], and dietary supplements [28,29], as well as electromagnetic [30] or laser [31] stimulation, and acupuncture [32] are not recommended [24,25]. Psychological therapies such as cognitive behavioral therapy (CBT) [33,34] are recommended [24,25]. Tinnitus retraining therapy (TRT) [35], psychotherapy [36], relaxation and meditation [37,38], hypnosis [39], biofeedback [40], education-information [41], and stress management-problem solving [42], among others, can be helpful and reduce tinnitus [24,25]. In the absence of hearing loss, sound therapy, delivered via ear/headphones, may be recommended for bothersome tinnitus [25,43], and in the presence of hearing loss, hearing aids (HAs) are recommended [24,25]. In cases of severe hearing loss, cochlear implant (CI) appears to be superior to conventional treatments, including HAs, contralateral routing of sound HAs (CROS), and bone conduction hearing devices [44–46]. Consequently, CI was approved by the US Food and Drug Administration for SSD [47] and was recently considered as an indication for disabling tinnitus with SSD in France after insufficient effectiveness of conventional treatments [48].

To date, a number of studies have evaluated the effect of cochlear implantation in the treatment of disabling tinnitus in SSDs; however, only a few reviews are available [49,50]. In the first review, no studies with objective tinnitus assessment tools were included and the maximum follow-up period was up to 28 months [49]. In the second review, tinnitus assessment tools were also subjective and were limited to those using THI and/or VAS [50]. The present systematic review included all studies, published through December 2021, in which tinnitus was evaluated as a primary or non-primary complaint. Assessing tinnitus as a primary complaint reduces the risk of false-positive and false-negative errors [51]. Studies using subjective assessment methods, as well as those using objective assessment methods, were included. When it came to subjective methods, all validated questionnaires and scales were considered without any restrictions. Furthermore, the effect of cochlear implantation on tinnitus was not only analyzed in the short term, but also the long term.

The present systematic review aims to provide a comprehensive overview of the short- and long-term effects of cochlear implantation on disabling tinnitus in adults with single-sided deafness.

2. Materials and Methods

The review protocol is available on International prospective register of systematic reviews (PROSPERO) (ID: CRD42022353292). The Preferred Reporting Items for Systematic Reviews and Meta-Analysis (PRISMA) statement was used for this systematic review [52].

2.1. Search Strategy

A systematic search of published studies was performed in PubMed/MEDLINE and SCOPUS databases using the syntax (tinnitus [Title/Abstract]) AND single-sided deafness [Title/Abstract] AND Cochlear implant) and the different combinations (tinnitus

AND single-sided deafness), (tinnitus AND cochlear implant), and (cochlear implant AND single-sided deafness). The search was conducted in December 2021. All published studies available at this time were included in the review process. The search terms included combined expressions and synonyms of tinnitus, single-sided deafness, and CI. These include ear ringing, buzzing, unilateral hearing loss, and intracochlear electrical stimulation.

2.2. Study Selection

All studies on cochlear implantation in adult patients with SSD and disabling tinnitus, in which tinnitus was evaluated as a primary or non-primary complaint, were selected. Studies where tinnitus was evaluated pre- and post- operatively, using subjective and/or objective tools, in the short- or long-term, were eligible. During screening, duplicates, systematic reviews, and articles written in languages other than English were excluded. Case reports and studies with overlapping study population were not excluded. Lack of previous therapeutic trials was not an exclusion criterion. Two reviewers, S.A.I. and P.R., screened each study (title/abstract) independently. Disagreements were resolved by a third reviewer. Studies were divided into two groups according to whether the primary complaint was tinnitus.

2.3. Quality Assessment

Two authors, S.A.I and K.K.S.A., independently assessed the risk of bias (RoB). We used the ROBINS-I tool (Risk Of Bias In Non-randomized Studies—of Interventions) to evaluate risk of bias [53]. The tool consists of seven domains: confounding, selection of participants, classification of interventions, deviation from intended intervention, missing data, measurement of outcomes, and selection of reported results. The criteria were defined and adapted to our research question about cochlear implantation for SSD with disabling tinnitus. Items were scored as low risk of bias, moderate risk of bias, serious risk of bias, or unclear based on the guidelines of the ROBINS-I tool. Consensus was obtained after discussion between the two reviewers.

2.4. Data Extraction

All study characteristics and outcomes were extracted by S.A.I. and P.R. independently. The primary outcome was the difference between pre- and post-operative evaluation of tinnitus on validated multi-item tinnitus distress questionnaires and/or objective evaluation measurements. Additional outcomes were also extracted including hyperacusis, sound hypersensitivity, speech perception, sound localisation, word recognition, quality of life, work performance, and psychosocial comorbidities.

3. Results

3.1. Search Strategy and Study Selection

A total of 474 records were retrieved, and 31 studies were included in the systematic review (Figure 1). Post-implantation tinnitus suppression was analysed in 479 patients using various assessment methods. These studies were divided into two groups; 14 studies in which the primary complaint was tinnitus, and 17 studies in which tinnitus was not the primary complaint. Some studies had an overlap in their population samples [54–57].

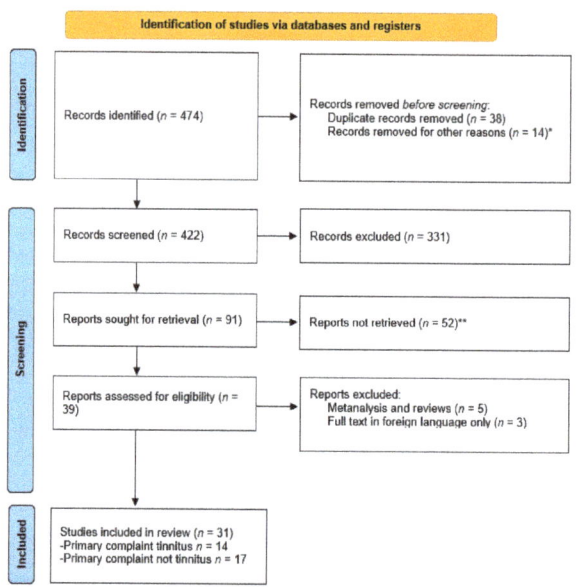

Figure 1. PRISMA 2020 flow chart diagram for updated systematic reviews which included searches of databases and study selection. Last date of search is December 2021. From: Page M J, et al. [52]. * not relevant to the topic, ** Full text not found.

3.2. Quality Assessment of Included Studies

The critical appraisal can be found in Tables 1 and 2 for studies where tinnitus was the primary complaint and those where tinnitus was not the primary complaint, respectively.

In studies where tinnitus was the primary complaint, only one study [58] defined appropriately its inclusion criteria. The remaining studies either did not provide information on contralateral ear [59] or included moderate hearing loss thresholds for inclusion criteria [54,55,60–62]. In addition, in several studies, the efficacy of conventional treatments was not tested before CI [56,63–68]. When selecting participants, inclusion and exclusion criteria were not well defined [55]. Two out of fourteen studies were retrospective [55,64]. Blinding was applied in only one study [62]. The population samples of two studies overlapped and the criteria for recruiting additional participants were not well defined [54,56]. The process of cochlear implantation and rehabilitation was not clear in all studies [60,64,67]. The intervention protocol was either unreported [55,58,59,63,64] or did not respect standard process [56,59,61,62,65,67]. Missing data, participant dropouts and withdrawal exceeding 10% [54,58,65] were justified in only one study [58].

Table 1. Quality assessment of studies in which tinnitus was the primary complaint.

ROBINS-I tool			Risk of Bias (RoB)						
Study	Study Design	Sample Size	Bias Due to Confounding	Bias in Selection of Participants	Bias in Classification of Interventions	Deviation from Intended Intervention	Bias Due to Missing Data	Bias in Measurement of Outcomes	Bias in Selection of Reported Result
Ahmed et al. [63]	PCS	13	●	O	O	Ø	Ø	◐	O
Arts et al. [62]	PCS	10	●	O	O	●	O	O	O
Holder et al. [64]	PCS	12	●	●	Ø	Ø	Ø	◐	O
Kleinjung et al. [60]	CR	1	●	NA	Ø	O	Ø	NA	Ø
Macias et al. [66]	PCS	16	●	O	O	O	O	◐	O
Mertens et al. [55]	RCT	23	●	●	●	Ø	Ø	◐	O
Mertens et al. [56]	PCS	11	●	O	O	●	Ø	◐	O
Poncet-Wallet et al. [65]	PCS	26	●	O	O	●	●	◐	◐
Punte et al. [59]	PCS	26	Ø	O	O	Ø	O	◐	●
Punte et al. [68]	PCS	7	●	O	O	●	O	◐	O
Ramos et al. [61]	PCS	6	●	O	O	●	O	◐	O
Song et al. [58]	PCS	9	O	O	O	Ø	●	◐	●
Van de Heyning et al. [54]	PCS	22	●	O	O	O	●	◐	◐
Zeng et al. [67]	CR	1	●	NA	Ø	●	Ø	NA	Ø

PCS: prospective cohort study; RCS: retrospective cohort study, CR: Case report. Confounding: O = no confounding (use of three inclusion criteria: SSD defined with (PTA (0.5, 1, 2, 4 kHz) > 70 dBs in one ear and <30 dBs in the other ear, severe tinnitus defined by TFI > 32, THI > 58, TQ > 42, VAS loudness or annoyance > 6/10, and failure of conventional treatment such as CROS, BCD, HA), ● = inclusion criteria not appropriately used, Ø = no information. Selection of participants (based on participant characteristics observed after the start of the intervention): O = no bias in selection of participants, ● = bias in selection of participants, NA: not applicable. Classification of interventions: O = intervention status well defined before application (CI), ● = intervention status defined retrospectively, Ø = no information. Deviation from intended intervention: O = standard cochlear implantation, activation and rehabilitation defined clearly in the protocol, ● = deviations to the intervention protocol, Ø = no information. Missing data: O = < 10% missing data, ● = ≥ 10% missing data, Ø = no information. Measurement of outcomes: O = similar measurement of outcomes between intervention groups AND blinding of the outcome assessors for intervention received by study participants, ◐ = similar measurement of outcomes between intervention groups AND no blinding of the outcome assessors for intervention received by study participants, ● = difference of measurement between groups AND no blinding of the outcome assessors for intervention received by study participants, NA: not applicable. Selection of reported results: O = primary outcomes reported according to the protocol, ◐ = primary outcomes reported for all groups (no subset) and explanation if missing data, ● = missing outcomes/data reported for a subset of measures, Ø: no information.

In studies where tinnitus was not the primary complaint, five studies defined appropriately its inclusion criteria [44,69–72]. When selecting participants, inclusion and exclusion criteria were not clearly provided [73,74], and blinding was not applied. Several studies were retrospective [71,72,74–76]. The CI intervention was not constantly described [57,77], and the majority of studies did not clarify if the standard CI protocol was adopted [44,69,71,72,74–76,78–81]. Missing data, participant dropouts and withdrawals exceeding 10% [71,74–76] were not constantly justified [75].

Table 2. Quality assessment of studies in which tinnitus was not the primary complaint.

	ROBINS-I Tool					Risk of Bias (RoB)			
Study	Study Design	Sample Size	Bias Due to Confounding	Bias in Selection of Participants	Bias in Classification of Interventions	Deviation from Intended Intervention	Bias Due to Missing Data	Bias in Measurement of Outcomes	Bias in Selection of Reported Result
Arndt et al. [44]	PCS	11	O	O	O	Ø	O	◐	O
Buechner et al. [73]	PCS	5	●	●	O	O	O	◐	O
Dillon et al. [8]	PCS	20	●	O	O	O	Ø	◐	O
Dorbeau et al. [82]	PCS	18	●	O	O	O	O	◐	O
Finke et al. [75]	RCS	14	●	O	●	Ø	●	◐	Ø
Friedman et al. [71]	RCS	16	O	O	●	Ø	●	◐	◐
Gartrell et al. [77]	CR	1	●	NA	Ø	Ø	Ø	NA	Ø
Harkonen et al. [80]	PCS	7	●	O	O	Ø	O	◐	O
Haubler et al. [72]	PCS	20	O	O	●	Ø	O	◐	O
Kitoh et al. [81]	PCS	5	●	O	O	Ø	●	◐	O
Macias et al. [78]	PCS	16	●	O	O	Ø	O	◐	O
Mertens et al. [57]	PCS	15	●	O	Ø	●	O	◐	O
Peters et al. [83]	PCS	28	●	O	O	O	O	◐	◐
Sladen et al. [74]	RCS	23	●	●	●	Ø	●	◐	◐
Sullivan et al. [76]	RCS	60	●	O	●	Ø	●	◐	◐
Tavora-Vieira et al. [69]	PCS	9	O	O	O	O	O	◐	O
Tavora-Vieira et al. [70]	PCS	28	O	O	O	O	O	◐	O

PCS: prospective cohort study; RCS: retrospective cohort study, CR: Case report. Confounding: O = no confounding (use of three criteria: SSD defined with (PTA (0.5,1,2,4 kHz) > 70 dBs in one ear and <30 dBs in the other ear, and failure of conventional treatment such as CROS, BCD, HA), ● = inclusion criteria not appropriately used. Selection of participants (based on participant characteristics observed after the start of the intervention): O = no bias in selection of participants, ● = bias in selection of participants, NA: not applicable. Classification of interventions: O = intervention status well defined before application (CI), ● = intervention status defined retrospectively, Ø = no information. Deviation from intended intervention: O = standard cochlear implantation, activation and rehabilitation defined clearly in the protocol, ● = deviations to the intervention protocol, Ø = no information. Missing data: O = < 10% missing data, ● = ≥10% missing data, Ø = no information. Measurement of outcomes: O = similar measurement of outcomes between intervention groups AND blinding of the outcome assessors for intervention received by study participants, ◐ = similar measurement of outcomes between intervention groups AND no blinding of the outcome assessors for intervention received by study participants, ● = difference of measurement between groups AND no blinding of the outcome assessors for intervention received by study participants, NA: not applicable. Selection of reported results: O = primary outcomes reported according to the protocol, ◐ = primary outcomes reported for all groups (no subset) and explanation if missing data, ● = missing outcomes/data reported for a subset of measures, Ø: no information.

3.3. Data Extraction and Study Outcomes

3.3.1. Tinnitus Evaluated as a Primary Complaint

In studies in which tinnitus was the primary complaint, pre- and post-operative tinnitus was evaluated, using numerous tools including validated questionnaires and scales, and objectives tests (Table 3). Validated self-reported instruments were used in all such studies, namely the Tinnitus Questionnaire (TQ) [10,11], THI [12], Tinnitus Reaction Questionnaire (TRQ) [13], VAS [14], Tinnitus Rating Score (TRS) [15], Subjective Tinnitus Severity Scale (STSS) [16], and/or Numeric Rating Scale (NRS) [17]. Objective measurements including electroencephalogram (EEG) along with functional imaging [58], and/or evoked and spontaneous cortical activities [67] were less frequently used. The follow-up period was variable studies and ranged between 12 min [67] to 36 months [55].

Table 3. Characteristics of studies investigating CI in SSD patients with disabling tinnitus in which tinnitus was the primary complaint.

Study	Patients' Criteria	n	Evaluation	Interval Studied	Results	Conclusion
Ahmed et al. [63]	CI in SSD and disabling tinnitus	13	*Questionnaires* - THI - TRS	3 months	- Significant improvement of THI and TRS	- CI is a treatment option of tinnitus suppression
Arts et al. [62]	CI in SSD and tinnitus (Intracochlear electrical stimulation vs. standard clinical CI).	10	*Tests* - VAS (tinnitus pitch and loudness matching) - RI *Questionnaires* - THI - TQ - HUI3 (HRQoL) - BDI (depression)	3 months	- Significant reduction of all tinnitus-related outcomes - Residual inhibition of tinnitus ranged from a few seconds to more than 30 min in 10 patients	- Significant reduction of tinnitus - No significant difference between intracochlear electrical stimulation and standard clinical CI on tinnitus outcomes - No significant difference between intracochlear electrical stimulation and standard clinical CI on QoL and depression outcomes
Holder et al. [64]	CI in SSD and tinnitus	12	*Tests* - CNC (word recognition). *Questionnaires* - THI	12 months	- Significant reduction of THI - Significant improvement of word recognition	- CI being an effective treatment option for SSD patients and tinnitus
Kleinjung et al. [60]	CI in SSD and severe tinnitus refractory to treatment	1	*Questionnaires* - VAS (tinnitus loudness and annoyance) - THI - TQ	3 months	- Distinct decrease in VAS, THI, and TQ - When CI is deactivated, tinnitus reoccurred only after presentation to loud noise	- Tinnitus completely disappeared 3 months after CI activation
Macias et al. [66]	CI in SDD and severe tinnitus	16	*Questionnaires* - VAS (tinnitus loudness) - THI - THS (hyperacusis) - HUI3 (QoL) - SSQ (Hearing)	12 months	- Significant decrease of VAS and THI - Significant decrease of hyperacusis handicap - Significant improvement of QoL and hearing - Residual inhibition of tinnitus was short-lasting with a median of less than 1 min	- Patients with SSD and concomitant severe tinnitus handicap were successfully treated with a CI
Mertens et al. [55]	CI in SSD and disabling tinnitus	23	*Questionnaires* - VAS (tinnitus loudness) - TQ - HQ (hyperacusis)	36 months	- Significant reduction of VAS and TQ - Significant difference of HQ scores - Residual inhibition of tinnitus is less than 1 min	- Tinnitus reduction remain stable up to 36 months
Mertens et al. [56]	CI in SSD and disabling tinnitus	11	*Questionnaires* - VAS (tinnitus loudness) - TQ	3 months	- Significant decrease of VAS and TQ	- CI can significantly reduce ipsilateral severe tinnitus in a subject with SSD.
Poncet-Wallet et al. [65]	CI in SSD and disabling tinnitus	26	*Tests* - Speech perception *Questionnaires* - VAS (tinnitus loudness and annoyance) - THI - TRQ - STSS	13 months	- Significant decrease of THI, TRQ, STSS, and VAS - Improvement of speech perception	- After 1 year of standard CI stimulation, 92% of patients reported a significant improvement in tinnitus

Table 3. Cont.

Study	Patients' Criteria	n	Evaluation	Interval Studied	Results	Conclusion
Punte et al. [59]	CI in SSD and severe tinnitus	26	Tests - TA (type, frequency, and loudness) Questionnaires - VAS (tinnitus loudness) - TQ (tinnitus distress)	6 months	- Significant reduction of VAS and TQ - When CI is deactivated, tinnitus reoccurred in 24 patients - Complete residual inhibition of tinnitus persists for at least 24 h ($n = 2$)	- Tinnitus loudness reduction remained stable over time - No difference on tinnitus reduction were observed according to tinnitus type - Tinnitus was completely abolished with CI activation in 3 patients
Punte et al. [68]	CI in SSD and severe tinnitus	7	Tests - TA (type, frequency, and loudness). Questionnaires - VAS (tinnitus loudness) - Psychoacoustic tinnitus loudness - TQ	6 months	- Significant decrease of VAS and TQ, and psychoacoustic tinnitus loudness after complete CI activation - When deactivated, tinnitus relapses and reoccurs to its original loudness in 6 patients - Complete residual inhibition of tinnitus persists for at least 24 h ($n = 1$)	- Tinnitus was completely abolished with CI activation in 1 patient - Limited reduction of VAS in 2 patients but coping with tinnitus is easier
Ramos et al. [61]	CI in SSD and disabling tinnitus refractory to prior treatment	6	Tests - TA (timbre, intensity, and minimum masking level) - HST (quantifying hyperacusis) - Hearing assessment Questionnaires - VAS - THI (perception and disability)	3 months	- Significant decrease or suppression of tinnitus perception and disability - Reduction of VAS - When CI is deactivated, improvement of tinnitus perception remained	- CI can reduce or suppress disabling tinnitus in patients with SSD
Song et al. [58]	CI in SSD and intractable tinnitus	9	Tests - EEG recording - sLORETA Questionnaires - NRS (tinnitus loudness) - TQ (subjective distress).	6 months	- Improvement in NRS and TQ	- Increased activities of AC and PCC, and increased functional connectivity between AC and PCC may be an unfavourable prognostic indicator after CI in patients with SSD
Van de Heyning et al. [54]	CI in SSD and severe intractable tinnitus unresponsive to treatment	22	Questionnaires - VAS (tinnitus loudness) - TQ (tinnitus distress)	24 months	- Significant reduction of VAS and TQ - When CI is deactivated, tinnitus reoccurred in 19 patients - Complete residual inhibition of tinnitus persists for at least 12 h ($n = 3$)	- Significant reduction in tinnitus when CI activated.

Table 3. *Cont.*

Study	Patients' Criteria	n	Evaluation	Interval Studied	Results	Conclusion
Zeng et al. [67]	CI in SSD and debilitating tinnitus refractory to treatment	1	*Tests* - Evoked and spontaneous cortical activities *Questionnaires* - VAS (tinnitus loudness)	720 s	- Low-rate low-level stimulus produced total tinnitus suppression - When stimulus is terminated, rebound in tinnitus was louder than baseline - Reduction of VAS	- Totally abolished tinnitus and restored normal brain activities

Abbreviations: AC (auditory cortex), BDI (Beck depression inventory), CI (cochlear implant), CNC (consonant-nucleus-consonant test), HQ (hyperacusis questionnaire), HST (hyperacusis test), HUI3 (health utilities index mark 3), NRS (numeric rating scale), PCC (posterior cingulate cortex), RI (residual inhibition), SHQ (sound hypersensitivity questionnaire), sLORETA (standardized low-resolution brain electromagnetic tomography), SSD (single-sided deafness), STSS (subjective tinnitus severity scale), TA (tinnitus analysis), THI (tinnitus handicap inventory), THS (test de Hipersensibilidad al sonido), TQ (tinnitus questionnaire), TRQ (tinnitus reaction questionnaire), TRS (tinnitus rating score), UHL (unilateral hearing loss), VAS (visual analogue scale).

In all studies in which tinnitus was the primary complaint, early after implant activation, electrical stimulation succeeded to significantly reduce, sometimes completely, tinnitus loudness and distress [60,68]. VAS, THI, and TQ were used in the majority of studies, but also similar results were obtained with other tools such as TRQ, TRS, and STSS [63,65]. No tinnitus aggravation was noted in any of the included studies. Long-term (>12 months) tinnitus suppression was reported in several studies [54,55,65]. Tinnitus suppression was less likely to persist when CI was turned off [54,59,60,68]; persistence of suppression after CI deactivation was only reported in one study [61]. While some studies reported complete residual inhibition of tinnitus that ranged between a minute to 30 min [55,62,66], others reported that residual inhibition persisted for 12 [54] and 24 h [59,68]. Taken together, these results confirm the effectiveness of CI as a treatment in disabling tinnitus (Table 3).

Zeng et al. [67] assessed tinnitus presence objectively by recording cortical potentials and tinnitus loudness subjectively using a VAS. Evoked and spontaneous cortical activity was recorded in "tinnitus-presence" and "tinnitus-suppressed" conditions. Complete suppression of tinnitus was obtained after a low-rate low-level electrical intracochlear stimulation and was associated re-established brain activities. These results were coherent with a reduction of tinnitus loudness (VAS). In another study, Song et al. [58] explored EEG waves and activated Auditory Cortex (AC) areas by brain electromagnetic tomography among patients with tinnitus and SSD pre- and post-cochlear implantation; those with pre-operative enhanced activity in different regions of the AC, higher delta and gamma bands, and an increased connectivity between different area of the AC, were less likely to improve after CI. These results matched with NRS and TQ scores (Table 3).

3.3.2. Tinnitus Evaluated as an Additional Complaint

In studies in which tinnitus was not the primary complaint, tinnitus was also investigated via validated questionnaires and scales including VAS, THI, TRQ, TQ, and/or tinnitus handicap questionnaire (THQ) (Table 4). No objective measurements were used.

All studies in which tinnitus was not the primary complaint reported tinnitus suppression. Among the 296 patients included in these studies, tinnitus was not suppressed in only one patient [75]. Tinnitus suppression remained stable over time [57,70,76,77]. When CI patients were compared to a control group, THI scores were significantly lower [83]. No objective measurements were applied for tinnitus in any of these studies (Table 4).

Table 4. Characteristics of studies investigating CI in SSD patients with disabling tinnitus in which tinnitus was not the primary complaint.

Study	Patients' Criteria	n	Evaluation	Interval Studied	Results	Conclusion
Arndt et al. [44]	CI in SSD and tinnitus refractory to conventional treatment	11	*Tests* - HSM sentence test (speech comprehension in noise) - OLSA sentence test (speech comprehension in noise and speech localization) *Questionnaires* - SSQ - HUI3 - IOI-HA (QoL and outcome with hearing devices) - VAS (tinnitus)	6 months	- Significant improvement of speech localization and comprehension - Significant improvement of QoL - Significant reduction or complete suppression of tinnitus when present	- CI improved hearing abilities and was superior to the alternative treatment options - CI use did not interfere with speech understanding in the normal hearing ear
Buechner et al. [73]	CI in SSD and tinnitus	5	*Tests* - FST and HSM sentence test (speech comprehension in noise) - OLSA sentence test (speech perception and localization). *Questionnaires* - Sound quality - VAS (tinnitus)	12 months	- Significant benefit of speech perception tests (NB = 3) - None of the participants judged CI sound quality as intolerable - Significant suppression (NB = 3) or reduction (NB = 2) of tinnitus	- CI improved hearing and tinnitus
Dillon et al. [8]	CI in SSD and tinnitus	20	*Questionnaires* - Speech localization and perception - Traditional scores and SSQ subscales (QoL) - APHAB (difficulty) - THI (tinnitus)	12 months	- Improvements in speech perception in noise, spatial hearing, and listening effort - Significant improvement of QoL and less perceived difficulty - Significant reduction of tinnitus severity	- CI may offer significant improvement in QoL, reduction in perceived tinnitus, and subjective improvement in speech perception and hearing
Dorbeau et al. [82]	CI in SSD and tinnitus	18	*Tests* - Sound localization - SRT in quiet and noise (speech understanding in noise) *Questionnaires* - SSQ - GBI (QoL) - THI (tinnitus)	12 months	- Significant improvement of speech localization - No significant SRTs difference when speech and noise were co-located, but significantly better SRTs when speech and noise spatially separated. - Significant improvement of SSQ - Significant improvement of QoL - Significant reduction of tinnitus severity	- Strong significant and consistent CI benefits were observed for localization, speech performance, tinnitus reduction, and QoL

Table 4. *Cont.*

Study	Patients' Criteria	n	Evaluation	Interval Studied	Results	Conclusion
Finke et al. [75]	CI in SSD and tinnitus	14	*Tests* - FST and HSM sentence test in quiet and noise (speech perception and sound localization). *Questionnaires* - Sound localization - Fear to lose the second ear - QoL - Tinnitus and noise sensitivity	53 months	- Significant improvement of sound localization and sound quality - Substantial change in QoL - Reduction of tinnitus ($n = 13$); only one patient stated that the CI failed to reduce tinnitus	- Overall sense of increased well-being explained by the four different core categories localization, tinnitus, fear of hearing loss and QoL
Friedman et al. [71]	CI in SSD and tinnitus	16	*Tests* - Sound localization - CNC monosyllabic words and AzBio sentences (speech perception) - BKB-SIN or HINT (hearing in noise) *Subjective assessments* - Integration ability - Tinnitus	12 months	- Significant improvement in speech perception - No significant difference in sound localization - Improvement in integration ability - Suppression of tinnitus	- CI improved speech perception and performance, integration ability, and tinnitus
Gartrell et al. [77]	CI in SSD and severe tinnitus refractory to medical therapies	1	*Tests* - Sound localization - Speech in noise test - Audiometric threshold - HINT (hearing in noise) - CNC (speech discrimination) - IEEE sentence test (speech quality) *Questionnaires* - TRQ - TQ - THI	18 months	- Significant improvement of sound localisation - Improved speech intelligibility - Marked tinnitus reduction and remained over 16 months	- CI improved sound localization accuracy when compared and reduced tinnitus handicap
Härkönen et al. [80]	CI in SSD and tinnitus	7	*Tests* - Sound localization - Bisyllabic Finnish words (speech in noise test) *Questionnaires* - GBI (QoL) - SSQ and VAS (QoH) - Working performance and work-related stress - VAS (tinnitus)	28 months	- Significant positive effect of sound localization, speech perception in noise, QoL, and QoH - Improved working performance - Decreased tinnitus perception	- CI improved QoL, QoH, sound localization, speech perception in noise, work performance, and tinnitus

Table 4. Cont.

Study	Patients' Criteria	n	Evaluation	Interval Studied	Results	Conclusion
Häußler et al. [72]	CI in SSD and tinnitus refractory to conventional treatment	20	Tests - Speech perception - Hearing ability. Questionnaires - NCIQ (health related QoL) - SF-36 (general QoL) - Psychological comorbidities - TQ (tinnitus)	36 months	- Significant improvement of speech perception - Significant improvement of heath related QoL - Significant decrease of anxiety symptoms - Significant reduction of tinnitus	- CI improved hearing, tinnitus, QoL, and psychological comorbidities
Kitoh et al. [81]	CI in SSD patients	5	Tests - Sound localization - Japanese monosyllable test (speech perception in quiet and noise) Questionnaires - THI (tinnitus disturbance)	12 months	- Improvement of speech perception and increased sound localization accuracy - Reduction of tinnitus	- CI improved speech perception, sound localization, and tinnitus
Macias et al. [78]	CI in SSD and disabling tinnitus and hyperacusis refractory to conventional treatment	16	Questionnaires - HUI3 (QoL) - SSQ (hearing quality) - SHQ (hyperacusis) - THI and VAS (tinnitus)	12 months	- Substantial reduction in sound intolerance - Increase QoL - Substantial decrease of tinnitus	- CI improved tinnitus, hyperacusis, and QoL
Mertens et al. [57]	CI in SSD and disabling tinnitus	15	Tests - SRT in noise in non-tinnitus ear in CI-on and CI-off conditions Questionnaires - VAS and TQ (tinnitus)	36 months	- Significant improvement of speech perception and SRT - Improvement of TQ and remained stable or became better for 3 years - Significant decrease of VAS	- CI improved speech perception and tinnitus
Peters et al. [83]	CI and bone conduction devices in SSD and tinnitus	28	Tests - Sound localization - USTARR (speech recognition in noise) Questionnaires - SSQ - APHAB - GBI (QoL) - TQ and THI (tinnitus)	6 months	- CI had better speech reception, sound localization, TQ and THI - All treatment options had an improvement of disease specific QoL - Significant decrease of tinnitus	- CI group had better sound localization and perception, and decreased tinnitus burden

Table 4. Cont.

Study	Patients' Criteria	n	Evaluation	Interval Studied	Results	Conclusion
Sladen et al. [74]	CI in SSD and tinnitus	23	Tests - CNC word and AzBio sentence in quiet and noise (speech perception) Other - Tinnitus assessment tool	6 months	- Significant improvement of both word and sentence scores in quiet - No significant improvement of speech recognition in noise - Reduction in tinnitus severity	- CI improved speech understanding and reduced tinnitus
Sullivan et al. [76]	CI in SSD patients and tinnitus	60	Tests - Sound localization - CNC word and AzBio sentence in quiet and noise (speech perception) - Adaptive HINT (binaural hearing) Questionnaires - THQ (tinnitus)	72 months	- Sound localization tended to improve - Significant improvement of speech perception - Improvement of tinnitus; kept stable for many years	- CI meaningfully improved word understanding, tend to gradually improve sound localization, and improve tinnitus
Tavora-Vieira et al. [69]	CI in SSD and tinnitus	9	Tests - BKB sentence in noise (speech perception). Questionnaires - SSQ (hearing perception) - TRQ (tinnitus)	3 months	- Improvement of speech perception in noise - Significant improvement of hearing perception - Improvement of tinnitus	- CI improved speech understanding in noise, hearing perception, and tinnitus control
Tavora-Vieira et al. [70]	CI in SSD with tinnitus	28	Tests - BKB-SIN (speech perception) 223 Questionnaires - SSQ (speech perception) - APHAB (hearing difficulties) - TRQ (tinnitus disturbance)	24 months	- Significant improvement of speech perception in noise - Significant improvement of hearing - Decreased disturbance caused by tinnitus; improvement was stable over time.	- CI use improved hearing and speech perception, and decreased tinnitus disturbance

Abbreviations: CI (cochlear implant), AHL (asymmetrical hearing loss), SSD (single-sided deafness), UHL (unilateral hearing loss), SSQ (speech, spatial and qualities of hearing scale), HSM (Hochmair–Schulz–Moser sentence test), CROS (contralateral routing of signal), BAHA (bone-anchored hearing aid), OLSA (Oldenburg sentence test), IOI-HA (international outcome inventory for hearing aids), HUI3 (health utilities index mark 3), VAS (visual analogue scale), THI (tinnitus handicap inventory), QoL (quality of life), APHAB (abbreviated profile of hearing aid benefit), FST (Freiburger numbers and monosyllabic test), TRQ (tinnitus reaction questionnaire), BKB-SIN (Bamford–Kowal–Bench sentence-in-noise), HINT (hearing in noise test), SRTs (speech reception thresholds), GBI (Glasgow benefit inventory), HADS (hospital anxiety depression scale), TTO (time trade off), HSM (Hochmair–Schulz–Moser sentences test), TQ (tinnitus questionnaire), SF-36 (36-Item *Short Form* Survey), AzBio test (Arizona biomedical institute sentence test), QoH (quality of hearing), NCIQ (Nijmegen cochlear implant questionnaire), PSQ (perceived stress questionnaire), COPE (Brief-COPE questionnaire), GAD-7 (generalized anxiety disorder questionnaire), OI (Oldenburg inventory), HRQoL (health-related quality of life), GFP (Gold field power), SHQ (sound hypersensitivity questionnaire), CAEPs (Cortical auditory evoked potentials), EQ-5D (European quality of life-five dimension), THQ (tinnitus handicap questionnaire), LIST (Leuven intelligibility sentence test), USTARR (Utrecht-sentence test with adaptive randomized roving levels), HINT (hearing in noise test), IEEE (Institute of Electrical and Electronics Engineers sentence test).

3.3.3. Effect of Cochlear Implant on Other Factors

Along with tinnitus suppression, other criteria were assessed including speech comprehension in quiet and in noise, spatial hearing, hearing quality, speech perception and localization, sound quality, hyperacusis, work performance, psychological comorbidities, and QoL. Most studies reported improvement of sound localization and speech perception. The improvement of speech perception remained inconstant and oscillated during the first 6 months after implantation [81]. Speech recognition threshold (SRT) was improved [57]. No deterioration of speech performance was noted in the better hearing side with electric and acoustic signals integration [71]. Communication leading to less fatigue after a long workday and better work performance was also reported [80]. In addition, hyperacusis, evaluated using sound hypersensitivity questionnaire (SHQ) [55,66], as well as sound intolerance [78] were decreased among patients with CI. Furthermore, intracochlear electric stimulation improved QoL indexes and psychological comorbidities [44,72,75,80,83]. Taken together, these findings suggest that CI reduced tinnitus, restored hearing aspects, and improved QoL in SSD patients (Tables 3 and 4).

4. Discussion

The present systematic review describes the effect of cochlear implantation on tinnitus in patients with SSD and disabling tinnitus. Reduction of tinnitus was reported in a relatively high number of studies (31 studies, 479 patients). No aggravation of tinnitus was reported in any patient. When compared to no treatment, CI was associated with better tinnitus suppression scores. These findings are encouraging in considering CI for SSD patients with disabling tinnitus, more specifically when conventional treatments fail to relieve the tinnitus. Although results are promising so far, the indication of CI for these patients is not yet widespread.

Most studies included in the present review assessed tinnitus using subjective tools; these are available in different languages, are not time consuming, and provide validated scores. VAS and THI were the most frequently used, followed by TQ. Although it could seem advantageous to not to be limited to a single tool, particularly since not all tools are validated for all languages, and some are more difficult to use than others, the heterogeneity of tools employed hampers comparison between studies. It is of note that objective tools were less likely to be used, which is possibly related to the difficulty of access to equipment required for electrophysiological and radiological assessments but also to the lack of available personnel with the skills to perform the assessments and interpret the results. These tools are, however, interesting in further understanding the mechanism of tinnitus reduction as well as the anatomical areas intervening in this process. It may also be helpful in identifying parameters that can predict prognosis. More generally, further research is needed to objectively assess treatment related physiological processes.

All SSD patients included in this review had disabling tinnitus, but the characteristics of their deafness were variable in terms of interval between onset and cochlear implantation, aetiology, and type of CI device. This makes it difficult to compare studies, but suggests treatment is successful independent of these factors. The risk of bias assessment showed a lack of precise inclusion criteria as well as a definition of the intervention in many studies. This emphasizes the need for a randomized clinical trial with clearly defined inclusion criteria and standard and clear intervention and rehabilitation protocols.

Whether tinnitus was evaluated as a primary complaint or not, CI succeeded to alleviate tinnitus. Studies in which tinnitus was evaluated as a primary complaint discussed several tinnitus characteristics including residual inhibition and recurrence of tinnitus after deactivation of implant. These studies were less likely to discuss hearing aspects or psychosocial benefits compared to studies where tinnitus was not the primary complaint.

Our review included all studies until December 2021. The present systematic review differs from previous published reviews in several ways. First, and to the best of our knowledge, this is the only review in which the listed studies have been divided into two groups depending on whether or not tinnitus was the primary complaint. The latter division permits reducing the risk of false-positive and false-negative errors. Second, the present review is not limited by the type of questionnaires used to assess tinnitus [50]: all validated multi-item questionnaires have been considered. In addition, studies using subjective assessment tools and studies using objective assessment tools were included. Audiological and neurophysiological levels of evidence were simultaneously considered when available. Last but not least, data on short- and long- term tinnitus suppression were analysed. The improvement of tinnitus, reflected by a significant reduction in various validated multi-item questionnaire scores, should strengthen considering CI in SSD with disabling tinnitus when conventional treatments are insufficient.

The present study has certain limitations; similar to the previously published systematic reviews, studies were mostly observational, and there was wide heterogeneity of tools used and a small sample size. This may preclude generalization of the results to a wider more heterogeneous population. Further studies with larger samples are needed to develop prediction models of tinnitus outcomes after cochlear implantation, where objective methods of tinnitus could be of interest.

5. Conclusions

In conclusion, this review included a large number of studies reporting the effectiveness of CI in suppressing disabling tinnitus in SSD patients when conventional treatment is insufficient. Tinnitus improvement is maintained in the long-term (>12 months). Considering the positive effect observed in all the studies, CI indication deserves to be more widely considered in such patients.

Author Contributions: H.T.-V. designed the plan of the article, contributed to the manuscript draft, and closely reviewed and revised the whole article critically for important intellectual content. S.A.I. made the literature review and data collection, wrote the manuscript draft, conceived and designed the tables and figures, and interpreted the data. M.M. and A.M. participated in the conception of the work, contributed to the article plan, and reviewed the article. P.R. participated in drafting the work and data collection. C.-A.J. contributed to data collection and analysis. K.K.S.A. participated in the quality assessment and reviewed the whole article. E.C.I. reviewed the whole article. All authors have made substantial contributions to this manuscript. They gave their final approval of the version to be published; and agreed to be accountable for all aspects of the work in ensuring that questions related to the accuracy or integrity of any part of the work are appropriately investigated and resolved. All authors have read and agreed to the published version of the manuscript.

Funding: This research received no external funding.

Acknowledgments: The authors acknowledge the support from the Paris Hearing Institute from Foundation pour l'Audition (FPA IDA09). They also thank Philip Robinson and Xuan Thai-Van for proofreading the article.

Conflicts of Interest: K.K.S.A. is employed at the Cochlear Technology Centre, Mechelen, Belgium. No further conflict of interest is reported by the authors.

References

1. Snapp, H.A.; Ausili, S.A. Hearing with one ear: Consequences and treatments for profound unilateral hearing loss. *J. Clin. Med.* **2020**, *9*, 1010. [CrossRef] [PubMed]
2. Iwasaki, S.; Sano, H.; Nishio, S.; Takumi, Y.; Okamoto, M.; Usami, S.I.; Ogawa, K. Hearing handicap in adults with unilateral deafness and bilateral hearing loss. *Otol. Neurotol.* **2013**, *34*, 644–649. [CrossRef] [PubMed]
3. Wie, O.B.; Pripp, A.H.; Tvete, O. Unilateral deafness in adults: Effects on communication and social interaction. *Ann. Otol. Rhinol. Laryngol.* **2010**, *119*, 772–781. [PubMed]
4. Douglas, S.A.; Yeung, P.; Daudia, A.; Gatehouse, S.; O'Donoghue, G.M. Spatial hearing disability after acoustic neuroma removal. *Laryngoscope* **2007**, *117*, 1648–1651. [CrossRef]
5. Marx, M.; Mosnier, I.; Venail, F.; Mondain, M.; Uziel, A.; Bakhos, D.; Lescanne, E.; N'Guyen, Y.; Bernardeschi, D.; Sterkers, O.; et al. Cochlear Implantation and Other Treatments in Single-Sided Deafness and Asymmetric Hearing Loss: Results of a National Multicenter Study including a Randomized Controlled Trial. *Audiol. Neurotol.* **2021**, *26*, 414–424. [CrossRef]

6. Henderson-Sabes, J.; Shang, Y.; Perez, P.L.; Chang, J.L.; Pross, S.E.; Findlay, A.M.; Mizuiri, D.; Hinkley, L.B.; Nagarajan, S.S.; Cheung, S.W. Corticostriatal functional connectivity of bothersome tinnitus in single-sided deafness. *Sci. Rep.* **2019**, *9*, 19552. [CrossRef]
7. König, O.; Schaette, R.; Kempter, R.; Gross, M. Course of hearing loss and occurrence of tinnitus. *Hear. Res.* **2006**, *221*, 59–64. [CrossRef]
8. Dillon, M.T.; Buss, E.; Rooth, M.A.; King, E.R.; Deres, E.J.; Buchman, C.A.; Pillsbury, H.C.; Brown, K.D. Effect of Cochlear Implantation on Quality of Life in Adults with Unilateral Hearing Loss. *Audiol. Neurotol.* **2017**, *22*, 259–271. [CrossRef]
9. Ciminelli, P.; Machado, S.; Palmeira, M.; Carta, M.G.; Beirith, S.C.; Nigri, M.L.; Mezzasalma, M.A.; Nardi, A.E. Tinnitus: The Sound of Stress? *Clin. Pract. Epidemiol. Ment. Health* **2018**, *14*, 264–269. [CrossRef]
10. Hallam, R.S.; Jakes, S.C.; Hinchcliffe, R. Cognitive variables in tinnitus annoyance. *Br. J. Clin. Psychol.* **1988**, *27*, 213–222. [CrossRef]
11. Zeman, F.; Koller, M.; Schecklmann, M.; Langguth, B.; Landgrebe, M.; Figueired, R.; Aazevedo, A.; Rates, M.; Binetti, C.; Elgoyhen, A.B.; et al. Tinnitus assessment by means of standardized self-report questionnaires: Psychometric properties of the Tinnitus Questionnaire (TQ), the Tinnitus Handicap Inventory (THI), and their short versions in an international and multi-lingual sample. *Health Qual. Life Outcomes* **2012**, *10*, 128. [CrossRef] [PubMed]
12. Newman, C.W.; Jacobson, G.P.; Spitzer, J.B.; Surgery, N.; Ford Hospital, H.; Newman, M. Development of the Tinnitus Handicap Inventory. *Arch. Otolaryngol. Head Neck Surg.* **1996**, *122*, 143–148. [CrossRef] [PubMed]
13. Wilson, P.; Henry, J.; Bowen, M.; Haralambous, G. Tinnitus reaction questionnaire: Psychometric properties of a measure of distress associated with tinnitus. *J. Speech Hear Res.* **1991**, *34*, 197–201. [CrossRef] [PubMed]
14. Raj-Koziak, D.; Gos, E.; Swierniak, W.; Rajchel, J.J.; Karpiesz, L.; Niedzialek, I.; Wlodarczyk, E.; Skarzynski, H.; Skarzynski, P.H. Visual analogue scales as a tool for initial assessment of tinnitus severity: Psychometric evaluation in a clinical population. *Audiol. Neurotol.* **2018**, *23*, 229–237. [CrossRef]
15. Croft, C.; Brown, R.F.; Thorsteinsson, E.B.; Noble, W. Development of the Tinnitus response scales: Factor analyses, subscale reliability and validity analyses. *Int. Tinnitus J.* **2013**, *18*, 45–56. [CrossRef]
16. Halford, J.; Anderson, S. Tinnitus severity measured by a subjective scale, audiometry and clinical judgement. *J. Laryngol. Otol.* **1991**, *105*, 89–93. [CrossRef]
17. Meikle, M.B.; Stewart, B.J.; Griest, S.E.; Henry, J.A. Tinnitus Outcomes Assessment. *Trends Amplif.* **2008**, *12*, 223–235. [CrossRef]
18. McCombe, A.; Baguley, D.; Coles, R.; McKenna, L.; McKinney, C.; Windle-Taylor, P. Guidelines for the grading of tinnitus severity: The results of a working group commissioned by the British Association of Otolaryngologists, Head and Neck Surgeons, 1999. *Clin. Otolaryngol. Allied Sci.* **2001**, *26*, 388–393. [CrossRef]
19. Han, B.I.; Lee, H.W.; Kim, T.Y.; Lim, J.S.; Shin, K.S. Tinnitus: Characteristics, causes, mechanisms, and treatments. *J. Clin. Neurol.* **2009**, *5*, 11–19. [CrossRef]
20. Auerbach, B.D.; Rodrigues, P.V.; Salvi, R.J. Central Gain Control in Tinnitus and Hyperacusis. *Front. Neurol.* **2014**, *5*, 206. [CrossRef]
21. Gomaa, M.A.M.; Elmagd, M.H.A.; Elbadry, M.M.; Kader, R.M.A. Depression, Anxiety and Stress Scale in patients with tinnitus and hearing loss. *Eur. Arch. Oto-Rhino-Laryngol.* **2014**, *271*, 2177–2184. [CrossRef]
22. Zirke, N.; Goebel, G.; Mazurek, B. Tinnitus und psychische Komorbiditäten. *HNO* **2010**, *58*, 726–732. [CrossRef] [PubMed]
23. Simões, J.P.; Neff, P.K.A.; Langguth, B.; Schlee, W.; Schecklmann, M. The progression of chronic tinnitus over the years. *Sci. Rep.* **2021**, *11*, 4162. [CrossRef] [PubMed]
24. Cima, R.F.F.; Mazurek, B.; Haider, H.; Kikidis, D.; Lapira, A.; Noreña, A.; Hoare, D.J. A multidisciplinary European guideline for tinnitus: Diagnostics, assessment, and treatment. *HNO* **2019**, *67*, 10–42. [CrossRef]
25. Tunkel, D.E.; Bauer, C.A.; Sun, G.H.; Rosenfeld, R.M.; Chandrasekhar, S.S.; Cunningham, E.R.; Archer, S.M.; Blakley, B.W.; Carter, J.M.; Granieri, E.C.; et al. Clinical practice guideline: Tinnitus. *Otolaryngol.–Head Neck Surg.* **2014**, *151*, S1–S40. [CrossRef]
26. Baldo, P.; Doree, C.; Lazzarini, R.; Molin, P.; McFerran, D.J. Antidepressants for patients with tinnitus. *Cochrane Database Syst. Rev.* **2012**, *2012*, CD003853. [CrossRef] [PubMed]
27. Hoekstra, C.E.L.; Rynja, S.P.; Van Zanten, G.A.; Rovers, M. Anticonvulsants for tinnitus. *Cochrane Database Syst. Rev.* **2011**, *2011*, CD007960. [CrossRef] [PubMed]
28. Sereda, M.; Xia, J.; Scutt, P.; Hilton, M.P.; El Refaie, A.; Hoare, D.J. Ginkgo biloba for tinnitus. *Cochrane Database Syst. Rev.* **2019**, *2019*, CD013514. [CrossRef]
29. Person, O.C.; Puga, M.E.; da Silva, E.M.; Torloni, M.R. Zinc supplementation for tinnitus. *Cochrane Database Syst. Rev.* **2016**, *11*, CD009832. [CrossRef]
30. Londero, A.; Bonfils, P.; Lefaucheur, J.P. Transcranial magnetic stimulation and subjective tinnitus. A review of the literature, 2014–2016. *Eur. Ann. Otorhinolaryngol. Head Neck Dis.* **2018**, *135*, 51–58. [CrossRef]
31. Ferreira, M.C.; De Matos, I.L.; De Toledo, I.P.; Honório, H.M.; Mondelli, M.F.C.G.; Gallun, F.E.; Rasetshwane, D. Effects of low-level laser therapy as a therapeutic strategy for patients with tinnitus: A systematic review. *J. Speech Lang. Hear. Res.* **2021**, *64*, 279–298. [CrossRef] [PubMed]
32. Rogha, M.; Rezvani, M.; Khodami, A.R. The effects of acupuncture on the inner ear originated tinnitus. *J. Res. Med. Sci.* **2011**, *16*, 1217–1223. [PubMed]

33. Jun, H.J.; Park, M.K. Cognitive behavioral therapy for tinnitus: Evidence and efficacy. *Korean J. Audiol.* **2013**, *17*, 101–104. [CrossRef]
34. Cima, R.F.F.; Maes, I.H.; Joore, M.A.; Scheyen, D.J.W.W.; El Refaie, A.; Baguley, D.M.; Anteunis, L.J.C.; Van Breukelen, G.J.P.; Vlaeyen, J.W.S. Specialised treatment based on cognitive behaviour therapy versus usual care for tinnitus: A randomised controlled trial. *Lancet* **2012**, *379*, 1951–1959. [CrossRef]
35. Scherer, R.W.; Formby, C.; Gold, S.; Erdman, S.; Rodhe, C.; Carlson, M.; Shade, D.; Tucker, M.; Sensinger, L.M.C.; Hughes, G.; et al. The Tinnitus Retraining Therapy Trial (TRTT): Study protocol for a randomized controlled trial. *Trials* **2014**, *15*, 396. [CrossRef] [PubMed]
36. Thompson, D.M.; Hall, D.A.; Walker, D.-M.; Hoare, D.J. Psychological Therapy for People with Tinnitus: A scoping review of treatment components. *Ear Hear.* **2017**, *38*, 149–158. [CrossRef] [PubMed]
37. Arif, M.; Sadlier, M.; Rajenderkumar, D.; James, J.; Tahir, T. A randomised controlled study of mindfulness meditation versus relaxation therapy in the management of tinnitus. *J. Laryngol. Otol.* **2017**, *131*, 501–507. [CrossRef] [PubMed]
38. Gunjawate, D.R.; Ravi, R. Effect of yoga and meditation on tinnitus: A systematic review. *J. Laryngol. Otol.* **2021**, *135*, 284–287. [CrossRef]
39. Attias, J.; Shemesh, Z.; Shoham, C.; Shahar, A.; Sohmer, H. Efficacy of self-hypnosis for tinnitus relief. *Scand. Audiol.* **1990**, *19*, 245–249. [CrossRef]
40. House, J.W. Treatment of severe tinnitus with biofeedback training. *Laryngoscope* **1978**, *88*, 406–412. [CrossRef]
41. Chen, J.; Zhong, P.; Meng, Z.; Pan, F.; Qi, L.; He, T.; Lu, J.; He, P.; Zheng, Y. Investigation on chronic tinnitus efficacy of combination of non-repetitive preferred music and educational counseling: A preliminary study. *Eur. Arch. Oto-Rhino-Laryngol.* **2021**, *278*, 2745–2752. [CrossRef] [PubMed]
42. Roland, L.T.; Lenze, E.J.; Hardin, F.M.; Kallogjeri, D.; Nicklaus, J.; Wineland, A.M.; Fendell, G.; Peelle, J.E.; Piccirillo, J.F. Effects of mindfulness based stress reduction therapy on subjective bother and neural connectivity in chronic tinnitus. *Otolaryngol.–Head Neck Surg.* **2015**, *152*, 919–926. [CrossRef]
43. Tyler, R.S.; Perreau, A.; Powers, T.; Watts, A.; Owen, R.; Ji, H.; Mancini, P.C. Tinnitus sound therapy trial shows effectiveness for those with tinnitus. *J. Am. Acad. Audiol.* **2020**, *31*, 6–16. [CrossRef] [PubMed]
44. Arndt, S.; Aschendorff, A.; Laszig, R.; Beck, R.; Schild, C.; Kroeger, S.; Ihorst, G.; Wesarg, T. Comparison of pseudobinaural hearing to real binaural hearing rehabilitation after cochlear implantation in patients with unilateral deafness and tinnitus. *Otol. Neurotol.* **2011**, *32*, 39–47. [CrossRef] [PubMed]
45. Marx, M.; Costa, N.; Lepage, B.; Taoui, S.; Molinier, L.; Deguine, O.; Fraysse, B. Cochlear implantation as a treatment for single-sided deafness and asymmetric hearing loss: A randomized controlled evaluation of cost-utility. *BMC Ear Nose Throat Disord.* **2019**, *19*, 1–10. [CrossRef]
46. Donato, M.; Santos, R.; Correia, F.; Escada, P. Single-sided deafness: Bone conduction devices or cochlear implantation? A systematic review with meta-analysis. *Acta Otorrinolaringol. Engl. Ed.* **2021**, *72*, 101–108. [CrossRef] [PubMed]
47. Nucleus 24 Cochlear Implant System—P970051/S205. Available online: https://www.fda.gov/medical-devices/recently-approved-devices/nucleus-24-cochlear-implant-system-p970051s205 (accessed on 3 March 2022).
48. *Recommandation pour la Pratique Clinique—Indications de L'implant Cochléaire chez L'adulte et chez L'enfant*; Société Française d'ORL Chirurgie la Face du Cou: France, 2018.
49. Peter, N.; Liyanage, N.; Pfiffner, F.; Huber, A.; Kleinjung, T. The Influence of Cochlear Implantation on Tinnitus in Patients with Single-Sided Deafness: A Systematic Review. *Otolaryngol.–Head Neck Surg.* **2019**, *161*, 576–588. [CrossRef] [PubMed]
50. Levy, D.A.; Lee, J.A.; Nguyen, S.A.; McRackan, T.R.; Meyer, T.A.; Lambert, P.R. Cochlear Implantation for Treatment of Tinnitus in Single-Sided Deafness: A Systematic Review and Meta-analysis. *Otol. Neurotol.* **2020**, *41*, e1004–e1012. [CrossRef] [PubMed]
51. Andrade, C. The primary outcome measure and its importance in clinical trials. *J. Clin. Psychiatry* **2015**, *76*, e1320–e1323. [CrossRef]
52. Page, M.J.; McKenzie, J.E.; Bossuyt, P.M.; Boutron, I.; Hoffmann, T.C.; Mulrow, C.D.; Shamseer, L.; Tetzlaff, J.M.; Akl, E.A.; Brennan, S.E.; et al. The PRISMA 2020 statement: An updated guideline for reporting systematic reviews. *Syst. Rev.* **2021**, *10*, 89. [CrossRef]
53. Sterne, J.; Hernán, M.A.; Reeves, B.C.; Savović, J.; Berkman, N.D.; Viswanathan, M.; Henry, D.; Altman, D.G.; Ansari, M.T.; Boutron, I.; et al. ROBINS-I: A tool for assessing risk of bias in non-randomised studies of interventions. *BMJ* **2016**, *355*, 4–10. [CrossRef] [PubMed]
54. Van De Heyning, P.; Vermeire, K.; Diebl, M.; Nopp, P.; Anderson, I.; De Ridder, D. Incapacitating unilateral tinnitus in single-sided deafness treated by cochlear implantation. *Ann. Otol. Rhinol. Laryngol.* **2008**, *117*, 645–652. [CrossRef] [PubMed]
55. Mertens, G.; De Bodt, M.; Van de Heyning, P. Cochlear implantation as a long-term treatment for ipsilateral incapacitating tinnitus in subjects with unilateral hearing loss up to 10 years. *Hear. Res.* **2016**, *331*, 1–6. [CrossRef] [PubMed]
56. Mertens, G.; Van Rompaey, V.; Van de Heyning, P. Electric-acoustic stimulation suppresses tinnitus in a subject with high-frequency single-sided deafness. *Cochlear Implants Int.* **2018**, *19*, 292–296. [CrossRef]
57. Mertens, G.; Punte, A.K.; De Ridder, D.; Van De Heyning, P. Tinnitus in a single-sided deaf ear reduces speech reception in the nontinnitus ear. *Otol. Neurotol.* **2013**, *34*, 662–666. [CrossRef]
58. Song, J.J.; Punte, A.K.; De Ridder, D.; Vanneste, S.; Van de Heyning, P. Neural substrates predicting improvement of tinnitus after cochlear implantation in patients with single-sided deafness. *Hear. Res.* **2013**, *299*, 1–9. [CrossRef]

59. Punte, A.K.; Vermeire, K.; Hofkens, A.; De Bodt, M.; De Ridder, D.; Van de Heyning, P. Cochlear implantation as a durable tinnitus treatment in single-sided deafness. *Cochlear Implants Int.* **2011**, *12* (Suppl. 1), S26–S29. [CrossRef]
60. Kleinjung, T.; Steffens, T.; Strutz, J.; Langguth, B. Curing tinnitus with a Cochlear Implant in a patient with unilateral sudden deafness: A case report. *Cases J.* **2009**, *2*, 7462. [CrossRef]
61. Ramos, Á.; Polo, R.; Masgoret, E.; Artiles, O.; Lisner, I.; Zaballos, M.L.; Moreno, C.; Osorio, Á. Cochlear Implant in Patients With Sudden Unilateral Sensorineural Hearing Loss and Associated Tinnitus. *Acta Otorrinolaringol. Engl. Ed.* **2012**, *63*, 15–20. [CrossRef]
62. Arts, R.A.G.J.; George, E.L.J.; Janssen, M.; Griessner, A.; Zierhofer, C.; Stokroos, R.J. Tinnitus suppression by intracochlear electrical stimulation in single sided deafness—A prospective clinical trial: Follow-up. *PLoS ONE* **2016**, *11*, e0153131. [CrossRef]
63. Ahmed, M.F.M.; Khater, A. Tinnitus suppression after cochlear implantation in patients with single-sided deafness. *Egypt. J. Otolaryngol.* **2017**, *33*, 61–66. [CrossRef]
64. Holder, J.T.; O'Connell, B.; Hedley-Williams, A.; Wanna, G. Cochlear implantation for single-sided deafness and tinnitus suppression. *Am. J. Otolaryngol.–Head Neck Med. Surg.* **2017**, *38*, 226–229. [CrossRef] [PubMed]
65. Poncet-Wallet, C.; Mamelle, E.; Godey, B.; Truy, E.; Guevara, N.; Ardoint, M.; Gnansia, D.; Hoen, M.; Saaï, S.; Mosnier, I.; et al. Prospective Multicentric Follow-up Study of Cochlear Implantation in Adults with Single-Sided Deafness: Tinnitus and Audiological Outcomes. *Otol. Neurotol.* **2020**, *41*, 458–466. [CrossRef] [PubMed]
66. Ramos Macías, A.; Falcón-González, J.C.; Manrique Rodríguez, M.; Morera Pérez, C.; García-Ibáñez, L.; Cenjor Español, C.; Coudert-Koall, C.; Killian, M. One-Year Results for Patients with Unilateral Hearing Loss and Accompanying Severe Tinnitus and Hyperacusis Treated with a Cochlear Implant. *Audiol. Neurotol.* **2018**, *23*, 8–19. [CrossRef] [PubMed]
67. Zeng, F.G.; Tang, Q.; Dimitrijevic, A.; Starr, A.; Larky, J.; Blevins, N.H. Tinnitus suppression by low-rate electric stimulation and its electrophysiological mechanisms. *Hear. Res.* **2011**, *277*, 61–66. [CrossRef] [PubMed]
68. Kleine Punte, A.; De Ridder, D.; Van De Heyning, P. On the necessity of full length electrical cochlear stimulation to suppress severe tinnitus in single-sided deafness. *Hear. Res.* **2013**, *295*, 24–29. [CrossRef]
69. Távora-Vieira, D.; Marino, R.; Krishnaswamy, J.; Kuthbutheen, J.; Rajan, G.P. Cochlear implantation for unilateral deafness with and without tinnitus: A case series. *Laryngoscope* **2013**, *123*, 1251–1255. [CrossRef]
70. Távora-Vieira, D.; Marino, R.; Acharya, A.; Rajan, G.P. The impact of cochlear implantation on speech understanding, subjective hearing performance, and tinnitus perception in patients with unilateral severe to profound hearing loss. *Otol. Neurotol.* **2015**, *36*, 430–436. [CrossRef]
71. Friedmann, D.R.; Ahmed, O.H.; McMenomey, S.O.; Shapiro, W.H.; Waltzman, S.B.; Thomas Roland, J. Single-sided deafness cochlear implantation: Candidacy, evaluation, and outcomes in children and adults. *Otol. Neurotol.* **2016**, *37*, e154–e160. [CrossRef]
72. Häußler, S.M.; Knopke, S.; Dudka, S.; Gräbel, S.; Ketterer, M.C.; Battmer, R.D.; Ernst, A.; Olze, H. Improvement in tinnitus distress, health-related quality of life and psychological comorbidities by cochlear implantation in single-sided deaf patients. *HNO* **2020**, *68*, 1–10. [CrossRef]
73. Buechner, A.; Brendel, M.; Lesinski-Schiedat, A.; Wenzel, G.; Frohne-Buechner, C.; Jaeger, B.; Lenarz, T. Cochlear implantation in unilateral deaf subjects associated with ipsilateral tinnitus. *Otol. Neurotol.* **2010**, *31*, 1381–1385. [CrossRef] [PubMed]
74. Sladen, D.P.; Frisch, C.D.; Carlson, M.L.; Driscoll, C.L.W.; Torres, J.H.; Zeitler, D.M. Cochlear implantation for single-sided deafness: A multicenter study. *Laryngoscope* **2017**, *127*, 223–228. [CrossRef] [PubMed]
75. Finke, M.; Bönitz, H.; Lyxell, B.; Illg, A. Cochlear implant effectiveness in postlingual single-sided deaf individuals: What's the point? *Int. J. Audiol.* **2017**, *56*, 417–423. [CrossRef] [PubMed]
76. Sullivan, C.B.; Al-Qurayshi, Z.; Zhu, V.; Liu, A.; Dunn, C.; Gantz, B.J.; Hansen, M.R. Long-term audiologic outcomes after cochlear implantation for single-sided deafness. *Laryngoscope* **2020**, *130*, 1805–1811. [CrossRef]
77. Gartrell, B.C.; Jones, H.G.; Kan, A.; Buhr-Lawler, M.; Gubbels, S.P.; Litovsky, R.Y. Investigating Long-Term Effects of Cochlear Implantation in Single-Sided Deafness. *Otol. Neurotol.* **2014**, *35*, 1525–1532. [CrossRef]
78. Ramos Macías, A.; Falcón González, J.C.; Manrique, M.; Morera, C.; García-Ibáñez, L.; Cenjor, C.; Coudert-Koall, C.; Killian, M. Cochlear implants as a treatment option for unilateral hearing loss, severe tinnitus and hyperacusis. *Audiol. Neurotol.* **2015**, *20*, 60–66. [CrossRef]
79. Tavora-Vieira, D.; De Ceulaer, G.; Govaerts, P.J.; Rajan, G.P. Cochlear Implantation Improves Localization Ability in Patients with Unilateral Deafness. *Ear Hear.* **2015**, *36*, e93–e98. [CrossRef]
80. Härkönen, K.; Kivekäs, I.; Rautiainen, M.; Kotti, V.; Sivonen, V.; Vasama, J.P. Single-Sided Deafness: The Effect of Cochlear Implantation on Quality of Life, Quality of Hearing, and Working Performance. *Orl* **2015**, *77*, 339–345. [CrossRef]
81. Kitoh, R.; Moteki, H.; Nishio, S.; Shinden, S.; Kanzaki, S.; Iwasaki, S.; Ogawa, K.; Usami, S.I. The effects of cochlear implantation in Japanese single-sided deafness patients: Five case reports. *Acta Otolaryngol.* **2016**, *136*, 460–464. [CrossRef]
82. Dorbeau, C.; Galvin, J.; Fu, Q.J.; Legris, E.; Marx, M.; Bakhos, D. Binaural Perception in Single-Sided Deaf Cochlear Implant Users with Unrestricted or Restricted Acoustic Hearing in the Non-Implanted Ear. *Audiol. Neurotol.* **2018**, *23*, 187–197. [CrossRef]
83. Peters, J.P.M.; van Heteren, J.A.A.; Wendrich, A.W.; van Zanten, G.A.; Grolman, W.; Stokroos, R.J.; Smit, A.L. Short-term outcomes of cochlear implantation for single-sided deafness compared to bone conduction devices and contralateral routing of sound hearing aids—Results of a Randomised controlled trial (CINGLE-trial). *PLoS ONE* **2021**, *16*, e0257447. [CrossRef] [PubMed]

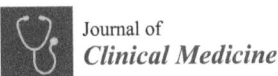

Journal of
Clinical Medicine

Article

Effect of Serious Gaming on Speech-in-Noise Intelligibility in Adult Cochlear Implantees: A Randomized Controlled Study

Pierre Reynard [1,2,3], Virginie Attina [3], Samar Idriss [3], Ruben Hermann [2,4,5], Claire Barilly [5], Evelyne Veuillet [1,2,3], Charles-Alexandre Joly [1,2,3] and Hung Thai-Van [1,2,3,*]

1. Institut de l'Audition, Institut Pasteur, Université de Paris, INSERM, 75012 Paris, France; pierre.reynard@hotmail.fr (P.R.); evelyne.veuillet@gmail.com (E.V.); charles-alexandre.joly01@chu-lyon.fr (C.-A.J.)
2. Faculty of Medicine, University Claude Bernard Lyon 1, 69100 Villeurbanne, France; ruben.hermann@chu-lyon.fr
3. Hospices Civils de Lyon, Hôpital Edouard Herriot, Service d'Audiologie et Explorations Otoneurologiques, 69003 Lyon, France; virginie.attina@gmail.com (V.A.); samar.a.idriss@hotmail.com (S.I.)
4. Lyon Neuroscience Research Center, INSERM U1028, CNRS UMR5292, Integrative, Multisensory, Perception, Action and Cognition Team (IMPACT), 69675 Bron, France
5. Hospices Civils de Lyon, Hôpital Edouard Herriot, Service d'ORL, Chirurgie Cervico-Faciale et d'Audiophonologie, 69003 Lyon, France; claire.barilly@gmail.com
* Correspondence: hthaivan@gmail.com or hung.thai-van@chu-lyon.fr

Citation: Reynard, P.; Attina, V.; Idriss, S.; Hermann, R.; Barilly, C.; Veuillet, E.; Joly, C.-A.; Thai-Van, H. Effect of Serious Gaming on Speech-in-Noise Intelligibility in Adult Cochlear Implantees: A Randomized Controlled Study. *J. Clin. Med.* **2022**, *11*, 2880. https://doi.org/10.3390/jcm11102880

Academic Editors: Giuseppe Magliulo and Nicolas Guevara

Received: 18 March 2022
Accepted: 17 May 2022
Published: 19 May 2022

Publisher's Note: MDPI stays neutral with regard to jurisdictional claims in published maps and institutional affiliations.

Copyright: © 2022 by the authors. Licensee MDPI, Basel, Switzerland. This article is an open access article distributed under the terms and conditions of the Creative Commons Attribution (CC BY) license (https://creativecommons.org/licenses/by/4.0/).

Abstract: Listening in noise remains challenging for adults with cochlear implants (CI) even after prolonged experience. Personalized auditory training (AT) programs can be proposed to improve specific auditory skills in adults with CI. The objective of this study was to assess serious gaming as a rehabilitation tool to improve speech-in-noise intelligibility in adult CI users. Thirty subjects with bilateral profound hearing loss and at least 9 months of CI experience were randomized to participate in a 5-week serious game-based AT program (*n* = 15) or a control group (*n* = 15). All participants were tested at enrolment and at 5 weeks using the sentence recognition-in-noise matrix test to measure the signal-to-noise ratio (SNR) allowing 70% of speech-in-noise understanding (70% speech reception threshold, SRT70). Thirteen subjects completed the AT program and nine of them were re-tested 5 weeks later. The mean SRT70 improved from 15.5 dB to 11.5 dB SNR after 5 weeks of AT ($p < 0.001$). No significant change in SRT70 was observed in the control group. In the study group, the magnitude of SRT70 improvement was not correlated to the total number of AT hours. A large inter-patient variability was observed for speech-in-noise intelligibility measured once the AT program was completed and at re-test. The results suggest that serious game-based AT may improve speech-in-noise intelligibility in adult CI users. Potential sources of inter-patient variability are discussed. Serious gaming may be considered as a complementary training approach for improving CI outcomes in adults.

Keywords: serious game; auditory rehabilitation; cochlear implant; listening-in-noise; speech reception threshold; re-test

1. Introduction

Since the early 1990s, cochlear implants (CI) have undoubtedly provided improvements in terms of the quality of life and auditory skills of both adults and children. However, some limitations remain [1]. Immediately after CI surgery, patients must adapt to perceiving new sounds, which they learn to recognize with the assistance of speech therapy. CI recipients need to learn how to treat sound flow and to mentally represent the relationships between the perceived sounds (signifier) and their meaning (signified) to improve their auditory skills.

Auditory training (AT) has been used since the early 1970s to teach a wide range of auditory skills, including detection (i.e., to be aware of the absence or presence of a target sound-alert function), discrimination (i.e., to distinguish between sounds), identification (i.e., to identify words, pseudo-words, syllables, phonemes), and comprehension (i.e., to make sense of the sounds heard, whether they are environmental (noise) or linguistic). In CI recipients, there is sparse evidence on the efficacy of AT, possibly due to the heterogeneity of training protocols, outcome measures, and demographic data [2].

Understanding in noise and suprasegmental speech parameter perception and interpretation (i.e., recognizing prosodic variations, rhythms, intonations) remain crucial in AT. The latter must focus on both verbal working memory abilities, and executive functions, such as attention (alertness, sustained attention, selective attention) and inhibition. Studies have found a correlation between verbal working memory abilities and speech comprehension in noise, meaning that knowledge and neurocognitive functions may influence the results of speech-in-noise intelligibility [2–4].

Speech recognition in a noisy environment is challenging for CI recipients, even for those with prolonged experience: speech recognition in CI listeners is more impaired by background noise than that of normal-hearing (NH) listeners [5]. Compared to NH listeners, CI recipients need a signal-to-noise ratio (SNR) at least 25 dB higher than NH listeners to reach the 50% speech reception threshold (SRT50), i.e., to be able to repeat 50% of the linguistic material delivered in the presence of noise [6]. As expected, speech recognition and sound localization in noisy environments is better in bilateral CI users compared to unilateral users [7,8]. Although AT has previously been reported to improve speech-in-noise intelligibility in subjects with hearing aids [9,10], this result is still debated. For instance, when Abrams et al. investigated the effect of computer-assisted AT (CAAT) on the listening skills in noise of a sample of subjects with newly fitted hearing aids, the authors found no significant improvement, which they believed was due to difficulties related to program compliance [11].

Despite technological advances, CI alone do not enable the satisfactory restoration of auditory skills and there is a consensus that speech re-education or AT is essential [12–15]. Traditionally, AT is provided in a face-to-face setting; however, there are some reports of computerized AT (CAT) programs for adult CI recipients, but not all are based on serious gaming [1,16–18]. AT programs can now be followed remotely, via computer or mobile applications [19,20]. The objective of AT is to stimulate the plasticity of rehabilitation, and research has shown that neurophysiological changes can occur after the placement of CI [21]. After activation of the implant, active rehabilitation strategies, based on explicit AT, show better results than passive strategies [22]. The period of auditory adaptation to ensure good post-implantation results varies for adult CI recipients. However, not all implanted subjects are offered active AT, not only because of its cost and the lack of speech therapists, but also due to the lack of consensus concerning therapeutic strategies [22]. It is, however, increasingly recognized that subjects need to be more involved in their aural rehabilitative process and that more options to personalize their rehabilitative program should be offered [23].

Serious gaming is an emerging applied field of research that focuses on the use of digital gaming platforms and technologies for more than just entertainment [24,25]. One suggested definition is "a mental contest, played with a computer in accordance with specific rules that uses entertainment to further government or corporate training, education, health, public policy, and strategic communication objectives" [26]. Serious games have been used in a variety of fields such as education, asthma education, psychotherapy, and even surgical training [27–31]. By offering a pleasant game experience, the use of serious game-based training is thought to significantly boost interest and motivation and thus reinforce the players' acquisitions in the trained domain [32]. Serious game-based programs may be adapted to the training needs specifically met by CI users.

To date, no study has evaluated the value of serious game-based AT in CI subjects. As speech comprehension in competitive listening situations remains a challenging improvement goal in CI adults, evaluating the effect of serious game-based AT on speech in noise intelligibility in this population is of great interest. The primary objective of the present study was to evaluate the efficacy of a 5-week digital gaming program in this regard. The secondary objective was to evaluate the maintenance of possible benefits over time.

2. Materials and Methods

2.1. Participants

A total of 30 adults with at least 9 months of CI experience were recruited at the department of audiology and otoneurology of the Edouard Herriot University Hospital, Lyon, France (Figure 1).

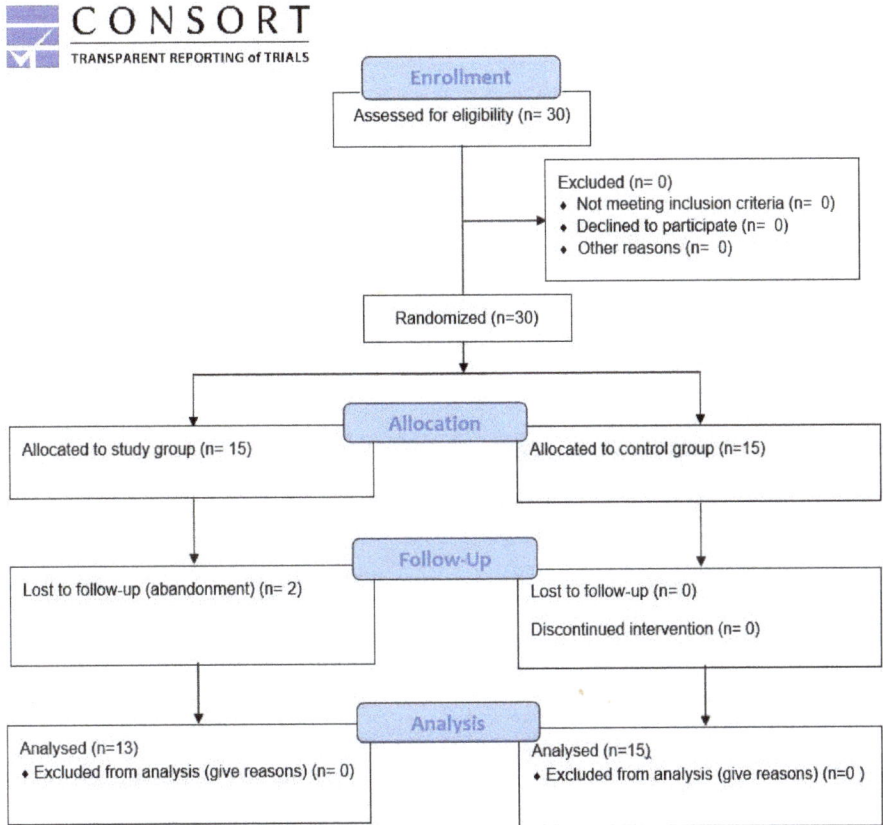

Figure 1. Flow chart.

Eligible subjects were over 18 years old, suffered from bilateral profound hearing loss, and had had unilateral or bilateral CI for at least 9 months (range 1 to 26 years). All participants reported auditory difficulties in a noisy environment. The study protocol was approved by the local ethics committee (CPP Sud-Est IV 14/034 ID RCB 2014-A00345-42). Written informed consent was obtained from all patients.

The CI subjects were randomized into two groups using a computer-generated randomization list: an intervention group, which was called the study group (n = 15, 7 males, 8 females; mean age, 48 years, range 24 to 76 years) and an untrained group (control group) (n = 15, 8 males, 7 females; mean age 60 years, range 45 to 75 years). None of the subjects followed any other AT program during the study.

2.2. Intervention

With the aim of providing innovative and translational therapeutic methods in CI adults, a dedicated serious game was developed with the support of the French government ("Neurosyllabic R&D project"). The design and development of the serious game were based on previously published criteria for an effective AT protocol [10]. These criteria included ease of access (achievable at home and suitable for the elderly), interactivity, tasks of increasing complexity (to maintain the interest and attention of the subject), feedback, and the ability to record performances at any time.

A simple serious game scenario was developed in order to enable most subjects to easily identify with an avatar (Figure 2). Participants underwent a 5-week training program including 6 activities. The first 2 consisted in detecting and discriminating target sounds (animal calls, instruments, everyday noises, and words) in noise. These 2 activities were the only ones available during the 1st week. Then, 4 other games were introduced in the 2nd week: 1 consisted in target sound identification, and the last 3 were word-based games during which the subject had to either discriminate words, identify their syllables, or categorize them according to their semantic.

The auditory material included 240 noises, 22 instrument sounds, 100 animal calls, 3135 words, 665 logatomes, and 600 syllables, while the video material contained 1400 illustrative images. Among all the sounds, syllables, and words used, 30% were selected from a dedicated database created for the study, 40% were recorded by professional actors, and 30% (especially ambient background sounds) were purchased from a database on the Internet. In order for training to remain close to real-life conditions, while allowing a progressive increase in difficulty, for the first 2 games, subjects could choose from 4 types of ambient sounds each of which had a variable signal-to-noise ratio (SNR): white noise, continuous noises (sound of rain, wind, etc.), discontinuous noises (such as the auditory environments of everyday life), or babbling noises.

The game was automatically adapted in terms of difficulty. The volumes of the target sounds and the ambient sound (SNR) were adjusted according to 20 levels of difficulty. For levels 1 to 10, the target sounds were set at 100%, while the volume of the ambient sound increased from 0 to 90%. For levels 11 to 20, the ambient sound was set at 100%, while the volume of the target sounds decreased from 100% to 10%. The level of difficulty could either be set manually (in which case, each game had a fixed duration of 2 min) or adapted automatically by an algorithm (the game then stopped after 4 errors). In case of automatic management, the level of difficulty was set according to the previous games: it increased after each correct answer and decreased after each error. Adaptive changes in the difficulty level depended on 3 factors:

The probability of reaching a correct answer by chance (for instance, the increment in difficulty was lower if there was 1 correct answer among 2 than if there was 1 among 5).

Elapsed time: the more time passed, the greater the increment in difficulty and the smaller the decrement. This ensured that each game did not last too long.

The number of errors and correct answers that already occurred. A sequence of several mistakes without any correct answer since the beginning of the game meant that the initial level of difficulty was too high and therefore needed to be adjusted more quickly. Conversely, a faultless course led to a faster increase in difficulty.

2.3. Experimental Protocol

The study group was instructed to undergo a minimum of 20 training sessions over a period of 5 weeks. One of the weekly sessions was performed at the hospital under the supervision of a board-certified audiologist. During the hospital session, the serious game parameters were constant, except for difficulty, which was increased as the patient progressed. The parameters of the 6 activities were unchanged. At home, the subjects carried out the other sessions by logging onto an online platform using their personal identifier. To ensure the regularity of the training, the home sessions were remotely controlled. Subjects were advised to sit comfortably in a quiet room; the noise level at the beginning of the game session was adjustable. As the speakers were often integrated into their computers, no further instructions regarding speaker placement were given. During the hospital sessions, the duration of each game was set at 2 min and the experimenter set the initial difficulty level (SNR) of tasks 1 and 2. In order to ensure that the level of difficulty was appropriate, the difficulty was determined automatically via an adaptive algorithm. To maintain a high level of motivation during the training sessions at home, the duration of the games could vary according to the performance of the participants. For each activity, gaming stopped as soon as the subject made 4 mistakes.

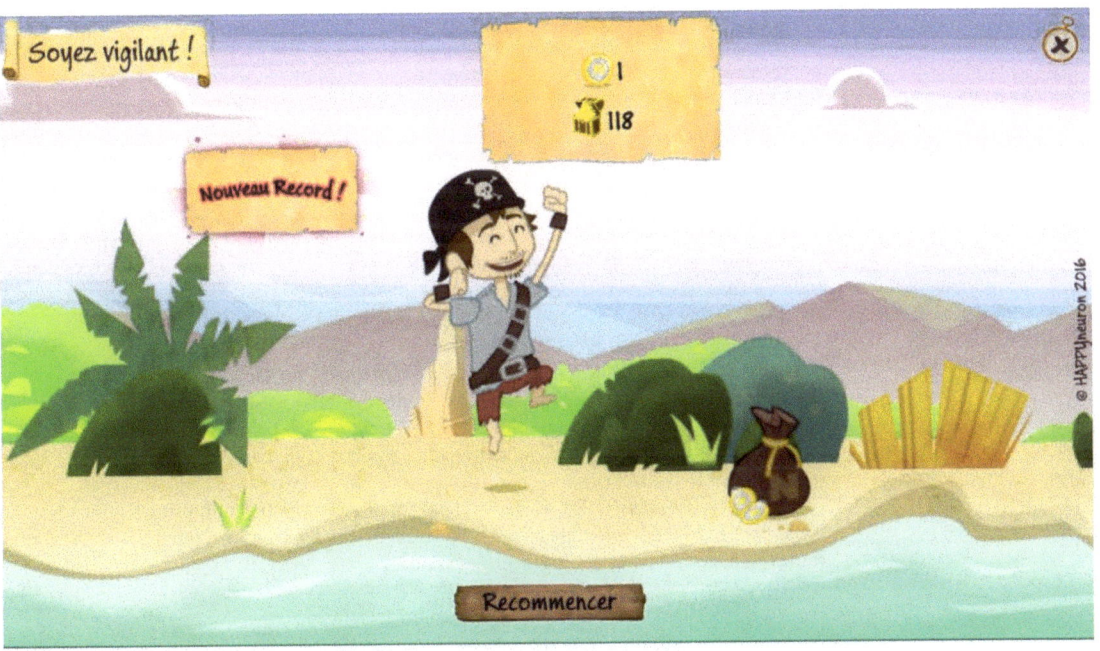

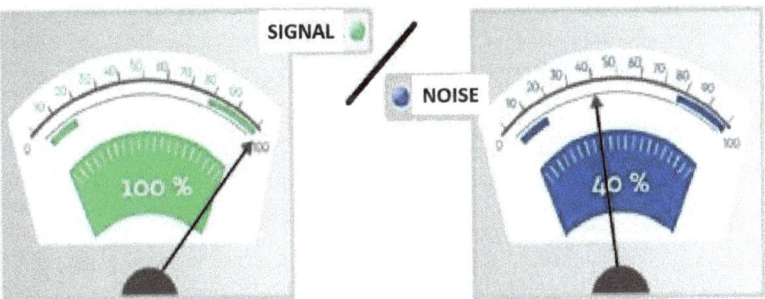

Figure 2. Serious game visuals with signal-to-noise ratio representation. As the player is detecting or identifying target sounds in the presence of background noise, the avatar is walking along a beach to collect coins. For each incorrect answer, the avatar falls and slightly regresses. After 4 incorrect answers or a pre-set time has elapsed, the game stops. The player is expected to collect as many coins as possible in 1 game with an updated score available on the screen at the end of each game. This playful mechanism encourages the player to immediately play again in an attempt to beat his/her personal record.

2.4. Data Logging

For each exercise carried out, the date, the total duration, and the actual playing duration were gathered on the online platform. This enabled the total number of exercises and the total playing time of all participants to be recorded.

2.5. Pre- and Post-Auditory Training Assessment of Speech-in-Noise

A pre- and post-AT assessment was conducted at enrolment (T1) and 5 weeks later (T2) using speech-in-noise audiometry for all participants. Additionally, 9 subjects from the study group agreed to be re-tested 5 weeks after the training period (T3) to evaluate if the benefit was maintained over time.

To assess speech-in-noise before and after training, the French version of the matrix test (Fr-matrix; adaptive procedure; system Ear 3.0, Auritec, Hamburg, Germany) was used since it exhibits high discriminative power, both in stationary and in fluctuating noise settings [33]. In this test, the speech reception threshold (SRT), which is the stimulus presentation level (relative to the noise level), is usually set to a recognition score of 50% (normative value: SRT 50 = -6.0 ± 0.6 dB SNR). The stimuli library contained 50 French words (10 names, 10 verbs, 10 numerals, 10 objects, and 10 colors) that were selected based on their phonetic content to represent the mean phonetic distribution in French spoken language. An advantage of this tool is the absence of any learning effect, which is particularly useful for repeated assessments [34].

Herein, following national guidelines for speech-in-noise testing in adults [35], the target threshold was fixed at 70% (SRT70) on purpose to avoid subjects experiencing a feeling of early failure, and was measured at T1, T2, and T3. To do so, 2 lists of words in a silent condition (20 randomly generated sentences) and 3 other lists with background noise (steady intensity of 60 dB) were played via 2 loudspeakers positioned 1 m in front of the patient in a soundproof booth. The examiner, a board-certified audiologist, was seated next to the patient in the booth.

The subjects in the study group underwent a semi-structured interview after the end of the training. They were asked: "Did you enjoy the training program?" and "Did the training improve your listening-in-noise skills?".

2.6. Statistical Analysis

Statistical analyses were performed using the SigmaStat® software (Systat Software, San Jose, CA, USA) and R version 4.1.2 (R Core Team 2021, R Foundation for Statistical Computing, Vienna, Austria). As they followed a normal distribution (confirmed by a Kolmogorov–Smirnov test), SRT70 values measured at T1 were compared between groups using a t-test. In each group, SRT70 values measured at T2 were compared to T1 values using paired t-tests.

To control for potential differences in demographics (age at testing, deafness duration prior to implant, years of implant experience) between groups, the t-test and Wilcoxon test were used. A possible correlation between demographics and SRT70 improvement between T1 and T2 was also tested.

In contrast, the total number of games played and the total duration of play were not normally distributed. The correlations of these 2 variables with each other and with SRT70 changes as a result of training were assessed using Spearman's correlation tests.

3. Results

Patient characteristics are summarized in Table 1.

Among all participants, two from the study group did not complete the training and were excluded (one moved, the other gave up), leaving 13/15 subjects (87%) who completed training and post-training Fr-matrix assessments. The time spent playing varied between 4 h 24 min and 39 h (mean 13 h) for a total of 141 to 973 exercises performed (mean 368); the number of games played was significantly correlated with the duration of play (Spearman rho = 0.951; $p < 0.001$).

Table 1. Demographic data for trained and untrained participants (CI = cochlear implant; HA = hearing aid; RE = right ear; LE = left ear; SNHL = sensori-neural hearing loss).

Patient	Age (Years)	Sex	Deafness Duration (Years)	Deafness Etiology	CI Experience (Years)	Side of CI and HA	CI Manufacturer
				Study group			
1	38	M	35	Progressive SNHL	3	CI: RE/CI: LE	Oticon Medical/Neurelec Digisonic SP
2	76	M	26	Presbycusis	5	CI: RE	Oticon Medical/Neurelec Digisonic SP
3	31	F	28	Meningitis	6	CI: LE/HA: RE	Oticon Medical/Neurelec Digisonic SP
4	56	F	26	Otosclerosis	3	CI: RE/CI: LE	Cochlear
5	70	M	15	Otosclerosis	1	CI: LE/HA: RE	AB Naida CI Q70
6	29	M	28	Meningitis	26	CI: RE/CI: LE	Cochlear
7	35	M	35	Progressive SNHL	1	CI: LE/HA: RE	AB Naida CI Q70
8	46	F	20	Progressive SNHL	7	CI: RE/CI: LE	Medel Concerto
9	76	F	16	Presbycusis	2	CI: RE/HA: LE	Medel Concerto
10	69	M	19	Otosclerosis	14	CI: RE	Neurelec
11	71	F	21	Presbycusis	1	CI: RE/HA: LE	Oticon Medical/Neurelec Digisonic SP
12	44	F	5	Meningitis	5	CI: RE	Medel Concerto
13	25	F	25	Genetic	19	CI: RE	Cochlear
14	37	F	36	Genetic	25	CI: RE/CI: LE	AB Naida CI Q70
15	24	M	24	Genetic	13	CI: RE/CI: LE	Cochlear
				Control group			
1	75	F	25	Progressive SNHL	7	CI: LE/HA: RE	Oticon Medical/Neurelec Digisonic SP
2	67	F	17	Progressive SNHL	3	CI: RE/HA: LE	Oticon Medical/Neurelec Digisonic SP
3	63	M	20	Otosclerosis	4	CI: RE/CI: LE	Oticon Medical/Neurelec Digisonic SP
4	45	M	39	Progressive SNHL	4	CI: RE	Oticon Medical/Neurelec Digisonic SP
5	68	M	5	Traumatic	4	CI: RE/CI: LE	Oticon Medical/Neurelec Digisonic SP
6	49	F	25	Genetic	6	CI: LE/HA: RE	Medel Concerto

Table 1. Cont.

Patient	Age (Years)	Sex	Deafness Duration (Years)	Deafness Etiology	CI Experience (Years)	Side of CI and HA	CI Manufacturer
7	55	F	30	Meningitis	5	CI: RE	Oticon Medical/Neurelec Digisonic SP
8	67	F	16	Progressive SNHL	8	CI: RE	Medel Concerto
9	67	M	15	Otosclerosis	8	CI: RE/CI: LE	Oticon Medical/Neurelec Digisonic SP
10	46	M	16	Iatrogenic	3	CI: LE/HA: RE	Cochlear
11	53	M	40	Genetic	9	CI: RE/CI: LE	Oticon Medical/Neurelec Digisonic SP
12	59	M	20	Menière	2	CI: LE/HA: RE	Medel Concerto
13	58	F	50	Genetic	19	CI: RE/CI: LE	Cochlear
14	73	M	23	Presbycusis	3	CI: RE/CI: LE	Oticon Medical/Neurelec Digisonic SP
15	63	F	55	Genetic	9	CI: RE/CI: LE	Oticon Medical

Before the intervention, the initial results from the Fr-matrix assessments were not significantly different between the study and control groups (t = 0.688 with 26 degrees of freedom; $p = 0.49$). Mean age differed between the study and control groups (t-test, $p = 0.039$). Age at testing, however, was not correlated with SRT70 improvement between T1 and T2 (Pearson test, $p = 0.525$). Moreover, neither deafness duration prior to implant (t-test, $p = 0.449$) nor the number of years of implant experience (Wilcoxon test, $p = 0.487$) differed between groups. Further, SRT70 improvement between T1 and T2 did not correlate with deafness duration (Pearson test, $p = 0.071$) nor with CI experience (Spearman test, $p = 0.360$).

In the control group, the mean difference in SRT70 between T1 (12.66 dB) and T2 (11.60 dB) was not significant ($t14df$-test = 0.655; $p = 0.523$, Table 2).

In the study group, a significant difference in speech-in-noise intelligibility was found between pre- and post-test assessments. The mean SRT70 in the study group was 15.5 dB at T1, and 11.5 dB at T2 ($t12df$-test = 4.521; $p < 0.001$; Figure 3). The mean SNR gain at SRT70 was −3.98 dB, with 6 of the 13 subjects evaluated having gained at least −4 dB SNR (Median = −2.8 dB SNR). All trained subjects improved their hearing abilities in noise, with decreased SRT70 after training, except Patient 5 (a 70-year-old male with 1 year of CI experience) whose SRT70 remained stable post-training (Table 2; Figure 3). The largest reduction in SRT70 was −10.2 dB SNR (Patient 12). Changes in SRT70 between T1 and T2 were not correlated with the number of games played (Spearman rho = −0.130; $p = 0.693$) nor with the total duration of play (Spearman rho = 0.033; $p = 0.915$).

Table 2. Individual and mean signal-to-noise ratio (SNR) results from Fr-matrix for the study and control groups at enrollment (T1), at 5 weeks (T2), and, for the study group, 5 weeks post-intervention (T3).

	Signal-to-Noise Ratio (dB) (Fr-Matrix Results)					
	Study group					
Patient	T1	T2	Δ T2−T1	T3	Δ T3−T1	Δ T3−T2
1	20.7	12.8	−7.9	15.7	−5.0	+2.9
2	7.9	5.1	−2.8	4.2	−3.7	−0.9
3	1.1	0.7	−0.4	−0.2	−1.3	−0.9
4	4.2	1.8	−2.4	2.8	−1.4	+1
5	3.6	3.7	+0.1	3.1	−0.5	−0.6
6	28.0	25.6	−2.4	24.3	−3.7	−1.3
7	23.1	16.2	−6.9	20.0	−3.1	+3.8
8	26.7	22.7	−4.0	32.9	+6.2	+10.2
9	16.8	12.8	−4.0	8.8	−8.0	−4.0
10	19.1	11.7	−7.4	NA		
11	6.2	3.7	−2.5	NA		
12	21.1	10.9	−10.2	NA		
13	22.8	21.8	−1.0	NA		
Mean	15.48	11.50	−3.98	12.40	−2.28	+1.13
SD	9.52	8.31		11.45		
SEM	2.64	2.71				
	Control group					
	Signal-to-noise ratio (dB) (Fr-matrix results)					
Patient	T1	T2	Δ T2−T1			
1	11.4	13.5	+2.1			
2	9.7	24.3	+14.6			
3	4.8	3.9	−0.9			
4	26.5	28	+1.5			
5	27.8	14.5	−13.3			
6	1.5	3.5	+2			
7	1.4	−1.2	−2.6			
8	8.6	4.7	−3.9			
9	30	24	−6			
10	8.8	1	−7.8			
11	5.2	8.3	+3.1			
12	15.9	10.1	−5.8			
13	0.1	−0.9	−1			
14	36.2	36.7	+0.5			
15	2	3.6	+1.6			
Mean	12.66	11.6	−1.06			
SD	11.86	11.67				
SEM	3.04	2.99				

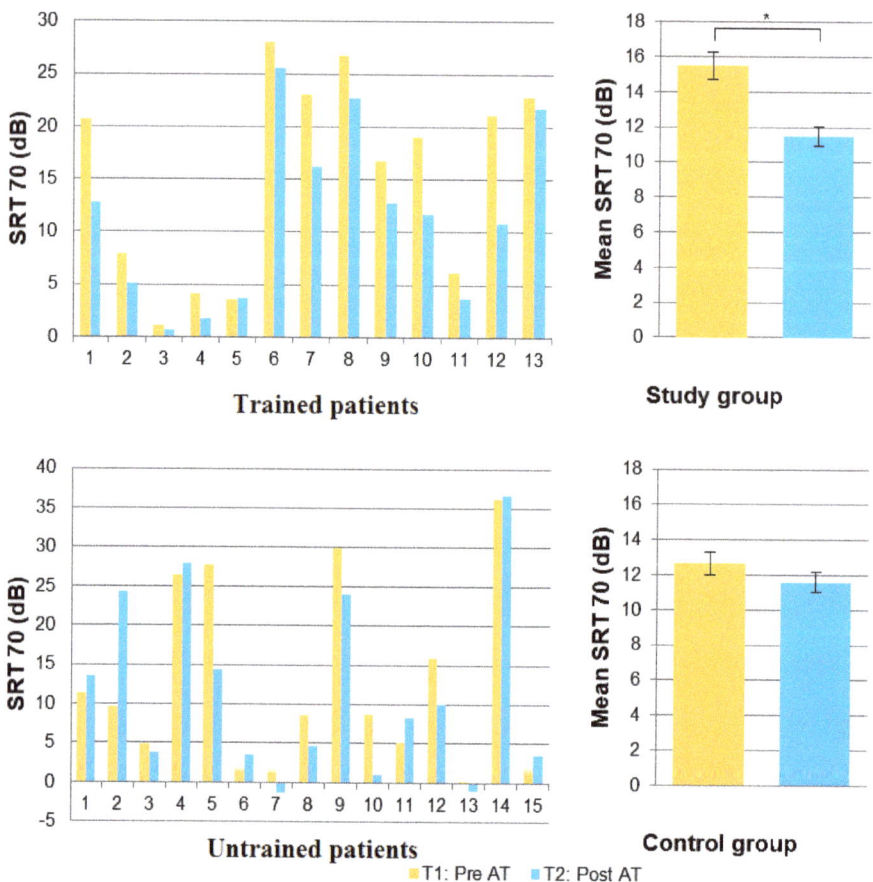

Figure 3. Changes over time in signal-to-noise ratio (dB) at a 70% speech reception threshold. Individual results are shown on the left and mean group results on the right in the study group (**top panel**) and control group (**bottom panel**); testing at enrollment (yellow) and at 5 weeks (blue). The difference is significant only in the study group (noted *).

All 13 participants in the study group responded 'Yes' to the two questions in the exit interview, i.e., "Did you enjoy the training program?" and "Did the training improve your listening-in-noise skills?".

At T3, eight out of the nine re-tested subjects still presented a decrease in SRT70 compared to T1, and the mean difference between T1 and T3 was of −2.28 dB. The mean SRT70 difference between T2 and T3 was +1.13, ranging from −4.0 in Patient 9 to +10.2 in Patient 8. Only one patient (Patient 5) did not show an overall improvement between T1 and T3 (Figure 4).

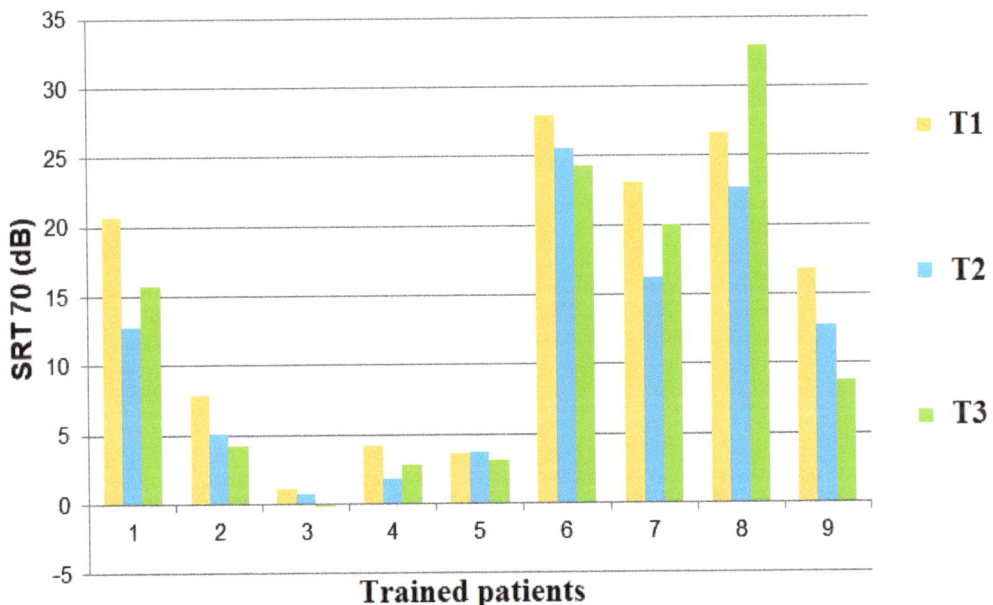

Figure 4. Changes over time in signal-to-noise ratio (dB) at a 70% speech reception threshold for nine subjects of the study group, 5 weeks after serious game-based AT (green).

4. Discussion

This study provides evidence of the impact of serious gaming on speech-in-noise intelligibility in adult CI users.

The Fr-matrix SRT70 was used as a measure of speech-in-noise intelligibility for assessing the effectiveness of a 5-week AT and its persistence. To remain as close as possible to real-life listening situations, the training assessment was performed using sentences and informational masking noise. Our group previously reported that, among speech-in-noise tests suitable for French-speaking populations, the Fr-matrix provides the lowest intra-subject variability (±0.6 dB for SRT50) [34,35].

Herein, the post-training improvement in SRT70 was measured at a mean of −3.98 dB, a result that cannot be attributed to either intra-individual variation or to procedural learning alone. The latter is, in fact, evaluated at 1.8 dB for the Fr-matrix test [33]. Moreover, the improvement in SRT70 was observed in 12 of the 13 trained subjects. In the patient who did not improve, the SRT70 degradation was minimal (+0.1 dB SNR). Conversely, the control group did not show an overall improvement. More precisely, eight subjects from the control group showed an improvement in SRT70 ranging from −0.9 to −13.3 dB SNR (mean −5.2 dB SNR), while seven showed a degradation ranging from +0.5 to +14.6 dB SNR (mean +3.6 dB SNR). Even when excluding the control patient with the highest SRT70 degradation after 5 weeks (+14.6 dB SNR), the mean SRT70 values after 5 weeks were still not significantly different from those measured initially (t13df = 1.733; $p = 0.107$). Among the participants' demographic characteristics, only mean age differed between the study and control groups. None of the demographic characteristics, including deafness duration and experience with the implant, were found to correlate with improvement in SRT70.

In the nine subjects of the study group re-tested 5 weeks after the end of the intervention, only one had a worse SRT70 than before training (difference T3-T1 = +6.2 dB SNR). For the other eight patients, the SRT70 remained better than before training: three subjects had a gain of between −0.5 and −2 dB SNR and five maintained a gain of greater than −3 dB. However, the mean difference in SRT70 (−2.28 dB SNR) measured between inclusion and re-test at 10 weeks was not significant. To date, only one study has measured the persistence of the efficacy of computer-assisted AT on speech-in-noise intelligibility in CI users [16]. These authors showed that, in 10 adult CI subjects, the benefit of AT on SRT50 could be observed up to 4 weeks after the end of the training with a gain of 2dB SNR. Future studies should more systematically integrate follow-up evaluation sessions to assess the long-term benefits of AT [36].

The serious game we used was developed specifically for this study. The software and its content had not been subject to a previous validation study. During the procedure, participants performed one training session face-to-face in the laboratory each week to ensure that the game's instructions were understood and well-followed during training, and to collect the user's experience over the previous week. The rest of the training was carried out remotely via the online gaming platform. In order to preserve the playful nature of AT, the duration of the training, the choice of activities among the six available options, and the initial difficulty level were left to the participant's will. However, an adaptive training procedure was used, in order to minimize the potential effect of inter-individual differences in initial SNR values.

Each participant was instructed to do a minimum of four training sessions per week, which was the case for each of them. The number of games played per session, however, was left up to the players in order to encourage their adherence. The relationship between the magnitude of improvement and the cumulative duration, in hours, over the 5 weeks of training could be assessed, since training logs were collected. Although the duration of training was highly variable between subjects, it was not associated with SRT70 improvement. The patient who participated the most showed an improvement at T2 (-6.9 dB SNR) compared to T1, which was higher than the mean SRT70 improvement. However, other subjects with less total training time (Patients 1, 10, and 12) showed a higher improvement (-7.9, -7.4, and -10.2, respectively) even though they had completed fewer games than the mean number of games played (336, 162, and 141, respectively). Furthermore, the patient with the highest improvement was the one who played the least. This result indicates that, while training had an overall beneficial effect and was measurable in almost all participants, there were large inter-individual disparities in the magnitude of SRT70 improvement, which prevailed over the total training time. While a weekly training schedule was set in the present study, only one study, to our knowledge, has evaluated the impact of AT schedule on speech recognition performance in degraded listening situations [37]. By training NH adults to recognize modulated vowels via a CI simulator, the authors did not find any influence of the pace of the training sessions on recognition improvement.

All or part of the inter-individual variability observed in speech-in-noise intelligibility improvement could be due to differences in the supraliminal abilities of the participants. Meta-analyses conducted in adult CI users provided evidence that demographic factors such as deafness duration or age at onset were predictive of CI outcomes, although they only explained 20% of the variance [38–40]. Furthermore, the sole SRT70 as a supraliminal measure does not account entirely for the patient's ability to recognize speech in noise. A recent meta-analysis identified the involvement of particular cognitive domains associated with speech-in-noise intelligibility, namely, processing speed, inhibitory control, working and episodic memory, and crystallized intelligence [41]. However, taken together, these cognitive abilities explain less than 10% of the inter-individual variability. A more recent review underlined the relationship between profound deafness of genetic origin and the occurrence of central auditory processing disorders in mice [42]. This is in full agreement with the fact that for a given degree of hearing loss, supraliminal auditory performance may considerably vary from one subject to another. Further studies on serious game-based AT are needed in order to better control cognitive biases potentially affecting speech comprehension in noise.

Author Contributions: Conceptualization, H.T.-V., V.A., E.V.; methodology, E.V., H.T.-V.; software, C.B., V.A.; validation, P.R., E.V., H.T.-V.; formal analysis, P.R., C.-A.J., V.A.; investigation, V.A., P.R.; resources, P.R.; data curation, P.R.; writing—original draft preparation, P.R.; writing—review and editing, C.-A.J., S.I., H.T.-V.; visualization, P.R., R.H.; supervision, H.T.-V.; project administration, H.T.-V.; funding acquisition, H.T.-V. All authors have read and agreed to the published version of the manuscript.

Funding: This study is part of a larger project (Neurosyllabic) that has been funded by a grant to Hung Thai-Van from the French Fonds Unique Interministériel. The funders had no role in the study design, data collection and analysis, decision to publish, or preparation of the manuscript.

Institutional Review Board Statement: The study was conducted according to the guidelines of the Declaration of Helsinki, and approved by the Institutional Review Board (local ethics committee (CPP Sud-Est IV 14/034 ID RCB 2014-A00345-42). The study protocol was registered on ClinicalTrials.gov (NCT02323256).

Informed Consent Statement: Informed consent was obtained from all subjects involved in the study. Written informed consent has been obtained from the subjects to publish this paper.

Data Availability Statement: The data presented in this study are available on request from the corresponding author. The data are not publicly available due to ethical, legal and privacy issues.

Acknowledgments: The authors acknowledge the support to the Paris Hearing Institute from Fondation pour l'Audition (FPA IDA09). They would like to thank all the subjects who accepted to participate in this study, and are grateful to Verena Landel for carefully proofreading the manuscript.

Conflicts of Interest: The authors declare no conflict of interest.

References

1. Ingvalson, E.M.; Lee, B.; Fiebig, P.; Wong, P.C.M. The Effects of Short-Term Computerized Speech-in-Noise Training on Postlingually Deafened Adult Cochlear Implant Recipients. *J. Speech Lang Hear. Res.* **2013**, *56*, 81–88. [CrossRef]
2. Henshaw, H.; Ferguson, M.A. Efficacy of Individual Computer-Based Auditory Training for People with Hearing Loss: A Systematic Review of the Evidence. *PLoS ONE* **2013**, *8*, e62836. [CrossRef] [PubMed]
3. Lunner, T. Cognitive Function in Relation to Hearing Aid Use. *Int. J. Audiol.* **2003**, *42* (Suppl. 1), S49–S58. [CrossRef] [PubMed]
4. Arehart, K.H.; Souza, P.; Baca, R.; Kates, J.M. Working Memory, Age and Hearing Loss: Susceptibility to Hearing Aid Distortion. *Ear Hear.* **2013**, *34*, 251–260. [CrossRef]
5. Kokkinakis, K.; Azimi, B.; Hu, Y.; Friedland, D.R. Single and Multiple Microphone Noise Reduction Strategies in Cochlear Implants. *Trends Amplif.* **2012**, *16*, 102–116. [CrossRef]
6. Turner, C.W.; Gantz, B.J.; Vidal, C.; Behrens, A.; Henry, B.A. Speech Recognition in Noise for Cochlear Implant Listeners: Benefits of Residual Acoustic Hearing. *J. Acoust. Soc. Am.* **2004**, *115*, 1729–1735. [CrossRef]
7. Laske, R.D.; Veraguth, D.; Dillier, N.; Binkert, A.; Holzmann, D.; Huber, A.M. Subjective and Objective Results after Bilateral Cochlear Implantation in Adults. *Otol. Neurotol.* **2009**, *30*, 313–318. [CrossRef]
8. Tyler, R.S.; Dunn, C.C.; Witt, S.A.; Noble, W.G. Speech Perception and Localization With Adults With Bilateral Sequential Cochlear Implants. *Ear Hear.* **2007**, *28*, 86S–90S. [CrossRef]
9. Humes, L.E.; Skinner, K.G.; Kinney, D.L.; Rogers, S.E.; Main, A.K.; Quigley, T.M. Clinical Effectiveness of an At-Home Auditory Training Program: A Randomized Controlled Trial. *Ear Hear.* **2019**, *40*, 1043–1060. [CrossRef]
10. Sweetow, R.W.; Sabes, J.H. The Need for and Development of an Adaptive Listening and Communication Enhancement (LACE) Program. *J. Am. Acad. Audiol.* **2006**, *17*, 538–558. [CrossRef]
11. Abrams, H.B.; Bock, K.; Irey, R.L. Can a Remotely Delivered Auditory Training Program Improve Speech-in-Noise Understanding? *Am. J. Audiol.* **2015**, *24*, 333–337. [CrossRef] [PubMed]
12. Olson, A.D. Options for Auditory Training for Adults with Hearing Loss. *Semin. Hear.* **2015**, *36*, 284–295. [CrossRef] [PubMed]
13. de Melo, Â.; Mezzomo, C.L.; Garcia, M.V.; Biaggio, E.P.V. Computerized Auditory Training in Students: Electrophysiological and Subjective Analysis of Therapeutic Effectiveness. *Int. Arch. Otorhinolaryngol.* **2018**, *22*, 23–32. [CrossRef] [PubMed]
14. Moberly, A.C.; Bates, C.; Harris, M.S.; Pisoni, D.B. The Enigma of Poor Performance by Adults with Cochlear Implants. *Otol. Neurotol.* **2016**, *37*, 1522–1528. [CrossRef] [PubMed]
15. Fu, Q.-J.; Galvin, J.J. Computer-Assisted Speech Training for Cochlear Implant Patients: Feasibility, Outcomes, and Future Directions. *Semin. Hear.* **2007**, *28*, 142–150. [CrossRef]
16. Oba, S.I.; Fu, Q.-J.; Galvin, J.J. Digit Training in Noise Can Improve Cochlear Implant Users' Speech Understanding in Noise. *Ear Hear.* **2011**, *32*, 573–581. [CrossRef]
17. Fu, Q.-J.; Galvin, J.; Wang, X.; Nogaki, G. Moderate Auditory Training Can Improve Speech Performance of Adult Cochlear Implant Patients. *Acoust. Res. Lett. Online* **2005**, *6*, 106–111. [CrossRef]
18. Fu, Q.-J.; Nogaki, G.; Galvin, J.J. Auditory Training with Spectrally Shifted Speech: Implications for Cochlear Implant Patient Auditory Rehabilitation. *J. Assoc. Res. Otolaryngol.* **2005**, *6*, 180–189. [CrossRef]
19. Charfeddine, S.; Chahed, H.; Besbes, G.; Dziri, S. Surdités sévères à profondes bilatérales de l'adulte: Étiologies et indications thérapeutiques. *J. Réadaptation Médicale Prat. Form. Médecine Phys. Réadaptation* **2016**, *36*, 173–184. [CrossRef]

20. British Society of Audiology Adult Rehabilitation—Common Principles in Audiology Services. Available online: https://www.thebsa.org.uk/resources/common-principles-rehabilitation-adults-audiology-services/ (accessed on 8 February 2022).
21. Tremblay, K.L.; Shahin, A.J.; Picton, T.; Ross, B. Auditory Training Alters the Physiological Detection of Stimulus-Specific Cues in Humans. *Clin. Neurophysiol.* **2009**, *120*, 128–135. [CrossRef]
22. Harris, M.S.; Capretta, N.R.; Henning, S.C.; Feeney, L.; Pitt, M.A.; Moberly, A.C. Postoperative Rehabilitation Strategies Used by Adults With Cochlear Implants: A Pilot Study. *Laryngoscope Investig. Otolaryngol.* **2016**, *1*, 42–48. [CrossRef]
23. Laplante-Lévesque, A.; Hickson, L.; Worrall, L. What Makes Adults with Hearing Impairment Take up Hearing AIDS or Communication Programs and Achieve Successful Outcomes? *Ear Hear.* **2012**, *33*, 79–93. [CrossRef]
24. Susi, T.; Johannesson, M.; Backlund, P. *Serious Games: An Overview*; Technical Report HS- IKI -TR-07-001; School of Humanities and Informatics, University of Skvde: Skvde, Sweden, 2007.
25. Ritterfeld, U.; Shen, C.; Wang, H.; Nocera, L.; Wong, W.L. Multimodality and Interactivity: Connecting Properties of Serious Games with Educational Outcomes. *Cyberpsychol. Behav.* **2009**, *12*, 691–697. [CrossRef]
26. Zyda, M. From Visual Simulation to Virtual Reality to Games. *Computer* **2005**, *38*, 25–32. [CrossRef]
27. Kapralos, B.; Cristancho, S.; Porte, M.; Backstein, D.; Monclou, A.; Dubrowski, A. Serious Games in the Classroom: Gauging Student Perceptions. *Stud. Health Technol. Inf.* **2011**, *163*, 254–260.
28. Sawyer, B. From Cells to Cell Processors: The Integration of Health and Video Games. *IEEE Comput. Graph Appl.* **2008**, *28*, 83–85. [CrossRef]
29. Drummond, D.; Monnier, D.; Tesnière, A.; Hadchouel, A. A Systematic Review of Serious Games in Asthma Education. *Pediatr. Allergy Immunol.* **2017**, *28*, 257–265. [CrossRef]
30. Eichenberg, C.; Schott, M. Serious Games for Psychotherapy: A Systematic Review. *Games Health J.* **2017**, *6*, 127–135. [CrossRef]
31. Cowan, B.; Sabri, H.; Kapralos, B.; Moussa, F.; Cristancho, S.; Dubrowski, A. A Serious Game for Off-Pump Coronary Artery Bypass Surgery Procedure Training. *Stud. Health Technol. Inf.* **2011**, *163*, 147–149.
32. Garris, R.; Ahlers, R.; Driskell, J.E. Games, Motivation, and Learning: A Research and Practice Model. *Simul. Gaming* **2002**, *33*, 441–467. [CrossRef]
33. Jansen, S.; Luts, H.; Wagener, K.C.; Kollmeier, B.; Rio, M.D.; Dauman, R.; James, C.; Fraysse, B.; Vormès, E.; Frachet, B.; et al. Comparison of Three Types of French Speech-in-Noise Tests: A Multi-Center Study. *Int. J. Audiol.* **2012**, *51*, 164–173. [CrossRef]
34. Reynard, P.; Lagacé, J.; Joly, C.-A.; Dodelé, L.; Veuillet, E.; Thai-Van, H. Speech-in-Noise Audiometry in Adults: A Review of the Available Tests for French Speakers. *Audiol. Neurotol.* **2022**, *27*, 185–199. [CrossRef]
35. Joly, C.-A.; Reynard, P.; Mezzi, K.; Bakhos, D.; Bergeron, F.; Bonnard, D.; Borel, S.; Bouccara, D.; Coez, A.; Dejean, F.; et al. Guidelines of the French Society of Otorhinolaryngology-Head and Neck Surgery (SFORL) and the French Society of Audiology (SFA) for Speech-in-Noise Testing in Adults. *Eur Ann. Otorhinolaryngol. Head Neck Dis.* **2022**, *139*, 21–27. [CrossRef]
36. Schumann, A.; Serman, M.; Gefeller, O.; Hoppe, U. Computer-Based Auditory Phoneme Discrimination Training Improves Speech Recognition in Noise in Experienced Adult Cochlear Implant Listeners. *Int. J. Audiol.* **2015**, *54*, 190–198. [CrossRef]
37. Nogaki, G.; Fu, Q.-J.; Galvin, J.J. Effect of Training Rate on Recognition of Spectrally Shifted Speech. *Ear Hear.* **2007**, *28*, 132–140. [CrossRef]
38. Blamey, P.; Arndt, P.; Bergeron, F.; Bredberg, G.; Brimacombe, J.; Facer, G.; Larky, J.; Lindström, B.; Nedzelski, J.; Peterson, A.; et al. Factors Affecting Auditory Performance of Postlinguistically Deaf Adults Using Cochlear Implants. *Audiol. Neurootol.* **1996**, *1*, 293–306.
39. Blamey, P.; Artieres, F.; Başkent, D.; Bergeron, F.; Beynon, A.; Burke, E.; Dillier, N.; Dowell, R.; Fraysse, B.; Gallégo, S.; et al. Factors Affecting Auditory Performance of Postlinguistically Deaf Adults Using Cochlear Implants: An Update with 2251 Patients. *Audiol. Neurootol.* **2013**, *18*, 36–47. [CrossRef]
40. Lazard, D.S.; Vincent, C.; Venail, F.; Van de Heyning, P.; Truy, E.; Sterkers, O.; Skarzynski, P.H.; Skarzynski, H.; Schauwers, K.; O'Leary, S.; et al. Pre-, per- and Postoperative Factors Affecting Performance of Postlinguistically Deaf Adults Using Cochlear Implants: A New Conceptual Model over Time. *PLoS ONE* **2012**, *7*, e48739. [CrossRef]
41. Dryden, A.; Allen, H.A.; Henshaw, H.; Heinrich, A. The Association Between Cognitive Performance and Speech-in-Noise Perception for Adult Listeners: A Systematic Literature Review and Meta-Analysis. *Trends Hear.* **2017**, *21*, 233121651774467. [CrossRef]
42. Michalski, N.; Petit, C. Central Auditory Deficits Associated with Genetic Forms of Peripheral Deafness. *Hum. Genet.* **2022**, *141*, 335–345. [CrossRef]

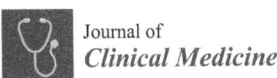

Article

Ecological Momentary Assessment to Obtain Signal Processing Technology Preference in Cochlear Implant Users

Matthias Hey [1,*], Adam A. Hersbach [2], Thomas Hocke [3], Stefan J. Mauger [4], Britta Böhnke [1] and Alexander Mewes [1]

[1] Audiology, ENT Clinic, UKSH, 24105 Kiel, Germany; britta.boehnke@uksh.de (B.B.); alexander.mewes@uksh.de (A.M.)
[2] Research and Development, Cochlear Limited, Melbourne, VIC 3000, Australia; ahersbach@cochlear.com
[3] Research, Cochlear Deutschland, 30625 Hannover, Germany; thocke@cochlear.com
[4] Research, Seer Medical, East Melbourne, VIC 3002, Australia; stefan.mauger@seermedical.com
* Correspondence: hey@audio.uni-kiel.de; Tel.: +49-431-500-21857

Abstract: Background: To assess the performance of cochlear implant users, speech comprehension benefits are generally measured in controlled sound room environments of the laboratory. For field-based assessment of preference, questionnaires are generally used. Since questionnaires are typically administered at the end of an experimental period, they can be inaccurate due to retrospective recall. An alternative known as ecological momentary assessment (EMA) has begun to be used for clinical research. The objective of this study was to determine the feasibility of using EMA to obtain in-the-moment responses from cochlear implant users describing their technology preference in specific acoustic listening situations. Methods: Over a two-week period, eleven adult cochlear implant users compared two listening programs containing different sound processing technologies during everyday take-home use. Their task was to compare and vote for their preferred program. Results: A total of 205 votes were collected from acoustic environments that were classified into six listening scenes. The analysis yielded different patterns of voting among the subjects. Two subjects had a consistent preference for one sound processing technology across all acoustic scenes, three subjects changed their preference based on the acoustic scene, and six subjects had no conclusive preference for either technology. Conclusion: Results show that EMA is suitable for quantifying real-world self-reported preference, showing inter-subject variability in different listening environments. However, there is uncertainty that patients will not provide sufficient spontaneous feedback. One improvement for future research is a participant forced prompt to improve response rates.

Keywords: cochlear implant; signal processing; hearing in noise; EMA; ecological momentary assessment; acoustic environment; BEAM; ForwardFocus

1. Introduction

Cochlear implantation is an established treatment option for patients with severe to profound, or moderate sloping to profound, bilateral sensorineural hearing loss [1,2]. To assess patients hearing ability and the success of cochlear implantation, speech perception is assessed through well-established tests performed in controlled conditions of the laboratory. Initially, speech perception was assessed with sentences in quiet [3,4], but assessment was complemented or replaced by more difficult word in quiet tests as cochlear implant (CI) patient performance increased [4,5]. Nowadays, monosyllabic or phoneme scores are an accepted measure used to identify and refer candidates for cochlear implantation [6,7] as well as for predicting and evaluating cochlear implant outcomes [8–10].

Speech perception in noise tests have also become a common outcome assessment, due to continued performance improvement in cochlear implant performance brought about by algorithms able to improve the signal-to-noise-ratio [11–16]. These tests also support further development and evaluation of new algorithms involved in cochlear implant processing, the access of CI recipients to sound processor upgrades through demonstrated performance improvements [14,17,18], and the individualization of settings in sound processors [12]. The assessment of the potential benefit of recent algorithms such as ForwardFocus (Cochlear Limited, Sydney, Australia) [18] expand the boundaries of current clinical audiometry practice.

Algorithms like ForwardFocus are designed to improve speech perception in complex real-world listening environments, where the target speech is in front of the listener and multiple and dynamic competing signals are towards the side and/or the rear [11,17–20]. These are challenging environments to simulate in a test booth, as they require significantly more dedicated hardware and software than commonly available in clinical audiometry practice. Questionnaires can assess the therapeutic effect through preoperative and postoperative comparison for a CI treatment or processor upgrade and can provide suitably complex listening environments for the evaluation of sound processor programs, which could include algorithms such as ForwardFocus [21]. However, data from questionnaires rely on retrospective recall of events and experiences and therefore reflect cumulative effects, are possibly biased by the interlocked effects of long-term memory and inference [22], and can therefore be inaccurate. Questionnaires also do not capture the variation of the sound environment across the day, a particular disadvantage in assessing algorithms designed for particular acoustic situations.

Clinical research in a variety of fields [23], and more recently in hearing research [24,25], has begun using a methodology called Ecological Momentary Assessment (EMA) to collect real-time situational responses from patients [26]. This method has the advantage of being conducted in real time in complex real-world situations, mitigating the limitations of common hearing research clinical outcome assessments. While EMA has been used in studies with hearing aid users [24,25,27], this method has not been widely used in studies with cochlear implant patients.

Most signal processing algorithms and fitting strategies in CI users are investigated in the lab and averaged over a group of patients. They do not take into account the individual needs and the time-dependent character of judging a given hearing program [28]. This evokes the need to validate these findings in real life. EMA methods have several advantages, for example, improved ecological validity due to data assessment in the real world; accounting for variations over time; being less vulnerable to recall bias [28]. Nevertheless, it has to be noted that this method is demanding and time consuming for subjects. Consequently, results may have variable reliability, as feedback is given without the presence of an investigator [28]. On the other hand, EMA methods allow the collection of time-dependent data, providing more detailed insights into the acoustic reality of CI patients in contrast to the questionnaire-based assessment when investigating in the clinic.

The audiometric clinical routine shows limitations in transferring the acoustic reality into an audiometric booth [27,29]. Additionally, it was shown that signal processing in sound processors should be individualized [12]. However, so far there is no method and no gold standard known to provide further detailed insights into patients views without extensive audiometric testing. To summarize, the evaluation of the individual benefit of signal processing algorithms expands the boundaries of current clinical audiometry practice [30].

The goal of this study was to investigate the feasibility of EMA in a CI population. The ability to capture specific data on the acoustic environment as well as patient-specific preference data on sound processing algorithms should be investigated. The individual preference of the new ForwardFocus algorithm [21], known to provide benefits in complex dynamic noise environments found in the real-world, is compared to the well-established Beamformer.

2. Materials and Methods

2.1. Research Subjects

This investigation included eleven (five unilateral and six bilateral) CI subjects. The patients were recruited from the clinic's patient pool. The investigation was approved by the local ethics committee (D 467/16), and all procedures were in accordance with the ethical standards of the institutional and national research committee and with the 1964 Helsinki declaration and its later amendments or comparable ethical standards.

CI subjects were recruited who were at least 18 years of age, with post-lingual onset of deafness and implantation with a Nucleus CI24RE or CI500 series cochlear implant (Cochlear Limited, Sydney, Australia), and who were current users of a CP900 series sound processor (Nucleus 6®). All subjects had at least six months' experience with their CI system. Bilateral implantation was not an exclusion criterion. Demographic information of these patients is provided in Table 1. This study cohort contained a subset of 20 subjects reported in Hey et al., 2019, who also took part in this additional EMA investigation. The signal processing algorithm ForwardFocus was evaluated in the laboratory in a range of noise types (stationary and fluctuating) as well as different spatial conditions (signal and noise from front; signal from front and noise from the posterior hemisphere) [21]. Reference for further comparison was the known BEAM algorithm [15,17]. It was shown that ForwardFocus was able to significantly improve speech comprehension in a wide range of acoustic scenes constructed in the laboratory.

Table 1. Biographical data of recipients.

Patient ID	Age (Years)	Usage of CI (Years)	Side	Gender	Rate (pps)	Maxima
#1	75.7	1.5	r	m	1200	12
#1	75.7	1.0	l	m	1200	12
#4	73.7	10.7	r	m	1200	8
#6	43.3	8.2	r	f	1200	12
#6	43.3	2.1	l	f	1200	12
#7	56.0	7.3	r	f	1200	12
#7	56.0	8.6	l	f	1200	12
#9	47.4	3.4	r	m	1200	12
#9	47.4	2.5	l	m	1200	12
#10	64.9	1.5	r	f	1200	12
#12	61.1	6.1	r	f	500	8
#12	61.1	8.7	l	f	500	10
#13	56.0	3.0	r	f	900	8
#14	65.0	10.9	r	f	500	12
#14	65.0	9.1	l	f	500	12
#15	73.4	2.6	l	m	900	10
#17	55.8	9.5	r	m	1200	12

2.2. Programming the Sound Processor Settings

During an initial session, participants were provided with two programs of the sound processor. The first program (subsequently named as "BEAM") consisted of default Nucleus 6 SmartSound® iQ technologies (ADRO, SNR-NR and ASC), with the addition of BEAM (adaptive directional microphone) [12,31]. The second program ("FF") contained the same Nucleus 6 SmartSound iQ technologies, with the addition of the ForwardFocus technology [21] implemented for research. All other fitting parameters were the same for both programs. The patients' MAPs were not changed for the study. Programs were randomized between the two program slots, and subjects were blind to the program slot allocation. To change programs and capture EMA data, a CI remote control (Nucleus® CR230; Figure 1) was provided to each patient for the take-home period. Programs were simply labelled "1" and "2" in order of the program slots used.

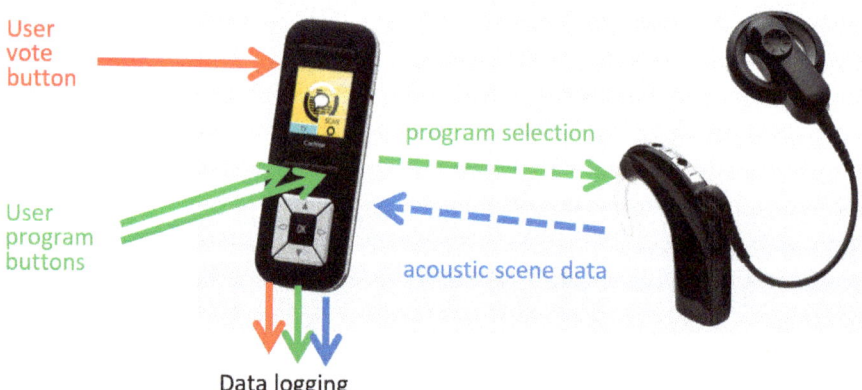

Figure 1. The CP900 sound processor and CR230 remote control used to capture EMA data.

2.3. EMA Data Capture and Analysis

The CR230 remote-control device allowed subjects control over sound processor volume and sensitivity, as is typical for daily use (Figure 1). It also displayed the current listening environment class [32]. A large side button (conventionally used to enable the telecoil feature) was repurposed and used as a vote button. The data logging capability of the CR230 allowed the listening environment (Quiet, Speech, Speech in Noise, Noise, Wind, and Music) and listening program to be recorded as the user pressed the vote button. These features provided a suitable platform to capture EMA data. In this study, we investigated a sound processing program preference through subject voting between a BEAM program and a ForwardFocus program in real-world environments. For analysis, the listening environments relevant for communication were used, which excluded the Wind and Music classes.

Subjects were provided with two programs and a sound processor remote control for a two-week period. During this period, they were asked to change between programs during each day to experience both programs. Subjects were also instructed to complete at least one vote (data capture) each day in a range of their different listening environments across the two-week period. To vote, subjects were instructed to change between programs during normal use of the device, and after several changes back and forth, to vote for their preferred program by pressing the side button on the remote control.

Data capture of the patient's instantaneous listening environment was possible due to the SCAN scene classification algorithm available on the CP900 sound processor [32]. At each time instance, the environment is classified into one of six sound classes: Quiet, Speech, Speech in Noise, Noise, Music, and Wind. This algorithm is based on extracting acoustic features such as sound level, modulation, and frequency spectrum from the microphone signal, followed by a decision tree to determine the sound class [32,33]. A data-driven machine learning approach was used to train the decision tree using sound recordings labelled by humans with the appropriate sound class. In contrast to the commercially available CP900, during this study the classification system did not make any automatic changes to the sound processing or program selection but was only responsible for determining the sound class for the purpose of data logging.

At the end of the two-week period, data logs containing the vote events, scene classification data, and program selection were downloaded. Analysis was first performed to exclude accidental voting and exclude votes that did not show temporal coincidence with previous changes between both programs. In order to determine the sound class associated with each vote, the detected sound class was analyzed over the 10 s preceding the vote event. It was assumed that the evaluation of programs would likely have occurred over a period of time, possibly under different scene classifications. In cases where the sound class was variable, the vote was assigned according to the dominant sound class over the 10 s preceding the vote event, and in the case of an equal distribution, to the most recently detected sound class. The preferred listening program was determined from the listening program that was selected at the time the vote button was pressed.

For each subject, raw vote data were aggregated separately for each acoustic scene and represented in a program verse scene matrix, where each element represented the number of votes for each program.

Statistical analysis was performed in R statistics package version 4.1.1. Program preference (vote) was modelled as a binomial dependent variable using repeated measures logistic regression by fitting generalized linear models (glms) with the logistic link function.

3. Results

EMA Results

A total of 205 valid votes were cast in total across the study group over the two-week period. The median number of votes cast by each subject was 15 and ranged from a minimum of seven to a maximum of 50. Six subjects voted at least once per day on average over the 2-week period, while five subjects voted less often. Votes were spread across the different acoustic scenes, the distribution of which is provided in Figure 2 for the entire subject pool. The scene with the fewest votes cast was Speech with 19 votes, while the other three classes had an approximately equal number of votes, with 55, 54 and 45 votes cast in the Quiet, Speech in Noise, and Noise class respectively. The median number of votes cast per subject in each scene was 6, 1, 4 and 4 for the Quiet, Speech, Speech in Noise, and Noise classes, respectively.

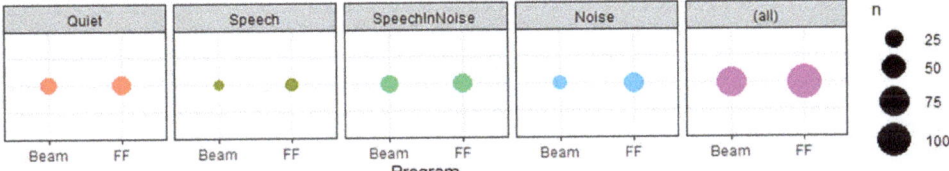

Figure 2. Program preference accumulated across entire subject group separated by sound class. Size of data point indicates number of votes. "BEAM" specifies the program consisting of the algorithms ADRO, SNR-NR, ASC and BEAM. "FF" indicates the second program containing the ForwardFocus microphone technology.

The number of votes cast by each individual subject is presented in Figure 3 using bubble plots. The location of the bubble on the x-axis indicates the program preference, the size of the bubble indicates the number of votes that contributed to that data point and the color indicates the sound class to which the votes were allocated.

Overall preference was analyzed by aggregating data across all scenes. A glm was fitted with program preference as the dependent variable and subject as the independent variable. The resulting chi-squared analysis of variance on the glm showed the effect of subject was highly significant ($p < 0.001$). P-values indicating the significance of preference for each subject are presented in Table 2. Two subjects had a significant preference for FF labelled as category A: subject #7 ($p = 0.004$) and #15 ($p < 0.001$). The remaining nine subjects showed no significant overall preference for either program.

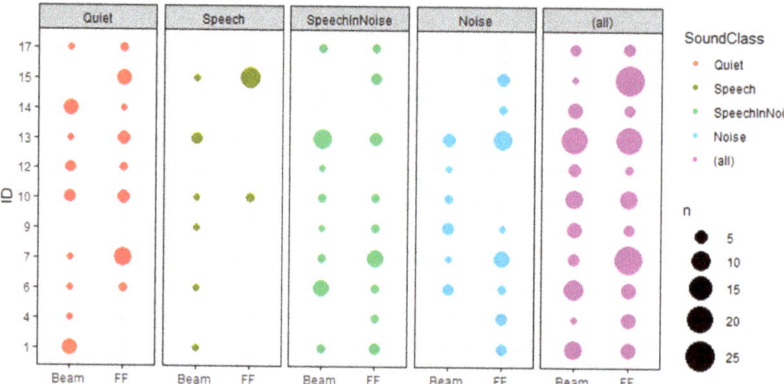

Figure 3. Individual program preference separated by sound class. Size of data point indicates number of votes.

Table 2. Summary of statistical analysis, indicating those subjects with an overall preference (A), those subjects whose preference varied with SoundClass (B), and those subjects where no preference could be determined (C). # xx – patient ID; * means significant test result.

Subject	Total Votes Cast	Logistic Regression of Preference with Subject (p-Value)	Logistic Regression of Preference with SoundClass (p-Value)	Category	Comments
#13	40	0.509	0.011 *	B	Preference varied with SoundClass
#7	28	0.004 *	0.807	A	Overall preference for FF
#15	27	<0.001 *	0.682	A	Overall preference for FF
#6	18	0.692	0.419	C	No conclusive preference
#10	18	0.566	0.358	C	No conclusive preference
#1	15	0.442	0.004 *	B	Preference varied with SoundClass
#9	9	0.744	0.268	C	No conclusive preference
#14	9	0.744	0.017 *	B	Preference varied with SoundClass
#4	7	0.068	0.057	C	No conclusive preference
#12	7	0.605	0.439	C	No conclusive preference
#17	7	0.455	0.658	C	No conclusive preference

To analyze the effect that sound class had on preference, a mixed-effects glm was fitted. The dependent variable was program preference and independent variable was sound class, while subject was considered as a random effect in the model.

The effect of SoundClass (fixed effect) was tested by comparing the mixed-effects glm to a model that excluded the SoundClass (fixed effect) and only included the random effect (subject). The resulting chi-squared analysis of variance showed SoundClass fixed effect was not significant ($p = 0.191$), indicating a lack of association between program preference and sound class for the group of subjects as a whole.

The effect of subject (random effect) was tested by comparing the mixed-effect glm to a model that excluded the random effect (Subject) and only included the fixed effect

(SoundClass). The resulting chi-squared analysis of variance confirmed that Subject (random effect) was highly significant ($p < 0.001$), indicating that individual subjects voting preferences varied amongst the group. For each individual subject, the logistic regression of preference with SoundClass was fitted, and the resulting p-values are shown in Table 1. Three subjects showed logistic regression that was significant, indicating that those subjects voting preference was dependent on the SoundClass (#1 $p = 0.004$, #13 $p = 0.011$, #14 $p = 0.017$), labelled as category B.

Six subjects (#4, #6, #9, #12, #14, #17) were labelled as category C, for which no conclusive preference could be determined. Four of those subjects voted less than once per day on average over the 2-week period.

4. Discussion

The automatic scene classifier in the cochlear implant sound processor offers the ability to characterize the surrounding with respect to its acoustics characteristics, such as speech and noise. It is known that signal pre-processing in cochlear implant systems should be chosen depending on the acoustic environment to improve speech comprehension [32]. Such conclusions were derived from in-lab investigations. So far, there is limited knowledge available on the patient's everyday real-world program preference using such algorithms.

The technical realization of the remote control of modern cochlear implant systems, as used as a scene-dependent voting tool in this study, can be used for the EMA in a cochlear implant population. The integration of the assessment tool into the patient's sound processor proved to be useful. The resulting link of the patients' input to the captured acoustic scene class potentially allows for the investigation of patients' individual preferences with respect to program settings and/or specific algorithms in different acoustic environments. Additionally, in cases of data mismatch to clinical expectations or ongoing inactivity, this method may provide new insight into individual preferences. This pilot study showed a significant difference in voting patterns across the group of subjects: for instance, two patients (#15, #7) had an overall preference for ForwardFocus that persisted regardless of the acoustic scene, three subjects (#1, #13, #14) had a scene specific algorithm preference, and the remaining six subjects (#4, #6, #9, #10, #12, #17) had no conclusive preference.

Our methodology complements the use of EMA in hearing science to date, where studies have prompted surveys where participants assess their acoustic environment and rate their hearing experience [24,25,27]. These methodologies provide in-the-moment responses to complex real-world situations, which is a significant improvement to surveys confounded by retrospective recall. In addition, our approach enables in-the-moment rating of signal pre-processing technology for real-world environments.

A significant advantage of this EMA methodology is the objective acoustic scene classification. By using the available scene classification of the sound processor [31], an accurate environmental measure is captured without further patient interaction. This ability is expected to be useful for sound processing algorithms that are designed and expected to provide benefit in specific noise environments. Research algorithms are being developed for specific noise scenes, such as constant noise [34] or babble noise [35]. To complement the in-booth speech understanding results, this method could provide real-world preference results for each of the available scene classes.

This study also aimed to investigate the feasibility of EMA to provide data on sound processing algorithms. Two sound processing algorithms were compared, with one being the adaptive directional microphone BEAM, and the other being ForwardFocus, known to provide significant speech understanding over BEAM in dynamic noise environments. Although these technologies were chosen because they were expected to provide differences, particularly in noisy listening environments, no clear general or scene-specific difference was determined from the group. This is not unexpected, due to the patient numbers and the numbers of votes collected. What was found was some evidence of individualized general or scene-specific voting patterns. In future, such EMA studies should therefore consider the proportion of votes expected in each scene. For instance, in this study, patients were far less likely to vote in Wind, Music, or Speech in Noise scenes spontaneously. For a prompted methodology, the proportion of time, on average, in each scene would be important to consider and could be found from the sound processor data logs [36,37]. These insights will provide at least a basis to determine study design to power and capture data for direct scene-specific algorithm comparisons.

Compared to BEAM, the ForwardFocus algorithm shows its advantages in speech understanding, especially in fluctuating noise [21]. Several consequences can result from this. The acoustic scenes of Noise and Speech in Noise are not only characterized with respect to the signal-to-noise ratio, but a characterization of the temporal properties of the noise is additionally performed: stationary or fluctuating. This can be the basis to introduce ForwardFocus as an algorithm that is activated in specific listening scenes, such as determined by the automatic classification algorithm SCAN [18,32].

Study Limits and Future Improvements

Subjects were asked to vote at least one time per day during the two-week take-home period. A total of 205 votes were recorded from the 11 patients, resulting in over one vote per subject per day, on average. All patients were able to use the remote control for data capture, successfully demonstrating the feasibility of EMA within a CI population. However, our self-initiated data capture method had some limitations. Six of the eleven patients provided at least one vote per day, while the remaining five subjects voted less often (averaged over the two-week period). Due to the low number of votes, four of those subjects had preference outcomes that were non-conclusive. In future such EMA studies, it would be beneficial to include a forced patient prompt, to request patients to conduct a comparison and vote. Additionally, an incentive, e.g., progress bars and gamification, for the study participant may help to minimize missing votes. Furthermore, the recipients should have the chance to withdraw an accidental vote. To support this, a possible review by the participants themselves of all votes might be worth considering for future studies. To summarize, most of the above-mentioned deficits cannot be addressed within a feasibility study.

The problem of obtaining an adequate number of responses is also described by Wu et al. [38]. The prompting frequency, take-home duration, number of acoustic scenes captured, and number of subjects need to be optimized to achieve sufficient data for subsequent statistical analysis. Nevertheless, a sufficient number of valid votes were collected in this study, showing the feasibility of EMA as well as this methodology in CI recipients.

The current fitting philosophy is to provide beneficial sound processing algorithms for each listening scene, which has been shown to provide benefits to a group, on average [31,39]. However, it may be that individual algorithm selection could provide further individual benefit [12]. These varying individual performance benefits or preferences can provide input for a machine learning approach [40] to select individualized sound processing algorithm options for specific listening scenes.

A central question for clinical application remains: is the individual scene-specific preference aligned with the benefits shown in speech-audiometry tests. The EMA methodology is expected to elucidate such real-world individualized patient algorithm preferences and may help to fit speech processing algorithms better to the individuals' needs.

5. Conclusions

This study found that program preference varied significantly among subjects. Some demonstrated an overall program preference, others demonstrated scene-specific preferences, and others demonstrated no conclusive preference. The data collection tool was integrated into the patient's cochlear implant system and was suitable for real-world self-assessment. To improve data collection, future research should encourage participants to realize a higher response rate.

Author Contributions: Conceptualization, A.A.H., S.J.M., M.H.; methodology, S.J.M., M.H., B.B.; software, A.A.H., S.J.M.; validation, B.B., A.M., M.H.; formal analysis, A.A.H., investigation, B.B., A.M., M.H.; resources, M.H.; data curation, B.B., M.H.; writing—original draft preparation, S.J.M., A.A.H., M.H., T.H.; writing—review and editing, all authors; visualization, A.A.H.; supervision, S.J.M., M.H.; project administration, M.H.; funding acquisition, M.H. All authors have read and agreed to the published version of the manuscript.

Funding: This research was funded by Cochlear Europe, grant number IIR-Ki15.

Institutional Review Board Statement: The study was conducted in accordance with the Declaration of Helsinki and approved by the CAU Ethics Committee (D467/16 1 June 2016).

Informed Consent Statement: Informed consent was obtained from all subjects involved in the study.

Data Availability Statement: Not applicable.

Acknowledgments: We wish to cordially thank all the patients who kindly took time to participate in the investigations. Our special thanks go to the medical-technical assistants at the Kiel University ENT Clinic, who conducted measurements for this study.

Conflicts of Interest: A.A.H., S.J.M. and T.H. are/were employees of Cochlear. The funders had no role in the design of the study; in the collection, analyses, or interpretation of data; in the writing of the manuscript, or in the decision to publish the results.

References

1. Buchman, C.A.; Gifford, R.H.; Haynes, D.S.; Lenarz, T.; O'Donoghue, G.; Adunka, O.; Biever, A.; Briggs, R.J.; Carlson, M.L.; Dai, P.; et al. Unilateral Cochlear Implants for Severe, Profound, or Moderate Sloping to Profound Bilateral Sensorineural Hearing Loss: A Systematic Review and Consensus Statements. *JAMA Otolaryngol. Head Neck Surg.* **2020**, *146*, 942–953. [CrossRef] [PubMed]
2. Hoppe, U.; Hast, A.; Hocke, T. Audiometry-Based Screening Procedure for Cochlear Implant Candidacy. *Otol. Neurotol.* **2015**, *36*, 1001–1005. [CrossRef] [PubMed]
3. Clark, G.M.; Tong, Y.C.; Martin, L.F.A.; Busby, P.A. A multiple-channel cochlear implant: An evaluution using an open-set word test. *Acta Otolaryngol.* **1981**, *91*, 173–175. [CrossRef]
4. Lehnhardt, E.; Battmer, R.D.; Nakahodo, K.; Laszig, R. Cochlear implants. *HNO* **1986**, *34*, 271–279.
5. Clark, G.M.; Tong, Y.C.; Martin, L.F.A. A multi-channel cochlear implant: An evaluation using open-set cid sentences. *Laryngoscope* **1981**, *91*, 628–634. [CrossRef]
6. Gifford, R.H.; Dorman, M.F.; Shallop, J.K.; Sydlowski, S.A. Evidence for the expansion of adult cochlear implant candidacy. *Ear Hear.* **2010**, *31*, 186–194. [CrossRef]
7. De Raeve, L.; Wouters, A. Accessibility to cochlear implants in Belgium: State of the art on selection, reimbursement, habilitation, and outcomes in children and adults. *Cochlear Implant. Int.* **2013**, *14*, S18–S25. [CrossRef]
8. Blamey, P.; Artieres, F.; Başkent, D.; Bergeron, F.; Beynon, A.; Burke, E.; Dillier, N.; Dowell, R.; Fraysse, B.; Gallégo, S.; et al. Factors affecting auditory performance of postlinguistically deaf adults using cochlear implants: An update with 2251 patients. *Audiol. Neurotol.* **2012**, *18*, 36–47. [CrossRef]
9. Holden, L.K.; Finley, C.C.; Firszt, J.B.; Holden, T.A.; Brenner, C.; Potts, L.G.; Gotter, B.D.; Vanderhoof, S.S.; Mispagel, K.; Heydebrand, G.; et al. Factors affecting open-set word recognition in adults with cochlear implants. *Ear Hear.* **2013**, *34*, 342–360. [CrossRef]
10. Hoppe, U.; Hocke, T.; Hast, A.; Iro, H. Cochlear Implantation in Candidates With Moderate-to-Severe Hearing Loss and Poor Speech Perception. *Laryngoscope* **2021**, *131*, E940–E945. [CrossRef]
11. Hersbach, A.A.; Arora, K.; Mauger, S.J.; Dawson, P.W. Combining directional microphone and single-channel noise reduction algorithms: A clinical evaluation in difficult listening conditions with cochlear implant users. *Ear Hear.* **2012**, *33*, e13–e23. [CrossRef] [PubMed]
12. Hey, M.; Hocke, T.; Mauger, S.; Müller-Deile, J. A clinical assessment of cochlear implant recipient performance: Implications for individualized map settings in specific environments. *Eur. Arch. Oto-Rhino-Laryngol.* **2016**, *273*, 4011–4020. [CrossRef] [PubMed]
13. James, C.J.; Blamey, P.J.; Martin, L.; Swanson, B.; Just, Y.; Macfarlane, D. Adaptive dynamic range optimization for cochlear implants: A preliminary study. *Ear Hear.* **2002**, *23*, 49S–58S. [CrossRef]
14. Mosnier, I.; Marx, M.; Venail, F.; Loundon, N.; Roux-Vaillard, S.; Sterkers, O. Benefits from upgrade to the CP810TM sound processor for Nucleus® 24 cochlear implant recipients. *Eur. Arch. Oto-Rhino-Laryngol.* **2014**, *271*, 49–57. [CrossRef] [PubMed]
15. Patrick, J.F.; Busby, P.A.; Gibson, P.J. The Development of the Nucleus® Freedom ^{TM} Cochlear Implant System. *Trends Amplif.* **2006**, *10*, 175–200. [CrossRef] [PubMed]
16. Wolfe, J.; Parkinson, A.; Schafer, E.C.; Gilden, J.; Rehwinkel, K.; Mansanares, J.; Coughlan, E.; Wright, J.; Torres, J.; Gannaway, S. Benefit of a commercially available cochlear implant processor with dual-microphone beamforming: A multi-center study. *Otol. Neurotol.* **2012**, *33*, 553–560. [CrossRef]

17. Dillier, N.; Lai, W.K. Speech Intelligibility in Various Noise Conditions with the Nucleus® 5 Cp810 Sound Processor. *Audiol. Res.* **2015**, *5*, 69–75. [CrossRef]
18. Hey, M.; Böhnke, B.; Mewes, A.; Munder, P.; Mauger, S.J.; Hocke, T. Speech comprehension across multiple CI processor generations: Scene dependent signal processing. *Laryngoscope Investig. Otolaryngol.* **2021**, *6*, 807–815. [CrossRef]
19. Lazard, D.S.; Vincent, C.; Venail, F.; van de Heyning, P.; Truy, E.; Sterkers, O.; Skarzynski, P.H.; Skarzynski, H.; Schauwers, K.; O'Leary, S.; et al. Pre-, Per- and Postoperative Factors Affecting Performance of Postlinguistically Deaf Adults Using Cochlear Implants: A New Conceptual Model over Time. *PLoS ONE* **2012**, *7*, e48739. [CrossRef]
20. Spriet, A.; Van Deun, L.; Eftaxiadis, K.; Laneau, J.; Moonen, M.; Van Dijk, B.; Van Wieringen, A.; Wouters, J. Speech understanding in background noise with the two-microphone adaptive beamformer BEAM^{TM} in the nucleus Freedom^{TM} cochlear implant system. *Ear Hear.* **2007**, *28*, 62–72. [CrossRef]
21. Hey, M.; Hocke, T.; Böhnke, B.; Mauger, S.J. ForwardFocus with cochlear implant recipients in spatially separated and fluctuating competing signals–Introduction of a reference metric. *Int. J. Audiol.* **2019**, *58*, 869–878. [CrossRef] [PubMed]
22. Meis, M.; Krueger, M.; Gablenz, P.V.; Holube, I.; Gebhard, M.; Latzel, M.; Paluch, R. Development and Application of an Annotation Procedure to Assess the Impact of Hearing Aid Amplification on Interpersonal Communication Behavior. *Trends Hear.* **2018**, *22*, 1–17. [CrossRef]
23. Shiffman, S.; Stone, A.A.; Hufford, M.R. Ecological momentary assessment. *Annu. Rev. Clin. Psychol.* **2008**, *4*, 1–32. [CrossRef] [PubMed]
24. Galvez, G.; Turbin, M.B.; Thielman, E.J.; Istvan, J.A.; Andrews, J.A.; Henry, J.A. Feasibility of ecological momentary assessment of hearing difficulties encountered by hearing aid users. *Ear Hear.* **2012**, *33*, 497–507. [CrossRef]
25. Timmer, B.H.B.; Hickson, L.; Launer, S. The use of ecological momentary assessment in hearing research and future clinical applications. *Hear. Res.* **2018**, *369*, 24–28. [CrossRef]
26. Wu, Y.H.; Stangl, E.; Zhang, X.; Bentler, R.A. Construct validity of the ecological momentary assessment in audiology research. *J. Am. Acad. Audiol.* **2015**, *26*, 872–884. [CrossRef]
27. Holube, I.; von Gablenz, P.; Bitzer, J. Ecological Momentary Assessment in Hearing Research: Current State, Challenges, and Future Directions. *Ear Hear.* **2020**, *41*, 79S–90S. [CrossRef]
28. Myin-Germeys, I.; Oorschot, M.; Collip, D.; Lataster, J.; Delespaul, P.; Van Os, J. Experience sampling research in psychopathology: Opening the black box of daily life. *Psychol. Med.* **2009**, *39*, 1533–1547. [CrossRef]
29. Badajoz-Davila, J.; Buchholz, J.M. Effect of test realism on speech-in-noise outcomes in bilateral cochlear implant users. *Ear Hear.* **2021**, *42*, 1687–1698. [CrossRef]
30. Keidser, G.; Naylor, G.; Brungart, D.S.; Caduff, A.; Campos, J.; Carlile, S.; Carpenter, M.G.; Grimm, G.; Hohmann, V.; Holube, I.; et al. The Quest for Ecological Validity in Hearing Science: What It Is, Why It Matters, and How to Advance It. *Ear Hear.* **2020**, *41*, 5S–19S. [CrossRef]
31. Plasmans, A.; Rushbrooke, E.; Moran, M.; Spence, C.; Theuwis, L.; Zarowski, A.; Offeciers, E.; Atkinson, B.; McGovern, J.; Dornan, D.; et al. A multicentre clinical evaluation of paediatric cochlear implant users upgrading to the Nucleus 6 system. *Int. J. Pediatr. Otorhinolaryngol.* **2016**, *83*, 193–199. [CrossRef] [PubMed]
32. Mauger, S.J.; Warren, C.D.; Knight, M.R.; Goorevich, M.; Nel, E. Clinical evaluation of the Nucleus 6 cochlear implant system: Performance improvements with SmartSound iQ. *Int. J. Audiol.* **2014**, *53*, 564–576. [CrossRef] [PubMed]
33. Cristofari, E.; Cuda, D.; Martini, A.; Forli, F.; Zanetti, D.; Di Lisi, D.; Marsella, P.; Marchioni, D.; Vincenti, V.; Aimoni, C.; et al. A Multicenter Clinical Evaluation of Data Logging in Cochlear Implant Recipients Using Automated Scene Classification Technologies. *Audiol. Neurotol.* **2017**, *22*, 226–235. [CrossRef] [PubMed]
34. Ye, H.; Deng, G.; Mauger, S.J.; Hersbach, A.A.; Dawson, P.W.; Heasman, J.M. A wavelet-based noise reduction algorithm and its clinical evaluation in cochlear implants. *PLoS ONE* **2013**, *8*, e75662. [CrossRef]
35. Goehring, T.; Bolner, F.; Monaghan, J.J.M.; van Dijk, B.; Zarowski, A.; Bleeck, S. Speech enhancement based on neural networks improves speech intelligibility in noise for cochlear implant users. *Hear. Res.* **2017**, *344*, 183–194. [CrossRef]
36. Oberhoffner, T.; Hoppe, U.; Hey, M.; Hecker, D.; Bagus, H.; Voigt, P.; Schicktanz, S.; Braun, A.; Hocke, T. Multicentric analysis of the use behavior of cochlear implant users. *Laryngorhinootologie* **2018**, *97*, 313–320. [CrossRef]
37. Busch, T.; Vanpoucke, F.; van Wieringen, A. Auditory environment across the life span of cochlear implant users: Insights from data logging. *J. Speech Lang. Hear. Res.* **2017**, *60*, 1362–1377. [CrossRef]
38. Wu, Y.-H.; Stangl, E.; Oleson, J.; Caraher, K.; Dunn, C.C. Personal Characteristics Associated with Ecological Momentary Assessment Compliance in Adult Cochlear Implant Candidates and Users. *J. Am. Acad. Audiol.* **2021**, *9*, 065007. [CrossRef]
39. Mauger, S.J.; Arora, K.; Dawson, P.W. Cochlear implant optimized noise reduction. *J. Neural Eng.* **2012**, *9*, 065007. [CrossRef]
40. Balling, L.W.; Molgaard, L.L.; Townend, O.; Nielsen, J.B.B. The Collaboration between Hearing Aid Users and Artificial Intelligence to Optimize Sound. *Semin. Hear.* **2021**, *42*, 282–294. [CrossRef]

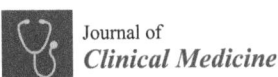

Article

Audiological Outcomes and Associated Factors after Pediatric Cochlear Reimplantation

Fabian Blanc [1,2], Catherine Blanchet [1], Marielle Sicard [1], Fanny Merklen [1], Frederic Venail [1,2] and Michel Mondain [1,2,*]

1. Department of Otolaryngology and Head and Neck Surgery, Gui de Chauliac Hospital, 80 Avenue Augustin-Fliche, 34090 Montpellier, France; fabian-blanc@chu-montpellier.fr (F.B.); c-blanchet@chu-montpellier.fr (C.B.); m-sicard@chu-montpellier.fr (M.S.); f-merklen@chu-montpellier.fr (F.M.); f-venail@chu-montpellier.fr (F.V.)
2. Institute for Neurosciences of Montpellier (INM), Institut National de la Santé et de la Recherche Médicale U1289, University of Montpellier, 80 Avenue Augustin-Fliche, BP 74103, CEDEX 5, 34091 Montpellier, France
* Correspondence: m-mondain@chu-montpellier.fr

Abstract: Cochlear implants are the most common and successful sensory neuroprosthetic devices. However, reimplantation can be required for medical reasons, device failure, or technological upgrading. Resolving the problem driving the intervention and offering stable or better audiological results are the main challenges. We aimed to analyze the success rate of this intervention and to identify factors influencing speech perception recovery after reimplantation in the pediatric population. We retrospectively collected the causes and the outcomes of 67 consecutive reimplantations in one cochlear implant center over 30 years. Reimplantation resolved the cause without recurrence for 94% of patients. The etiology of deafness, time since implantation, indication of reimplantation, sex, and age did not influence word discrimination test scores in silence, 3 years after surgery. However, adherence to a speech rehabilitation program was statistically associated with gain in perception scores: +8.9% [−2.2; +31.0%] versus −19.0% [−47.5; −7.6%] if no or suboptimal rehabilitation was followed ($p = 0.0037$). Cochlear reimplantation in children is efficient and is associated with predictable improvement in speech perception, 3 years after intervention. However, good adherence to speech rehabilitation program is necessary and should be discussed with the patient and parents, especially for the indication of reimplantation for technological upgrading.

Keywords: cochlear implant; reimplantation; audiological outcomes

1. Introduction

Sensorineural hearing loss is the most common sensory deficit [1]. A cochlear implant (CI) is a neuroprosthetic device that enables the restoration of sound perception for patients receiving little or no benefit from hearing aids. In children with severe and profound sensorineural hearing loss, cochlear implantation is the reference rehabilitation [2,3]. Cochlear implantation is a safe and effective procedure, and CIs are considered the most reliable neuroprosthetic device. However, in 1.3 to 11.2% [4–8], reimplantation can be required. The causes include medical complications and device malfunctions. Device malfunctions can be separated into hard device failure (acute and complete loss of connection between the external and internal device with abnormal electrophysiological testing) and soft device failure (audiological performance decrement and exclusion of detectable hardware or software-related causes) [9,10]. More recently, the indication of reimplantation for technological upgrading of older implants has been discussed [11,12].

Offering stable or better audiological results after reimplantation is a major challenge. We hypothesized that the audiological outcomes may be influenced by several intrinsic and extrinsic factors: sex, age, etiology of deafness, timing of intervention, electrode array insertion, or the speech rehabilitation followed after reimplantation.

In addition, few specific pediatric cohorts have been published regarding the percentage of success of this intervention. Cochlear reimplantation does not guarantee a resolution of the problem necessitating the intervention. Indeed, reimplantations sometimes fail to solve the medical problems or the suspected device malfunctions driving the intervention [6,9,13].

This study aimed to identify factors influencing speech perception recovery and evaluate the success rate of cochlear reimplantation in the pediatric population.

2. Materials and Methods

We retrospectively collected the indications and the outcomes of 67 consecutive reimplantations in one CI center over 30 years (1989–2019). We included all consecutive cochlear reimplantations concerning patients that received their first CI before 18 years old. Overall, the reimplantation rate was 8.6% during the period (67/781 cochlear implantations). Cumulative survival was measured for each indication; subjects were censored yearly, and reimplantation dates were considered events (see Supplementary Figure S1).

The mean age at implantation was 4.8 +/− 3 years, ranging from 12 months to 15 years. Thirty-one boys and thirty-five girls with an age of 15.3 +/− 6.9 years underwent reimplantation. The time since initial implantation was 10.6 +/− 6.6 years, ranging from 3 months to 28 years. Etiologies of deafness are detailed in Table 1. The majority of etiology was genetic-related (46%).

Table 1. Etiologies of deafness.

Etiologies of Deafness	n	%
Genetic		
Nonsyndromic	19	28
Syndromic [1]	12	18
Unknown	23	34
Meningitis	7	10
CMV	2	3
Labyrinthitis	2	3
Perinatal anoxia	1	2
Prematurity	1	2
Total	67	100

[1] Including 6 patients with Usher syndrome.

The primary outcome was the audiological performance, evaluated with open-set word testing in quiet of the phonetically balanced kindergarten words (PBK) [14]. The best scores obtained 1, 2, or 3 years after reimplantation were compared to the best results obtained before reimplantation. The consequence of reimplantation was thus expressed as a percentage decrease or increase in scores. Medical records were reviewed to identify the associated factors correlated with the evolution of word discrimination scores after reimplantation: sex, age, etiology of deafness, indication, best scores before reimplantation, time since the first implantation, difference in the angle of reinsertion of the electrode array (measured by cone-beam computed tomography according to Connor et al. [15]), and adherence to the speech rehabilitation program after re-implantation. Speech rehabilitation was systematically proposed to patients after cochlear reimplantation, on the same schedule than initial cochlear implantation. Participation in less than 50% of the speech rehabilitation sessions was considered "suboptimal" and represented 12% of the cohort.

No children with cochlear malformation underwent reimplantation in our cohort. Two children presented an enlarged vestibular aqueduct; complete reinsertion of the electrode array was possible in both cases.

Device failures were divided into hard failure 50% ($n = 32$), soft failure 30% ($n = 20$), and device failure in a context of head trauma 6% ($n = 4$). Medical indications included: infections in 7.5% ($n = 5$), 2 patients requiring deep brain stimulation to control severe dystonia (Mohr–Tranebjaerg syndrome), 1 patient presenting a displacement of the CI, and

3 patients presenting with non-auditory atypical symptoms during activation of the CI (headache, nausea, vomiting).

The success rate of reimplantation was assessed using specific criteria for each indication: better or stable audiological outcomes for the suspected device failures, recovery of the infection without recurrence of infections, and recovery of the non-auditive symptoms for the other causes.

Prism 9.0.2 (GraphPad Software LLC, San Diego, CA, United States of America) was used for statistical analysis. Statistical differences in the audiological outcomes were compared using a non-parametric test for paired data (Wilcoxon's rank test). The difference in the audiological outcomes as a function of the different putative associated factors were analyzed using a non-parametric test for unpaired data (Kruskal–Wallis and Mann–Whitney tests) whereas the correlation with quantitative associated factors were analyzed with the Spearman correlation coefficient.

All subjects gave their informed consent for inclusion before they participated in the study. The study was conducted in accordance with the Declaration of Helsinki.

3. Results

3.1. Audiological Outcomes

The median words recognition test score was better after reimplantation than before: 78% [47–90%] versus 85% [65–92%] for the best score 3 years after reimplantation (median, 1st and 3rd quartile, Wilcoxon's rank test for paired data, $p = 0.006$). The performances improved by over 10% in 46% ($n = 23$) of children, were similar (an increase or a decrease of less than 10% in scores between the implantation and the reimplantation) in 38% ($n = 20$), and showed a deterioration (decrease of more than 10%) in 16% ($n = 7$).

3.2. Factors Associated with Audiological Performance

We did not observe a statistically significant difference in the audiological outcomes regarding sex, etiology of deafness, or indication of reimplantation (Table 2). However, adherence to the speech rehabilitation program after the reimplantation was statistically associated with better audiological outcomes in the 3 years after reimplantation.

Table 2. Percentage decrease or increase in word discrimination scores depending on sex, etiology, indication of reimplantation, and adherence to speech rehabilitation program after cochlear reimplantation (median and 1st and 3rd quartile).

		Percentage Decrease/Increase in Word Discrimination	p
Sex	Female	+7.50 [−3.02–28.7]	0.96
	Male	+9.32 [−1.63–26.4]	
Etiology	Unknown	+15.1 [3.89–33.4]	0.5
	Genetic nonsyndromic	0 [−2.21–4.44]	
	Genetic syndromic	+5.00 [−8.82–38.8]	
	Meningitis	+16.9 [3.75–20.9]	
	Other	+4.17 [−27.1–35.4]	
Indication of reimplantation	Hard failure	+12.5 [2.38–42.9]	0.052
	Soft failure	+10.0 [−1.09–27.6]	
	Medical indication	−13.0 [−31.7–4.75]	
	Head trauma	−2.13 [−3.77–3.81]	
Adherence to speech rehabilitation	Optimal	+8.89 [−2.15–31.0]	<0.01
	Suboptimal	−19.0 [−47.5−−7.63]	

The scores before reimplantation were correlated with the scores after reimplantation, and followed an exponential non-linear curve (Figure 1a, correlation of fit: 0.685). Indeed, the patients with low scores before reimplantation presented a greater gain than the patients with high scores. Conversely, the patients with high scores tended to have stable audiological performance after reimplantation. However, the angle of reinsertion (Figure 1b), the age at reimplantation (Figure 1c), and the time since the initial implantation (Figure 1d) were not statistically correlated with better audiological outcomes.

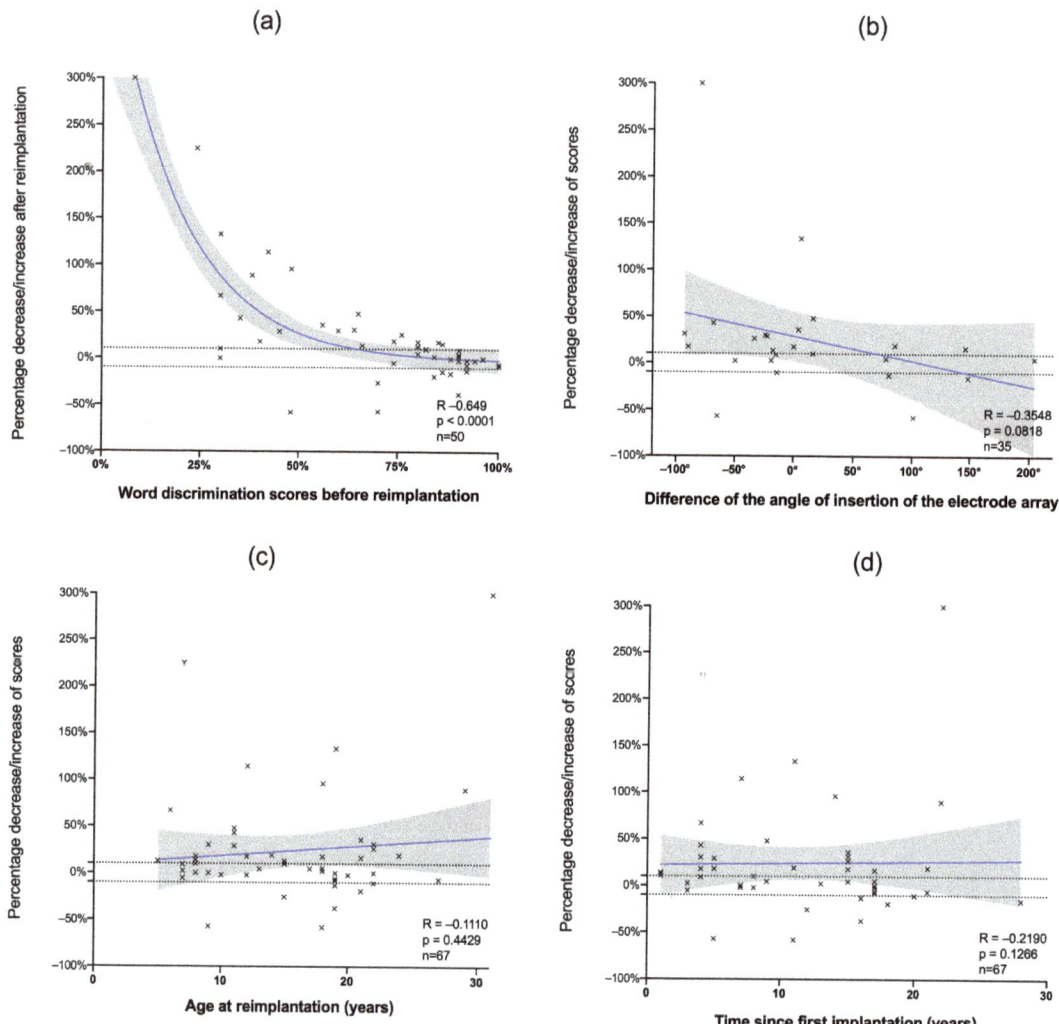

Figure 1. Correlation between the percentage increase or decrease in word discrimination and different factors: (**a**) Patients with low scores before reimplantation tend to have significantly increased scores in the 3 years after reimplantation, whereas patients with high scores tend to maintain audiological performance. The angle of insertion of the electrode array (**b**), the age at reimplantation (**c**), and the time since first implantation (**d**) were not correlated with the scores after reimplantation. Each patient cross represents a patient. Dotted lines: decrease or increase of 10% in word discrimination; blue line: simple linear regression; grey area: 95% confidence interval; R: Spearman coefficient of correlation.

3.3. Success of Reimplantation

Reimplantation resolved the problem driving the intervention in 94% of patients. Four patients did not benefit from reimplantation (Table 3). The main hypothesis explaining these results were suspicion of auditory neuropathy spectrum disorder, scala vestibuli insertion of the electrode array, suboptimal speech rehabilitation, and initial diagnostic error. Patient 2 presented with ossification of the basal portion of the scala tympani. The reinsertion of the electrode array in the scala tympani was not possible despite several attempts of cochleostomies. The new electrode array was thus inserted in the scala vestibuli (complete insertion), but presumably had led to the decrease in auditory performances (−26%). For two other patients, partial reinsertion into the scala tympani occurred (the etiology was post-meningitis in one case, and unknown for the other case). Aside from these patients, complete reinsertion in the scala tympani was achievable in 96% of the cohort. For patient 3, the speech rehabilitation program was not followed because of the presence of severe tinnitus after reimplantation. The tinnitus was associated with anxiety and depression-like symptoms.

Table 3. Description of patients receiving no benefit from the cochlear reimplantation. NSHL: non-sensory hearing loss; SHL: syndromic hearing loss.

	Etiology	Age	Time since Implantation	Indication	Surgical Findings	Word Discrimination Scores (after Reimplantation and Gain)	Comments
Patient 1	Perinatal anoxia [1]	18 years	11 years	Soft failure	Complete insertion	20% (−58%)	Suspicion of evolutive auditory neuropathy
Patient 2	NSHL	15 years	12 years	Head trauma	Scala vestibuli insertion	52% (−26%)	Scala vestibuli insertion of the electrode array
Patient 3	SHL [2]	21 years	18 years	Soft failure	Complete insertion	68% (−10%)	Suboptimal speech rehabilitation
Patient 4	NSHL	8 years	7 years	Medical reasons [3]	Complete insertion	96% (+0%)	Pain after reimplantation remains stable—suspicion of migraine

[1] Epilepsy and dysarthria; [2] Usher syndrome (type 1); [3] Pain around the processor.

4. Discussion

The present study showed that cochlear reimplantation in children was efficient and associated with a predictable overall increase in audiological performances. Adherence to the speech rehabilitation program was associated with better audiological outcomes.

According to our results, word discrimination scores improved or were stable in 84% of patients; the scores showed poorer performance (i.e., decrease of more than 10%) in only 16% of patients. These results are in line with other reports in the literature: deterioration of audiological performances in only 2.9% for Rivas et al. [16], 37% for Henson et al. [17], and 10% for van der Marel et al. and Orús Dotú [18,19]. We did not observe any statistical correlation of these poorer results with sex, age, etiology of deafness, indication, time since the first implantation, and angle of reinsertion of the electrode array, consistent with other studies [20–24]. However, the audiological performance before reimplantation was found to be associated with the audiological outcomes: the patients with low scores tended to have a significant gain (up to +300%), whereas patients with high scores maintained these good performances after reimplantation (variation of less or more than 10%). This is an encouraging result, as patients with CI offering good performances seemed not to be at risk of significant decrement after reimplantation. This outcome favors the feasibility of replacing the old CI for technological upgrading without risking audiological performance decrement [12]. However, we observed that patients with suboptimal speech rehabilitation presented a median decrease of −19% in their performances. This finding is new in the context of cochlear reimplantation. It is in line with similar reported results after cochlear implantation [3]. In our center, the therapy consisted of teaching the child to use their residual hearing with optimal amplification (listening therapy) allowing the additional use of speechreading and/or natural gestures. The goal of these visual cues was to aid the child to understand the spoken language. The program also aimed to foster parental involvement, and to teach them how to create an optimal listening learning and language environment in everyday life, child's daily routines, and play activities. Based on our findings, it seems that cochlear reimplantation should be associated with a thorough speech rehabilitation program to offer the best audiological outcomes after the intervention. Because of the retrospective design of our study, and the length of the cohort, it was difficult to quantify the speech rehabilitation program and analyze potential associated factors. We thus defined suboptimal rehabilitation as participation of less than 50% of the program. Non-adherence to the program (12% of the cohort) was because of the patient's unwillingness, other intercurrent conditions (severe epilepsy, depression), or because of severe tinnitus in one case. It can be discussed that these factors by themselves could interfere with the audiological performances, and further studies need to be designed to understand the specific role of each factor. Moreover, the number of patients was small, and the calculation of a relative risk was not meaningful in this context because the confidence interval was too wide.

In our cohort, cochlear reimplantation presented a high success rate (94%). Only few studies are available in the literature on the pediatric population. One recent study observed a similar rate of 85% [6]. As in our cohort, the failure of cochlear reimplantation has revealed a central origin in some patients. They suspected an evolutive auditory neuropathy spectrum disorder in one case, and cochlear nerve hypoplasia in another case. In young children, the diagnosis of soft failure is often challenging. The absence of language development after implantation or the audiological performance decrement can evoke a soft failure [9]. However, other diagnoses can have the same presentation. In this context, the absence of language development may correspond to auditory neuropathy spectrum disorder, whereas audiological performance decrement may correspond to a degenerative central pathology. Finally, neurological delay or psychiatric conversion disorder are other possible final diagnoses if the reimplantation fails to restore the audiological performance [22]. Hence, several studies agree to consider that in these situations, as electrophysiological tests fail to reliably determine internal component functional status, the only option is to propose explantation–reimplantation [6,9,10].

In our study, another possible reason for failure in one case was the insertion of the electrode array in the scala vestibuli because of an ossified scala tympani. This patient's score decrease by 26%. Audiological results after insertion into the scala vestibuli are reported to be worse, with an average score of word discrimination of 50% [25,26]. The insertion in the scala vestibuli could offer greater results if the scala media is not injured [27]. However, this technique presents a high risk of secondary degeneration of spiral ganglion neurons and remains a last chance option.

This study has several limitations. The retrospective design did not allow the analysis of certain data such as the quantification of the speech rehabilitation program. Moreover, it resulted in 47% of missing data, for the value of angle of insertion based on computed tomography. However, for our primary outcome, the audiological scores during 3 years after reimplantation were available for 75% of the cohort. Because of the indications of cochlear reimplantation, the cohort was also heterogeneous and of a relatively small size. However, its size remains average compared with the previously reported cohort [6,9,23]. Our long experience in cochlear implantation and the single-center design ensured that no major modification of the decision algorithm occurred during the study period. However, it may have introduced selection bias and may limit the possibility of generalizing these results.

5. Conclusions

Audiological performance improved after cochlear reimplantation in children. This intervention was highly efficient and tended to ensure stable performance in the patients with previously good audiological scores. Speech rehabilitation was an important factor associated with favorable audiological outcomes.

Supplementary Materials: The following supporting information can be downloaded at: https://www.mdpi.com/article/10.3390/jcm11113148/s1, Figure S1: Time after initial implantation (years).

Author Contributions: Conceptualization, M.M. and F.B.; methodology, M.M. and F.B.; formal analysis, F.B.; investigation, F.B., C.B., M.S. and F.M.; data curation, F.B., C.B., M.S. and F.M.; writing—original draft preparation, F.B.; writing—review and editing, M.M., C.B., F.V. and F.B.; supervision, M.M. All authors have read and agreed to the published version of the manuscript.

Funding: This research received no external funding.

Institutional Review Board Statement: The study was conducted in accordance with the Declaration of Helsinki.

Informed Consent Statement: Informed consent was obtained from all subjects involved in the study.

Data Availability Statement: Not applicable.

Acknowledgments: The authors thanks Adrien Caplot for the review of the statistical analysis.

Conflicts of Interest: The authors declare no conflict of interest.

References

1. World Health Organization Deafness and Hearing Loss. Available online: https://www.who.int/news-room/fact-sheets/detail/deafness-and-hearing-loss (accessed on 4 September 2019).
2. Lieu, J.E.C.; Kenna, M.; Anne, S.; Davidson, L. Hearing Loss in Children: A Review. *JAMA* **2020**, *324*, 2195–2205. [CrossRef] [PubMed]
3. Illg, A.; Haack, M.; Lesinski-Schiedat, A.; Büchner, A.; Lenarz, T. Long-Term Outcomes, Education, and Occupational Level in Cochlear Implant Recipients Who Were Implanted in Childhood. *Ear Hear.* **2017**, *38*, 577–587. [CrossRef] [PubMed]
4. Cullen, R.D.; Fayad, J.N.; Luxford, W.M.; Buchman, C.A. Revision Cochlear Implant Surgery in Children. *Otol. Neurotol.* **2008**, *29*, 214–220. [CrossRef] [PubMed]
5. Brown, K.D.; Connell, S.S.; Balkany, T.J.; Eshraghi, A.E.; Telischi, F.F.; Angeli, S.A. Incidence and Indications for Revision Cochlear Implant Surgery in Adults and Children. *Laryngoscope* **2009**, *119*, 152–157. [CrossRef] [PubMed]
6. Distinguin, L.; Blanchard, M.; Rouillon, I.; Parodi, M.; Loundon, N. Pediatric Cochlear Reimplantation: Decision-Tree Efficacy. *Eur. Ann. Otorhinolaryngol. Head Neck Dis.* **2018**, *135*, 243–247. [CrossRef] [PubMed]
7. Sterkers, F.; Merklen, F.; Piron, J.P.; Vieu, A.; Venail, F.; Uziel, A.; Mondain, M. Outcomes after Cochlear Reimplantation in Children. *Int. J. Pediatr. Otorhinolaryngol.* **2015**, *79*, 840–843. [CrossRef] [PubMed]
8. Bhadania, S.; Vishwakarma, R.; Keshri, A. Cochlear Implant Device Failure in the Postoperative Period: An Institutional Analysis. *Asian J. Neurosurg.* **2018**, *13*, 1066. [CrossRef]
9. Moberly, A.C.; Welling, D.B.; Nittrouer, S. Detecting Soft Failures in Pediatric Cochlear Implants: Relating Behavior to Language Outcomes. *Otol. Neurotol.* **2013**, *34*, 1648–1655. [CrossRef]
10. Sunde, J.; Webb, J.B.; Moore, P.C.; Gluth, M.B.; Dornhoffer, J.L. Cochlear Implant Failure, Revision, and Reimplantation. *Otol. Neurotol.* **2013**, *34*, 1670–1674. [CrossRef]
11. Roßberg, W.; Timm, M.; Matin, F.; Zanoni, A.; Krüger, C.; Giourgas, A.; Bültmann, E.; Lenarz, T.; Kral, A.; Lesinski-Schiedat, A. First Results of Electrode Reimplantation and Its Hypothetical Dependence from Artificial Brain Maturation. *Eur. Arch. Otorhinolaryngol.* **2021**, *278*, 951–958. [CrossRef]
12. Holcomb, M.A.; Burton, J.A.; Dornhoffer, J.R.; Camposeo, E.L.; Meyer, T.A.; McRackan, T.R. When to Replace Legacy Cochlear Implants for Technological Upgrades: Indications and Outcomes: CI Reimplantation for Technology Upgrade. *Laryngoscope* **2019**, *129*, 748–753. [CrossRef] [PubMed]
13. Kou, Y.-F.; Hunter, J.B.; Kutz, J.W.; Isaacson, B.; Lee, K.H. Revision Pediatric Cochlear Implantation in a Large Tertiary Center since 1986. *Cochlear Implant. Int.* **2020**, *21*, 353–357. [CrossRef] [PubMed]
14. Meyer, T.A.; Pisoni, D.B. Some Computational Analyses of the PBK Test: Effects of Frequency and Lexical Density on Spoken Word Recognition. *Ear Hear.* **1999**, *20*, 363–371. [CrossRef] [PubMed]
15. Connor, S.E.J.; Bell, D.J.; O'Gorman, R.; Fitzgerald-O'Connor, A. CT and MR Imaging Cochlear Distance Measurements May Predict Cochlear Implant Length Required for a 360° Insertion. *Am. J. Neuroradiol.* **2009**, *30*, 1425–1430. [CrossRef] [PubMed]
16. Rivas, A.; Marlowe, A.L.; Chinnici, J.E.; Niparko, J.K.; Francis, H.W. Revision Cochlear Implantation Surgery in Adults: Indications and Results. *Otol. Neurotol.* **2008**, *29*, 639–648. [CrossRef]
17. Henson, A.M.; Slattery, W.H.; Luxford, W.M.; Mills, D.M. Cochlear Implant Performance after Reimplantation: A Multicenter Study. *Am. J. Otol.* **1999**, *20*, 56–64.
18. van der Marel, K.S.; Briaire, J.J.; Verbist, B.M.; Joemai, R.M.S.; Boermans, P.-P.B.M.; Peek, F.A.W.; Frijns, J.H.M. Cochlear Reimplantation with Same Device: Surgical and Audiologic Results: Results of Cochlear Reimplantation. *Laryngoscope* **2011**, *121*, 1517–1524. [CrossRef]

19. Orús Dotú, C.; Venegas Pizarro, M.d.P.; De Juan Beltrán, J.; De Juan Delago, M. Reimplantación coclear en el mismo oído: Hallazgos, peculiaridades de la técnica quirúrgica y complicaciones. *Acta Otorrinolaringológica Esp.* **2010**, *61*, 106–117. [CrossRef]
20. Balkany, T.J.; Hodges, A.V.; Gómez-Marín, O.; Bird, P.A.; Dolan-Ash, S.; Butts, S.; Telischi Mee, F.F.; Lee, D. Cochlear Reimplantation. *Laryngoscope* **1999**, *109*, 351–355. [CrossRef]
21. Cote, M.; Ferron, P.; Bergeron, F.; Bussieres, R. Cochlear Reimplantation: Causes of Failure, Outcomes, and Audiologic Performance. *Laryngoscope* **2007**, *117*, 1225–1235. [CrossRef]
22. Migirov, L.; Taitelbaum-Swead, R.; Hildesheimer, M.; Kronenberg, J. Revision Surgeries in Cochlear Implant Patients: A Review of 45 Cases. *Eur. Arch. Otorhinolaryngol.* **2007**, *264*, 3–7. [CrossRef] [PubMed]
23. Durand, M.; Michel, G.; Boyer, J.; Bordure, P. Auditory Performance after Cochlear Reimplantation. *Eur. Ann. Otorhinolaryngol. Head Neck Dis.* **2021**, S1879729621002581, in press. [CrossRef] [PubMed]
24. Xu, Y.; Ren, H.-B.; Jiang, L.; Liu, L.-Y.; Han, F.-G.; Wang, S.-F. Reference Function of Old Electrical Stimulation Electrode in Cochlear-Reimplantation in Children. *Eur. Ann. Otorhinolaryngol. Head Neck Dis.* **2020**, *137*, 415–417. [CrossRef] [PubMed]
25. Adunka, O.; Kiefer, J.; Unkelbach, M.H.; Radeloff, A.; Gstoettner, W. Evaluating Cochlear Implant Trauma to the Scala Vestibuli. *Clin. Otolaryngol.* **2005**, *30*, 121–127. [CrossRef]
26. Aschendorff, A.; Kromeier, J.; Klenzner, T.; Laszig, R. Quality Control After Insertion of the Nucleus Contour and Contour Advance Electrode in Adults. *Ear Hear.* **2007**, *28*, 75S–79S. [CrossRef]
27. Shepherd, R.K.; Pyman, B.C.; Clark, G.M.; Webb, R.L. Banded Intracochlear Electrode Array: Evaluation of Insertion Trauma in Human Temporal Bones. *Ann. Otol. Rhinol. Laryngol.* **1985**, *94*, 55–59. [CrossRef]

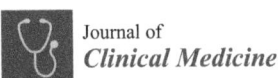

Article

Effect of Sound Coding Strategies on Music Perception with a Cochlear Implant

Gaëlle Leterme [1,2], Caroline Guigou [1,2,*], Geoffrey Guenser [1], Emmanuel Bigand [3] and Alexis Bozorg Grayeli [1,2]

[1] Otolaryngology, Head and Neck Surgery Department, Dijon University Hospital, 21000 Dijon, France; gaelle.leterme@chu-reunion.fr (G.L.); gg@histoiredentendre.fr (G.G.); alexis.bozorggrayeli@chu-dijon.fr (A.B.G.)
[2] ImVia Research Laboratory, Bourgogne-Franche-Comté University, 21000 Dijon, France
[3] LEAD Research Laboratory, CNRS UMR 5022, Bourgogne-Franche-Comté University, 21000 Dijon, France; emmanuel.bigand@u-bourgogne.fr
* Correspondence: caroline.guigou@chu-dijon.fr; Tel.: +33-615718531

Abstract: The goal of this study was to evaluate the music perception of cochlear implantees with two different sound processing strategies. Methods: Twenty-one patients with unilateral or bilateral cochlear implants (Oticon Medical®) were included. A music trial evaluated emotions (sad versus happy based on tempo and/or minor versus major modes) with three tests of increasing difficulty. This was followed by a test evaluating the perception of musical dissonances (marked out of 10). A novel sound processing strategy reducing spectral distortions (CrystalisXDP, Oticon Medical) was compared to the standard strategy (main peak interleaved sampling). Each strategy was used one week before the music trial. Results: Total music score was higher with CrystalisXDP than with the standard strategy. Nine patients (21%) categorized music above the random level (>5) on test 3 only based on mode with either of the strategies. In this group, CrystalisXDP improved the performances. For dissonance detection, 17 patients (40%) scored above random level with either of the strategies. In this group, CrystalisXDP did not improve the performances. Conclusions: CrystalisXDP, which enhances spectral cues, seemed to improve the categorization of happy versus sad music. Spectral cues could participate in musical emotions in cochlear implantees and improve the quality of musical perception.

Keywords: music perception; hearing function; cochlear implant; sound processing strategy; pitch perception; rhythm perception

Citation: Leterme, G.; Guigou, C.; Guenser, G.; Bigand, E.; Bozorg Grayeli, A. Effect of Sound Coding Strategies on Music Perception with a Cochlear Implant. *J. Clin. Med.* **2022**, *11*, 4425. https://doi.org/10.3390/jcm11154425

Academic Editors: Nicolas Guevara and Adrien Eshraghi

Received: 25 May 2022
Accepted: 26 July 2022
Published: 29 July 2022

Publisher's Note: MDPI stays neutral with regard to jurisdictional claims in published maps and institutional affiliations.

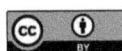

Copyright: © 2022 by the authors. Licensee MDPI, Basel, Switzerland. This article is an open access article distributed under the terms and conditions of the Creative Commons Attribution (CC BY) license (https://creativecommons.org/licenses/by/4.0/).

1. Introduction

The effects of music on the brain extend far beyond hearing [1,2] and positively affect quality of life [3]. The stimulating properties of music not only promote the development of the auditory system in children [4,5] and increase the capacity of speech discrimination in noise [6], but also reinforce many cognitive capacities involved in communication skills and social integration [7,8]. For the hard of hearing, music is a valuable tool for training [7–9] and for exploring the hearing loss in a complementary manner to conventional audiometry [10]. It is a source of joy even in patients with profound hearing loss and a cochlear implant (CI), and this may explain their motivation to engage in musical rehabilitation programs [11].

In adult CI patients, music perception is severely deteriorated [12]. Recognizing melodies remains a difficult task and shows high interindividual variability (25% success versus 88% in normal hearing patients) [13]. This handicap is mainly attributed to the limitations inherent to CI sound coding and processing strategies [14–16]. In addition, auditory nerve survival in the implanted ears, which can be suboptimal, is directly related to the number of functional channels eliciting different auditory sensations, the electrical dynamic range, and also the capacity of benefiting from high rates of stimulations [17].

Alterations in central sound processing mechanisms caused by auditory deprivation may additionally contribute to this poor perception [18]. Despite these limitations, many implantees enjoy music [11,19], and some can also perform well, especially after training [20]. When evaluating CI patients for basic music characteristics such as rhythm, melody, and timbre, typically, poor pitch discrimination and melody recognition are described but a near-normal performance in rhythm perception is reported [21,22]. The existence of a few star patients and the effect of training on timbre perception and melody recognition suggest that some patients can extract spectral cues to compensate for a lack of pitch resolution, that central auditory processing is probably subject to plasticity in this field, and finally, that patients learn to enjoy music based on cues different from those used by normal hearing individuals [23]. This idea is supported by the observation that recognizing a melody is influenced by the timbre of the instrument in CI users [24]. These spectral cues depend largely on coding and the sound processing strategies [13,24]. Pitch resolution refers to the smallest pitch interval detectable by the patients, which is coded by the place (electrode position) and time (pulse rate and pattern) cues for each electrode and is related to the number of functional channels in the CI [17]. Spectral differences can generate different activation patterns across several electrodes, and their distinction requires complex peripheral and central mechanisms [25,26].

To improve sound quality delivered by CI, several interconnected issues should be tackled. Alteration in pitch perception severely deteriorates harmonies and musical lines [27]. This phenomenon is largely due to the modified cochlear tonotopy after CI [28] and the drastic reduction in functional channels (number of electrodes eliciting a distinctive pitch) entailing a significant loss of frequency resolution [29]. Attempts to increase the number of functional channels by current steering (simultaneous current delivery by adjacent electrodes with variable ponderation) have shown some improvement in speech performance [30] but cannot compensate for the reduced number of nerve endings in the cochlea.

Another issue in music listening with CI is the loss of spectral information. Better encoding the sound envelope and providing the temporal fine structure have shown their efficacy in enhancing bass frequency discrimination and higher musical sound quality [31]. However, these relatively new coding strategies encounter a pathophysiological barrier, which is the channel interaction and overload [18]. Indeed, delivering electrical pluses at a higher rate on a larger number of electrodes requires performant and numerous functional channels [32] that many patients do not have [33]. These channel interactions are largely responsible for inter-individual performance variability [33]. Improvement in the acoustic dynamic range is another paramount obstacle not only for understanding speech in noise, but also for enjoying music [34]. Indeed, delivering sound intensity nuances of daily life or music while disposing of a restricted range of tolerable sound intensities is problematic in many patients with a long history of hearing deprivation. With the increasing processing capacity of hearing aids, new sound processing algorithms such as nonlinear frequency compression and adaptative dynamic range optimization have been developed in the field of hearing aids [35–37], and some of these solutions have been more recently implemented in CI technology [34,38]. CrystalisXDP strategy (Oticon Medical, Vallauris, France) focuses on rendering the spectral details of the entering signal with a lower distortion than the standard "main peak interleaved sampling" (MPIS) strategy. In addition, it provides possibly more comfortable listening through an adjustable compression system [38]. In a previous study, this sound processing strategy seemed to enhance speech perception in quiet and noise [38]. Its effect on music perception has not been evaluated to our knowledge.

The present study focuses on the emotional response to music, which is the most important aspect of everyday life music experience. Tempo and mode were found to be the most robust factors inducing joy and sadness in listeners [39]. A given musical piece will be perceived to be happier when played faster, and in major rather than in minor mode. Although the perception of tempo raises no difficulty in CI, the perception of mode remains a challenging issue. In contrast to the major mode, minor music contains intervals such as minor third intervals, which induce significant roughness or dissonance in the auditory filter [40]. Accordingly, we hypothesized that, with a poor pitch resolution, CI patients would have difficulty distinguishing happy from sad music using spectral cues, but that reducing the spectral distortion would enhance this capacity. The goal of this study was to evaluate the effect of reducing spectral distortion with the CrystalisXDP sound processing program on the ability of CI patients to distinguish happy from sad music based on rhythmical and/or modal cues, and to confront this performance to their subjective musical experience.

2. Materials and Methods

Twenty-one patients were included in this prospective double-blind and crossover study. Inclusion criteria in this study were the following: adult patients with bilateral profound hearing loss, unilateral or bilateral cochlear implants with at least one year of experience, Digisonic CI and Saphyr 2 sound processor (Oticon Medical) in their monaural or binaural versions, and a dissylabic word discrimination score (WDS) >20% with CI alone.

Among the 48 patients corresponding to these criteria in our center, we excluded 21 (44%) who did not wish to participate, 6 (13%) who had moved from our region and were lost to follow-up, and 1 who had poor speech recognition (WDS with CI alone: 14%). Twenty-one patients were included: five had a unilateral Digisonic DX10® (bearing 15 electrodes); t wore a unilateral and one a bilateral Digisonic SP® (20 electrodes); and three were rehabilitated by a binaural Digisonic® CI (12 electrodes on each side).

The protocol was reviewed and approved by the institutional ethical committee (CCP grand Est III). All patients were clearly informed and provided their oral and written consent for this study.

2.1. Study Design

At inclusion, the patient was examined, underwent a hearing test, and filled in a questionnaire on past and current musical experiences. The visit ended with a standard fitting session by the audiologist. Two programs (P1 and P2) were downloaded into the processor. During the study, the fitting parameters (frequency allocations, loudness) remained the same for the 2 strategies. CrystalisXDP and standard MPIS strategy were randomly assigned to P1 and P2 program slots in a double-blind manner to the patient and to the investigator who tested the hearing performances and the musical experience. The patient was asked to use P1 for one week. A second visit was then programmed. The patient participated in a musical test and responded to a questionnaire pertaining to experience with P1. Subsequently, P2 was activated. One week later, P2 was evaluated with the same tests. In bilateral and binaural cases, the programs were applied to both ears.

2.2. Population Characteristics

Twelve women and nine men participated in the test (Table 1). The mean age of the group was 55 ± 2.7 years (23–74). All presented with postlingual deafness. Patients had been implanted for a mean duration of 8 ± 1.2 years [3–19] before inclusion. The hearing deprivation period before implantation was 9 ± 3.1 years [1–48] and the mean age at implantation was 47 ± 2.6 years [19–65].

Seventeen patients (81%) had a unilateral CI (nine right and eight left), three (14%) had a binaural CI, and one (5%) had a bilateral CI. All patients wore their CI more than 12 h per day. Seven patients (33%) with a unilateral CI had a contralateral hearing aid. Before inclusion, 15 patients used CrystalisxDP and 6 used the standard MPIS strategy.

Etiologies of hearing loss were idiopathic in 11 patients (52%), Meniere's disease in 1 (5%), congenital in 4 (19%), advanced otosclerosis in 2 (10%), and traumatic in 2 cases (10%).

Table 1. Subject demographics. Age, hearing deprivation and CI experience are expressed in years. Hearing deprivation began by the abandonment of the ipsilateral hearing aid. Process.: Type of Saphyr processor, CI Exp: Cochlear implant experience, F: female, M: Male, L: Left, R: Right, BIN: binaural, BIL: bilateral. Number of active electrodes/total electrodes in BIN and BIL cases are indicated as Right + Left.

ID#	Sex	Age	Etiology	Hearing Deprivation	CI Exp.	CI Side	Process.	Active/Total Electrodes	Initial Strategy
1	M	50	Idiopathic	3	5	L	SP	18/20	Crystalis
2	M	53	Trauma	1	7	R	SP	18/20	Crystalis
3	M	47	Congenital	1	3	L	SP	18/20	Crystalis
4	M	23	Congenital	1	4	R	SP	20/20	Crystalis
5	F	51	Idiopathic	1	4	L	SP	17/20	Crystalis
6	F	62	Idiopathic	1	19	L	SP	9/15	Crystalis
7	M	67	Idiopathic	1	11	L	CX	15/15	Crystalis
8	M	62	Idiopathic	48	3	L	SP	19/20	Crystalis
9	F	67	Idiopathic	37	17	L	CX	12/15	MPIS
10	F	58	Otosclerosis	14	19	R	CX	9/15	MIPS
11	F	74	Otosclerosis	1	10	L	SP	16/20	MPIS
12	M	63	Idiopathic	1	4	R	SP	20/20	Crystalis
13	F	54	Idiopathic	1	5	BIN	SP	12/12 + 12/12	Crystalis
14	F	55	Idiopathic	8	6	BIN	SP	12/12 + 12/12	Crystalis
15	M	69	Meniere's	29	6	L	SP	16/20	Crystalis
16	F	56	Congenital	28	16	R	CX	11/15	MPIS
17	F	47	Idiopathic	3	3	R	SP	17/20	Crystalis
18	F	44	Idiopathic	2	2	L	SP	16/20	Crystalis
19	F	38	Congenital	1	6	BIN	SP	12/12 + 12/12	MPIS
20	F	38	Idiopathic	3	4	BIL	SP	16/20 + 18/20	MPIS
21	M	69	Trauma	1	4	R	SP	18/20	Crystalis

The ipsilateral pure tone average (PTA) was 108 ± 8.8 dB before implantation and 39 dB ± 3.1 in free-field with CI. The aided contralateral PTA was estimated as 79 ± 11.2 dB (n = 21) with no response above 1 kHz. The WDS was 6.5 ± 9.88% without CI and with lipreading only, 58.6 ± 22.01 with CI only, and 78.3 ± 19.25 with CI + lipreading.

2.3. Coding and Sound Processing Strategies

The main peak interleaved sampling (MPIS) strategy was used as the standard strategy in this study [41]. The speech processor (DigiSP) uses a Fourier Frequency Transform (FFT) to extract frequency peaks from the input signal spectrum in the 195–8003 Hz range. Available intracochlear electrodes, or channels (ranging from to 9–20 in this study), are selected for assignment of frequency bands to cover the 195–8003 Hz range using monopolar constant current stimulation. The signal level in each of the bandpass filters is assigned to the active electrodes. Loudness is coded by pulse duration, and pulse amplitude remains constant over time. Active electrodes associated with the highest signal level (spectral maxima) are stimulated in a basal to apical order. The number of transmitted peaks can be modified (default setting: 10 transmitted peaks out of 20 extracted peaks). The number of channels to be stimulated at each cycle is predetermined during fitting. Electrical stimulation rates range from 150 to 1000 pulses per second per electrode (pps/e). The default factory setting is 600 pps/e. Patients in this study used default settings. Only the number of available electrodes changed from one patient to another.

The digital signal processing of CrystalisXDP (Figures 1 and 2) is an evolution of the standard MPIS strategy specifically designed to enhance speech discrimination. It incorporates a multichannel back-end output compression function designated as XDP [38]. The Crystalis coding strategy enhances the FFT analysis by a window analysis in order to suppress artifacts and to extract not only the most salient but also the most relevant peaks to speech discrimination. The signal input spectrum is then processed by a noise reduction algorithm (Voicetrack®) that is based on a human voice reconnaissance and spectral subtraction. The signal is sent to the XDP transfer function module, which provides an adjustable compression of the electrical dynamic range as a function of the acoustic dynamic range. The knee point can be adjusted independently for four frequency bands: 195–846; 846–1497; 1497–3451; and 3451–8000 Hz, which groups electrodes with a similar energy spectrum for speech. Ninety-five percent of the speech information falls in the area under the knee point in each ambience considered. In this population, a medium preset for the knee point was used (average sound intensity at 70 dB SPL). In comparison to the standard MPIS strategy, CrystalisXDP improves the selection of the most relevant spectral peaks; it enhances the spectral contrast of the signal by a noise-reduction algorithm after the FFT analysis; and finally, it provides fine adjustment of the input–output compression function in order to contain everyday life sounds in a comfortable range.

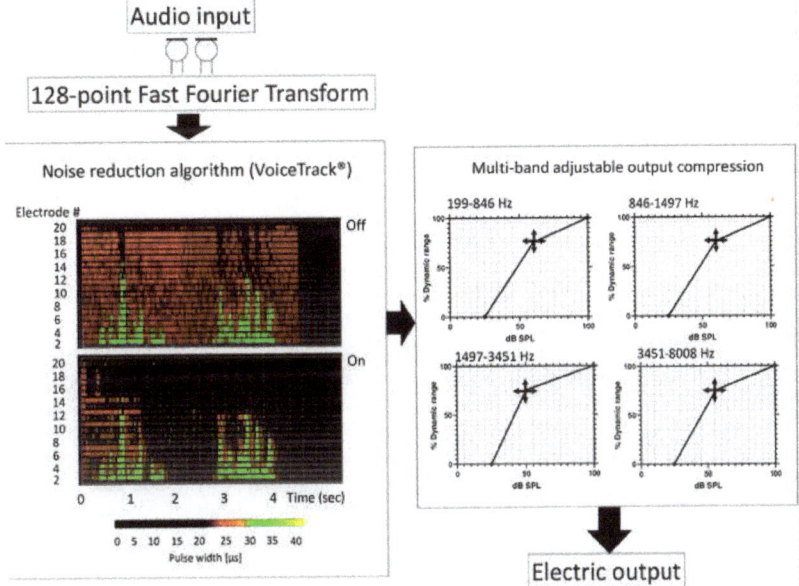

Figure 1. Functional Structure of CrystalisXDP. The system extracts the spectral features of the acoustic input by a 128-point Fast Fourier Transform (FFT). A noise reduction algorithm (VoiceTrack) based on spectral subtraction is then applied to enhance the spectral contrast. The 2 diagrams in the VoiceTrack panel show the simulated electrodograms of a human speech sample (dissyllabic word, 4 s), before (top) and after processing (below), generated by an in-house Oticon Medical simulation program as an example. Finally, the multi-band output compression provides adjustable output levels (Y-axis in % of electric dynamic range) as a function of acoustic input (X-axis, dB SPL) in 4 frequency bands.

2.4. Clinical Data

Clinical data regarding hearing loss (etiology, duration of deprivation, age at implantation) and audiometry data (pure-tone and speech performances with speech reception threshold, SRT and word discrimination score, WDS before and after implantation were recorded.

Audiometry was performed with a calibrated audiometer (AC40®, Interacoustics Inc., Middelfart, Denmark) in a standard audiometric booth. Preoperative tests were conducted with a headset. Postoperative tests were conducted in free-field conditions with 2 frontal loudspeakers and contralateral masking (headset and white noise). SRT and WDS were evaluated by French Fournier dissyllabic lists. WDS was tested at 60 dBA (SPL).

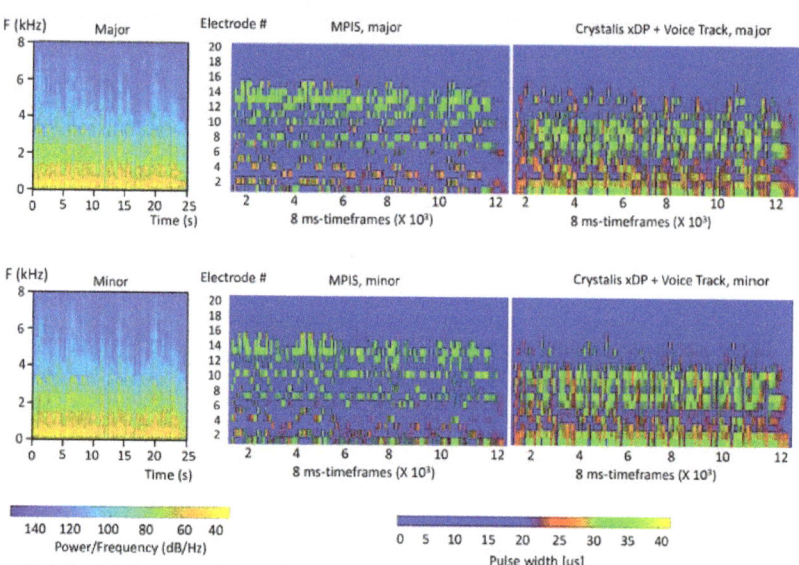

Figure 2. Spectrograms of the acoustic input, and electrodograms with standard MPIS and Crystalis xDP for 2 samples from test 3 with the same melody in major and minor modes. Spectrograms and electrodograms were simulated on Mathlab software using the same algorithms used in the processors by an in-house Oticon Medical program. For electrodograms, vertical axis shows electrode numbers (from 20 at the apex to 1 at the base) and the horizontal axis shows the number of analysis frames for the total duration of the sample (25 s). Each pixel represents an 8 ms frame sliding every 2 ms. Color codes represent pulse width (μs) coding for intensity for electrodograms and power/frequency (dB/Hz) for the spectrograms. Both strategies produced different electrodograms for minor and major modes. Crystalis xDP showed a richer electrodogram with more spectral cues. Differences between minor and major modes were translated by both temporal and spectral differences (i.e., different activation patterns across channels and within channels).

2.5. Questionnaires

The musical questionnaire was a simplified version of Munich Music Questionnaire (MMQ, 42) to limit the duration of each session. The questions concerned the musical experience in daily life through the average time of daily music listening, sound quality, instrument recognition, importance or implication of musical activities in the past and present (Table 2), and the sound and music perception by their CI before inclusion (Table 3). For this question, CI experience was compared to the period before implantation with still some degree of functional hearing for the progressive congenital or acquired diseases.

2.6. Music Test

We designed a music trial composed of 4 tests with increasing difficulty. The first 3 tests assessed emotional perception through music. In each of these tests, 6 melodies were played on piano in major (happy) and in minor (sad) modes, representing a total of 12 musical samples of 25 s each. The melodies were unknown to the general public in order to avoid cultural references. The melody line was accompanied by 1–4 note chords. Stimuli were equally tempered MIDI piano notes. All samples were recorded with a 44.1 kHz sampling rate at 16-bit depth. The participant could listen to these samples in a free order and as many times as desired. The subject was asked to categorize these samples as happy or sad with a forced two-choice task. No feedback was given. In the first test (easiest), in addition to the mode difference, happy samples were played faster than sad excerpts with a large difference in tempo (vivace, 140 beats/min for happy versus andante,

80 beats/min for sad). In the second test (intermediate), there was only a small difference in tempo (moderato, 100 versus 90 beats/min). In the third test (most difficult), the tempo was identical (moderato, 90 beats/min) and only the mode difference could allow the distinction. Test 4 evaluated the dissonance perception. Ten melody samples, with ($n = 5$) or without ($n = 5$) dissonance, were presented and the patient had to categorize them as "dissonant" or "harmonious". Melodies had the same characteristics as in the first 3 tests and were played with a moderato tempo (100 beats/min.). All tests were finally marked out of 10. The test interface was a laptop computer screen (Powerpoint 2010, Microsoft Inc. Redmond, VI, USA) where the patient could click on the musical sample to listen and to drag-and-drop the file into the proposed categories represented by happy and sad emojis. Samples were presented on 2 frontal loudspeakers (Sony, SRS-Z510, Tokyo, Japan) at a comfortable level judged by the patient. All tests were conducted in CI-only mode. In patients with residual hearing, the hearing aid was deactivated, and a sound reduction ear plug was placed in the ear. The patient used the interface independently and was only assisted by the investigator for technical issues.

Table 2. Musical Questionnaire Part 1: Musical Habits. Numbers indicate the number of choices among proposed responses and the number of positive responses ($n = 21$). Propositions for type of music were not exclusive. For the first question, the numbers indicate mean ± standard error of mean of Likert score [range]. MPIS ($n = 6$) and Crystalis XDP ($n = 15$) refer to the usual strategies used by the patients. HL: hearing loss, CI: cochlear implant.

Item		Before HL	Before CI	MPIS ($n = 6$)	CrystalisXDP ($n = 15$)
How important is music in your life?		-	-	3.7 ± 0.42	3.6 ± 0.34
Do you attend musical events?		-	-	2	9
Do you look for new musical releases?		-	-	3	2
Do you read publications on music?		-	-	2	6
How often do you listen to music?	Often	-	10	2	3
	Sometimes	-	7	4	9
	Never	-	4	0	3
How much music daily?	<30 min	5	16	2	8
	30–60 min	11	2	3	6
	1–2 H	1	2	0	0
	>2 H	3	0	1	0
	All day long	1	1	0	1

At the end, an auto questionnaire allowed the participant to rate the clarity of sound, the enjoyment of the melody, and the ease of each test (Likert scale 1–10), and to answer to the question, "which program did you prefer?" in a blinded manner (program 1 or 2, at the end of the second session).

2.7. Statistical Tests

Data were managed with Excel software (Office 2010, Microsoft Inc. Redmond, VI, USA) and Graphpad prism (v.6, Graphpad Inc., San Diego, CA, USA). Continuous variables were presented as mean ± standard error of mean (SEM) [min.-max.] and nominal variables were noted as n (%). Comparison of continuous parameters in 2 groups was studied by paired or unpaired t-tests. Continuous variables in multiple groups were tested by one- or two-way ANOVA. Music test scores were compared to the random level (score 5 out of 10) for each test by a one-sample t-test. A p-value < 0.05 was considered as significant. Linear regression analysis was conducted by F-test for the slope of the regression line and R for goodness of fit. Correlations were considered significant when $R > 0.5$ and $p < 0.05$. Test–retest reliability was tested by Cronbach's alpha. A value in the range of [0.8–0.9] was considered as good and >0.9 as excellent. To control for the effect of the usual strategy used by the patients in their music test performances, a mixed-model analysis was used to compare the results of the 4 music tests with the CystalisXDP versus MPIS program as a function of their usual strategy. A separate model was mixed employed for the global music score.

Table 3. Musical Questionnaire part 2: Music Perception with Cochlear Implant. Numbers indicate the number of choices among propositions, positive responses or Likert scores (mean ± standard error of mean, range, $n = 21$). MPIS ($n = 6$) and Crystalis XDP ($n = 15$) refer to the usual strategies used by the patients. CI: cochlear implant.

Item	Subitems/Choices	MPIS ($n = 6$)	Crystalis XDP ($n = 15$)
How does music sound with CI?	0:Unnatural-5:Natural	4.0 ± 0.26 [3,5]	2.9 ± 0.28 [1,5]
	0:Unpleasant-5:Pleasant	4.5 ± 0.22 [4,5]	3.5 ± 0.31 [1,5]
	0:Unclear-5:Clear	3.0 ± 0.4 [1,4]	2.6 ± 0.24 [1,4]
	0:Metallic-5:Not metallic	3.33 ± 0.56 [1,5]	3.1 ± 0.31 [1,5]
How do you listen to music?	As background	2	1
	Active listening	2	8
	Both	3	4
	Neither	1	0
Why do you listen to music? (answers not exclusive)	Pleasure	6	12
	Emotion	0	4
	Good mood	1	2
	Dance	3	6
	During work	2	3
	Relaxing	3	5
	Staying awake	0	1
	None of the above	0	1
When did you listen to music after CI?	Never	0	1
	<1 week after	2	4
	1–6 months	3	5
	7–12 months	1	3
	>12 months	0	2
Do you enjoy listening to solo instruments or orchestra?	Solo	1	5
	Orchestra	0	1
	Both	2	8
	None	3	1
What do you hear best or most? (answers not exclusive)	Pleasant sounds	5	10
	Rhythm	6	13
	Unpleasant sounds	1	3
	Melodies	6	12
	Voices	2	9
Can you detect wrong notes?		2	5
- detect false rhythms?		2	8
- compare performances?		5	10
- recognize a known melody?		4	14
- identify musical style?		4	11
- recognize the lyrics?		2	10
- recognize the singer?		2	9
- distinguish male/female singer?		3	13
- sing in tune?		2	3
- sing in public?		1	1
Did you train with music and CI?		5	8

The population size was estimated for test–retest reliability by setting $\alpha = 0.05$, $\beta = 0.1$, k (number of test items) = 4, the value of Cronbach's alpha at null hypothesis = 0, and the expected value of Cronbach's alpha = 0.75. The required number was evaluated as 17 subjects according to Bonnett [42] and increased to 21 to account for potential loss to follow-up at the retest.

3. Results

3.1. CI and Sound Processing Strategies

The number of active electrodes was 15 ± 0.7 ($n = 21$): 11 ± 2.5 for patients with Digisonic DX10 ($n = 5$), 18 ± 1.5 for unilateral Digisonic SP ($n = 12$), 12 on each side for binaural CI ($n = 3$), and 16 and 18 for the bilateral Digisonic SP. Before inclusion, 6 patients were fitted with the standard program (MPIS) and 15 already used CrystalisXDP. Patients using CrystalisXDP before inclusion performed similarly to those with a standard program as assessed by WDS ($78 \pm 6.5\%$ $n = 15$, versus 60 ± 13.9, $n = 6$, not significant, unpaired t-test followed by Bonferroni). Speech performances were not related to the number of active electrodes in this group (WDS: $83 \pm 5.8\%$, $n = 15$, versus 48 ± 10.5, $n = 6$, respectively, not significant, unpaired t-test, followed by Bonferroni correction).

3.2. Musical Experience

At inclusion, the questionnaire revealed that music was important in the daily life of this group (average Likert score 3.6 ± 1.20, with 18 patients (86%) scoring >3 out of 5, Table 2). The implantation did not change the frequency of music listening (response to "How often?", not significant, chi-2 test), or the type of music (not significant, chi-2 test). The majority (18, 86%) continued to listen for pleasure (Table 3) and practiced active music listening (17, 81%). While most declared being capable of recognizing a known melody (18, 86%), the musical style (15, 71%), and even the lyrics (15, 71%), only a few declared being capable of detecting a wrong note (6, 29%), singing in tune (5, 24%) or singing in public (2, 10%) underlining the inherent CI limitations in frequency discrimination.

CI negatively impacted music activities in this group. After implantation, many patients stopped musical activity such as music lessons (6 out of 7), playing an instrument (3 out of 6) or singing (3 out of 9). However, most declared training themselves with music after CI (13, 62%).

3.3. Music Test

Scores decreased with increasing levels of difficulty from tests 1 to 4 for both CrystalisXDP and standard programs (Figure 3). Scores for tests 1, 2 and 3 were above chance level (8.81 ± 0.25 for test 1, $p < 10^{-4}$, 6.87 ± 0.25, for test 2, $p < 10^{-4}$, and 5.43 ± 0.20, $p < 0.05$ for test 3, $n = 42$, one-sample test). In contrast, the average score for test 4 was not different from the chance level (5.02 ± 0.31, $n = 42$, not significant, one sample test, Figure 3).

The short period of adaptation could have advantaged CrystalisXDP over the standard program in those who already used CrystalisXDP and represented the majority (15 out of 21). A mixed-model analysis (restricted maximum likelihood approach) comparing the results for music tests 1 to 4 with CrystalisXDP and standard strategies in patients who regularly used CrystalisXDP versus those who regularly benefited from the standard program showed a significant effect of the test levels (DFn = 3, DFd = 76, F = 32.15, $p < 0.001$) and the strategy during the test (higher scores for CrystalisXDP versus standard, DFn = 1, DFd = 76, F = 5.76, $p < 0.05$). However, the usual strategy used by the patients before inclusion did not have a significant effect on the test results (CrystalisXDP versus standard, DFn = 1, DFd = 76, F = 0.12, not significant). There was no interaction between these factors (test level*tested strategy: DFn = 3, DFd = 76, F = 1.52, $p = 0.214$; test level *initial strategy: DFn = 3, DFd = 76, F = 1.31, not significant; Tested strategy*usual strategy: DFn = 1, DFd = 76, F = 0.021; not significant; test level*tested strategy*initial strategy: DFn = 3, DFd = 76, F = 0.081, not significant). A Tukey's multiple comparison test applied to this model showed a higher level of scores for test 1 in comparison to all other tests ($p < 10^{-4}$), a higher score for T2 in comparison to test 4 ($p < 0.001$), and higher scores for T3 versus T4 ($p < 0.05$).

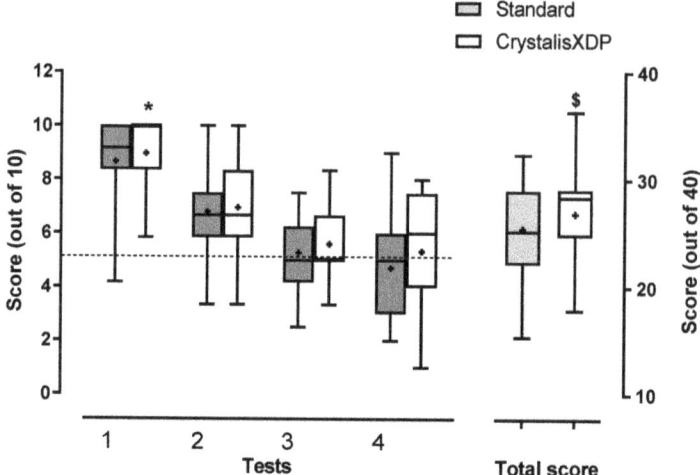

Figure 3. Scores for music tests with standard (MPIS) and CrystalisXDP sound processing strategies. Each test was marked out of 10, and the total score out of 40. Bars represent mean ± SEM ($n = 21$). Scores decreased with the difficulty level (*: $p < 0.001$, mixed model analysis). Patients performed better with CrystalisXDP than with standard program ($p < 0.05$) regardless of their usual strategy (effect not significant). Total scores were also higher with CrystalisXDP than with MPIS regardless of the patients' usual strategy ($: $p < 0.05$, mixed-effects analysis). Box and Whiskers plot represents first and third quartiles, median, and range. Mean is depicted by (+). Dashed line represents chance level.

As assessed by the total score, patients also performed better with CrystalisXDP than with the standard program regardless of their usual strategy (mixed-effects analysis, DFn = 1, DFd = 38, F = 4.98, and $p < 0.05$ for the effect of the tested strategy; F = 0.644, not significant for the effect of usual strategy, and F = 0.046 not significant for tested strategy*usual strategy, Figure 3). Higher scores with CrystalisXDP suggested that patients exploit some spectral-based cues in addition to the rhythm to distinguish between happy and sad music.

There was no statistical difference between the total scores at the first and second sessions, suggesting that there was no effect of order (global scores 30.5 ± 5.19 vs. 31.2 ± 5.23, respectively, mean of differences: 1.52, not significant, paired-*t*-test, $n = 21$). The test–retest reliability of the total score was good between the two sessions (Cronbach alpha = 0.87, average R = 0.77).

Musical background was significant in this population. Ten patients used to sing in their childhood (47%). Among these, five continued singing during adulthood and even after CI. Seven declared playing an instrument in their childhood: drums ($n = 1$), flute ($n = 1$), piano ($n = 3$), accordion ($n = 1$), and clarinet ($n = 1$). Only four pursued their hobby as an adult. Five singers also played an instrument. Singing before CI tended to improve scores regardless of strategy ($p = 0.05$, 2-way ANOVA, Table 4), but there was no effect of playing an instrument or training with CI on the scores (not significant, 2-way ANOVA).

Table 4. Music test scores as a function of musical experience and training. Total scores for music tests are presented as Mean score ± standard error of mean [range] for each subgroup.

	Total Score with MPIS		Total Score with Crystalis XDP	
	Yes	No	Yes	No
Player before CI (Yes: $n = 7$; No: $n = 14$)	24.9 ±1.34 [18.7–29.2]	25.7 ± 1.36 [15.3–32.3]	27.1 ± 1.03 [22.5–30.5]	26.7 ± 1.40 [17.8–36.3]
Singer before CI (Yes: $n = 10$; No: $n = 11$)	26.7 ± 0.92 [23–31.7]	24.2 ± 1.67 [15.3–32.3]	28.4 ± 1.14 [22.5–36.3]	25.4 ± 1.46 [17.8–31.8]
Musical training with CI (Yes: $n = 13$; No: $n = 8$)	25.5 ± 1.09 [18.7–32.3]	25.3 ± 2.03 [15.3–31.7]	26.9 ±0.90 [19–30.5]	26.8 ± 2.22 [17.8–36.3]

Total music scores were correlated with WDS (Figure 4). Total music scores appeared to be influenced by the number of active electrodes. Although there was no correlation between the number of electrodes and the total score (Figure 5), patients with more than 15 electrodes ($n = 14$) performed better with CrystalisXDP sound processing programs (28 ± 5.89, $n = 7$ for patients with <15 electrodes versus 33 ± 3.93, $n = 14$, t(19) = 2.18, $p = 0.042$, unpaired t-test). With the standard MPIS program, this difference also tended to be significant (26.6 ± 4.12, $n = 7$ versus 30.8 ± 5.10, $n = 14$, t(19) = 2.07, $p = 0.052$, unpaired t-test).

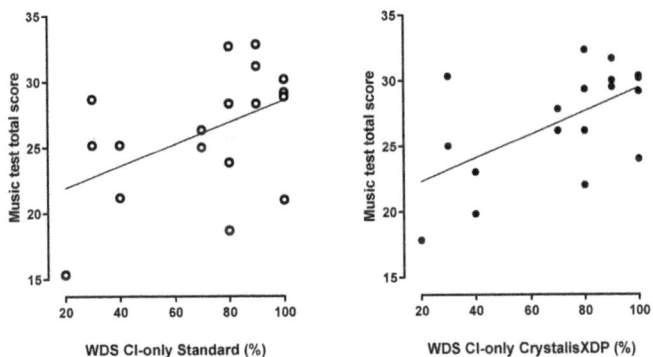

Figure 4. Correlation between musical test total scores and word discrimination scores (WDS) with cochlear implant (CI) only with standard (MPIS) and CrystalisXDP sound processing strategies. WDS tended to be correlated with total scores in standard condition (right panel, Y = 0.08 * X + 20.2, R = 0.47, $p < 0.05$, F test) and was significantly correlated to total scores in CrystalisXDP condition (left panel, Y = 0.09 * X + 20.5, R = 0.58, $p < 0.01$, F-test).

Total scores obtained by patients with unilateral CI were not different from those with binaural or bilateral CI (31.8 ± 4.57, $n = 17$ versus 29.6 ± 5.04, $n = 4$, with CrystalisXDP, and 29.5 ± 7.68 versus 28.5 ± 6.14 without CrystalisXDP, not significant, unpaired t-test). Patients with bimodal hearing did not perform better than those with one or 2 CIs in this population (29.1 ± 3.81, $n = 7$ versus 25.5 ± 1.55, $n = 14$, respectively, with standard program, not significant, unpaired t-test, data not shown for CrystalisXDP). Similarly, patient who reported musical training during rehabilitation with CI did not perform better than others according to the total score or the scores obtained for each test (data not shown). Patients performed well at tests 1 and 2 and these scores were highly correlated, suggesting the prominence of rhythmical cues even for small differences in tempo in test 2 (Y = 1.00 + 0.67 X, R = 0.73, $p < 0.001$, and Y = −0.31 + 0.81 X, R = 0.67, $p < 0.001$ for standard and CrystalisXDP were Y: test 2 and X: test 1).

In contrast, only nine (43%) patients could categorize above the random level (score > 5) in test 3 (sad versus happy based only on mode) with the standard or CrystalisXDP programs (average scores 6.4 ± 0.59 and 6.9 ± 0.93, respectively, $p < 0.001$, one-sample test for both). In this group, CrystalisXDP, significantly improved the score in comparison to the standard strategy ($p < 0.05$, paired t-test, followed by Bonferroni correction). Similarly, only a few patients could distinguish dissonance above chance level (score >5 at test 4): 6 (29%) with standard program (average score 7.0 ± 1.27, $p < 0.05$, one-sample test) and 11 (52%) with CrystalisXDP (average score: 7.0 ± 1.00, $p < 0.0001$, one-sample test). In this group, CrystalisXDP did not improve the scores (not significant, paired t-test, followed by Bonferroni correction).

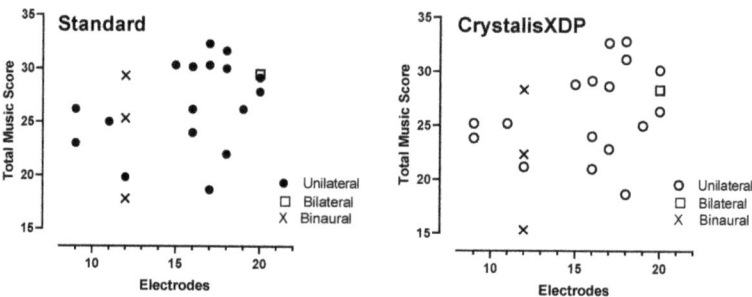

Figure 5. Total music scores as a function of the number of active electrodes with standard (MPIS) and CrystalisXDP strategies. Bilateral and binaural cases are depicted with the number of electrodes in one ear (20 and 12, respectively).

Performances for tests 3 (sad/happy only based on mode) and 4 (dissonance) were similar (5.4 ± 0.24 versus 5.0 ± 0.40, respectively, $n = 21$, average of two programs, unpaired t-test, not significant), but not correlated (data not shown), suggesting that these two tasks explored different domains. The duration of the hearing deprivation influenced the scores for test 3: patients with a score >5 with CrystalisXDP had a hearing deprivation period <10 years in all cases ($n = 8$), while those who performed poorer had longer deprivation periods (6 out of 12 with deprivation >10 years, $p < 0.05$, chi-2 test). Performances in test 4 were not related to hearing deprivation period (data not shown). Additionally, scores >5 in tests 3 and 4 were not related to age, sex, number of active electrodes, contralateral hearing aid, or previous training (data not shown).

These poor performances contrasted with the questionnaire results in which the majority (18, 86%) declared hearing the melody most (or best) (Table 3). The performances in tests 3 and 4 were not higher in those who declared detecting wrong notes than others (data not shown).

The subjective ease scores decreased with the level of difficulty (Figure 6). Sound processing programs did not influence the ratings of ease, sound clarity or liking (Figure 6). There was a significant correlation between the total music score and the level of ease rated by the participant for the first test (first trial: Y = 2.58 + 0.17X, R = 0.5, $p < 0.05$, second trial: Y = 0.45 + 0.33X, R = 0.6, $p < 0.01$, F-test, X: score, Y: level of ease), but for more difficult levels involving modes and dissonances (tests 2 to 4), this correlation did not exist (data not shown). Clarity and liking ratings were not correlated with total music scores (data not shown) and were not modified by the program (not significant, unpaired t-test, Figure 6).

Interestingly, test 3 (happy versus sad based on mode) was rated as easier than test 4 regardless of the program (3.3 ± 0.16 for test 3 versus 2.6 ± 0.20 for test 4, average scores for 2 programs, $n = 21$, $p < 0.01$, paired t-test), while the performances were similarly poor for both tests. Finally, most patients ($n = 16$, 76%, $p < 0.05$, binomial test) preferred CrystalisXDP to the standard MPIS. Among patients ($n = 15$) who used CystalisXDP before the study, 12 kept their usual program and 3 chose the standard program. In the group using MPIS regularly ($n = 6$), three conserved their program and three switched to CystalisXDP.

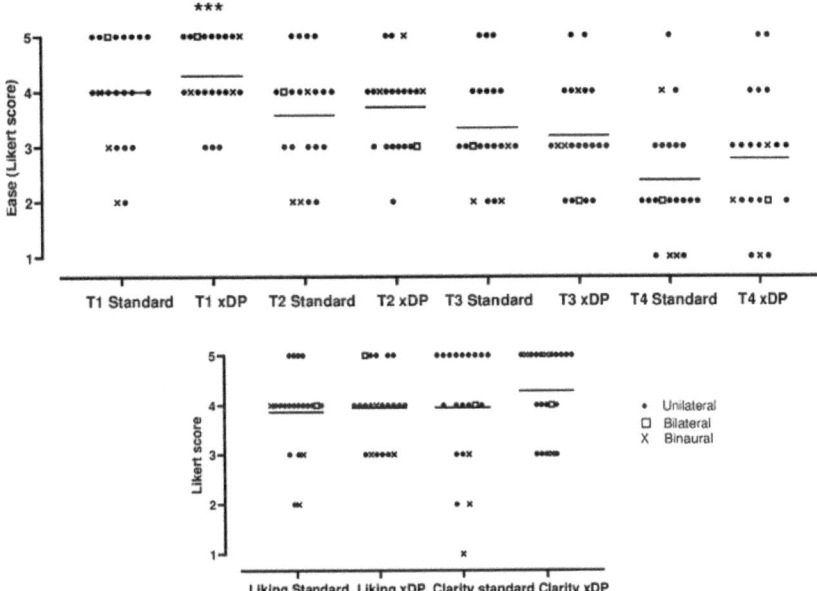

Figure 6. Musical test ratings in terms of ease, clarity and melody liking. Patients scored each item on an auto questionnaire at the end of each test on a Likert scale (1 to 5). Symbols (***) represent individual values ($n = 21$) and bars represent mean. Ease scores decreased with the difficulty level, but programs (standard or MPIS versus CrystalisXDP) did not influence ratings ($p < 0.001$ for test levels and not significant for programs, 2-way ANOVA), unpaired t-test versus standard.

4. Discussion

In this study, we showed that music represents a significant daily activity for cochlear implantees. Our original music test, which assessed the hearing performances and explored the emotional aspect of the music, yielded a total score correlated to word discrimination score. It had a good test–retest reliability and did not have a floor or ceiling effect. It was positively influenced by a higher number of active electrodes. As expected, the test revealed a good detection of rhythmical cues but poor performances in detecting dissonances and musical modes. CrystalisXDP improved the musical test results based on both rhythm and spectral cues. Since MPIS and CrystalisXDP have the same basic coding strategy providing the same rhythmical information, and the fitting parameters were identical for both strategies, the results suggest that this improvement is related to modifications in spectral cues.

Musical experience is difficult to describe and analyze since it deals with several intricate factors such as rhythm, pitch, timbre, melody, cultural references, and complex capacities, such as musical sophistication [44]. The latter parameter is defined by the frequency of exerting musical skills or behaviors and the ease, the accuracy or the effect of musical behaviors, and a varied repertoire of musical behavior patterns can be a source of inter individual variability in music tests [44].

Most of the reported music tests evaluate basic features such as pitch, timbre, and rhythm perception [19,45,46]. However, considering the gap between poor musical hearing performances with a CI and a relatively high music enjoyment [47–49], it is interesting to explore higher levels of music perception such as emotions since it can a lead to better understanding of coping mechanisms and neural plasticity in cochlear implantees [50,51].

The effect of Western musical modes on emotions is well known and appears to be effective even in individuals with little or no musical background [for review, see 52]: the major mode evokes dynamism, joy, hope, force and tenderness, and oppositely, the minor mode elicits passivity, despair, sadness, pain, mystery and obscurity. To control the overall difficulty of the trial, we organized the tests in a gradually increasing order of complexity. The rhythmic cue, known to be largely exploited by the CI patients [53], was employed to mitigate the difficulty of the pitch and mode discrimination. As expected, the performances and the level of ease rated by the participants decreased with a lower contribution of rhythm in the categorization. Without this hint, the average score dropped from excellent to chance level for tests 3 (happy versus sad only based on mode) and 4 (dissonance in a melody). This poor performance was in line with the questionnaire in which only 29% of the patients declared being capable of detecting a wrong note. It is noteworthy that CrystalisXDP, which improves spectral cues but provides rhythmical information similar to MPIS, enhanced the happy versus sad categorization performances based on both musical modes and rhythmical information. Previous reports have shown that in cochlear implantees, both place (i.e., electrode position in the cochlea and its assigned frequency band) and temporal cues (i.e., stimulation pulse pattern and rate) are closely related to each other for pitch perception [54,55]. In our study, while place cues remained the same, temporal cues were modified through spectral modifications by CrystalisXDP. The optimization of the temporal cues might influence the pitch perception and provide a possible explanation for the enhancement of sad versus happy categorization.

However, interestingly, a few patients performed relatively well (scores > 5) for these tasks despite the inherent limitations of CI. Better scores for test 3 (happy versus sad based on only mode) were obtained by patients who had a short time of hearing deprivation (<10 years), suggesting the need for an efficient auditory central pathway in music processing [16]. Scores for tests 3 and 4 were not correlated, while scores for tests 1 and 2 (categorization mainly or partly based on rhythm) were highly correlated. This observation suggests that musical modes may involve a different auditory processing task than the detection of a dissonance in a melody. Another important factor, which may explain high performances in tests 3 and 4, is the above-average spectral and pitch resolution related to a higher neural survival in the implanted ear. The quantity of preserved neurons directly influences the number of functional channels, the channel interactions, and the neural capacity to be stimulated at high rates [17,31–33,56].

The distinction of consonant from dissonant notes from a musical instrument or human voices is directly related to the interval between their fundamental frequencies and mainly detected at the cochlear level [57,58]. A dissonant note with fundamental frequency (F0) too close to the reference note to be resolved by the cochlea produces a rapid variation in total amplitude and a sensation of roughness or beating which can be evidenced on the spectrogram [59]. A dissonant note easily distinguishable by the cochlea from the reference has component frequencies that cannot aggregate with those of the reference note producing an inharmonic spectrum. The participation of central auditory processing in this distinction has been suggested based on observation of subjects with amusia [59], but the exact role of peripheral auditory system and the auditory centers are extremely hard to separate in this process. To this end, CI patients represent an interesting pathophysiological model. Observations on CI patients with contralateral normal hearing are in line with this mechanistic explanation. CI patients appear to be sensitive to dissonance by the perception of roughness, and the information related to the temporal envelope plays an important role in distinguishing harmonicity from dissonance [40]. In our study, reducing the spectral distortions without altering the rhythmic information by CrystalisXDP sound processing strategy improved total scores, leading to the hypothesis that by providing discrete cues on roughness and beating, it could enhance global music perception. This phenomenon may be explained by the reduction in spectral smearing and undesired channel interactions in CI patients. Spectral information directly influences the temporal coding within channels. This possible explanation is in line with the observation that reducing the number of harmonics increases the musical enjoyment in both normal-hearing and CI subjects [60].

Despite their poor performances in tests 3 and 4, patients attributed an above-average score to the clarity and the liking of the melodies, and this discrepancy underlines the difference between performance and enjoyment, an observation that has also been reported by others [45,46]. With time, CI patients develop other musical esthetic criteria, and choose types of music which are easier to listen to (more rhythmical cues, less polyphony, and harmonics) as coping strategies [61]. To enjoy music with CI, postlingually deaf patients need time and effort to gather musical experience with new sensations and auditory landmarks. Pleasant music is a skilled mix of predictable events, which drive expectations, and sparse unpredictable developments leading to surprises, and these expectations are related to the experience of musical pleasure [62,63]. Alterations in timber perception and low pitch resolution deteriorate the melody reconnaissance in CI patients [13] and probably also the predictability. With training, these auditory expectations and surprises can be developed in CI patients [7–9]. Another issue is that musical pleasure seems to increase with stimulus complexity (e.g., musical lines, harmonics, timber) up to an intermediate level, and then to decrease with even more complex sounds [64]. Achieving such a level of performance to detect complexity appears possible in some CI patients, since in our population, 9 declared listening to classical music and 5 to opera, reputed as relatively complex, and 15 declared being capable of even comparing performances. However, this ability probably requires a high number of functional channels in the cochlea and a performant central auditory pathway [24,65].

Many variables, such as number of active electrodes, insertion depth, or duration of hearing deprivation may have an impact on the music perception in CI patients [66] and explain the heterogeneity of the results. However, when attempting to control all variables in a very homogeneous population, one might argue that the observations do not apply to other groups of CI patients and the effect is marginal. In addition, one might oppose the fact that other variables such as sex, age, body laterality, ethnicity and cultural background could still interfere. Moreover, it would be difficult, if not impossible, to control parameters such as electrode insertion depth and electrode position or even musical background and experience in such a population. Consequently, we compared sound processing strategies in a paired cross-over design to limit the potential effect of these factors in the outcome. Despite the heterogeneity, which corresponds to the every-day audiology practice, we could observe a quite significant effect of spectral cue enhancement on the music scores. Using only one or both ears could influence the results. However, interestingly, total scores obtained by patients with unilateral CI did not differ from those with binaural or bilateral CIs. Patients with bimodal hearing had marginal acoustic hearing and were tested in CI-only mode; they did not perform better than those with one or 2 CIs in this population. This is consistent with the experimental conditions, which did not disadvantage monaural patients (twin frontal loudspeakers).

In our study, the adaptation period to new sound processing strategies was relatively short. This could have masked the effect or created a bias. However, CrystalisXDP is not a radical change in strategy in comparison to the standard program. It improves the already installed strategy by a better selection of spectral peaks to code, by increasing the spectral contrast, and by fine-tuning the output compression. There is no change in the frequency-place function, frequency band allocation, the loudness or even the basic strategy, which is the MPIS. A previous publication on this sound processing algorithm had shown a rapid adaptation of the patients with significant improvements of WDS in 30 days [38]. This is consistent with the improvement of music scores with CrystalisXDP, which were correlated with WDS in this study. The short adaptation period could have advantaged CrystalisXDP in the majority who used this strategy before inclusion. However, a mixed-model analysis showed that the strategy used regularly before the inclusion did not affect the results.

To our knowledge, there is no validated test for evaluating the emotional aspects of music or musical experience in cochlear implantees. The Munich Music questionnaire has not been validated but was previously published as a relevant tool to evaluate musical perception in CI patients [42]. This questionnaire appeared to provide coherent and consistent results in cochlear implantees from different countries and cultural backgrounds [42,67–69].

This lack of validation imposes precaution in the interpretation of the results related to this tool. In contrast, Likert scales have been largely used as a validated method for the psychometric evaluation of music perception [70] and auditory handicap [71] and provided coherent information regarding the ease of the tests.

In conclusion, the categorization of happy versus sad music samples only based on musical mode or the distinction of melodies with dissonant notes from harmonious ones did not exceed the chance level. CrystalisXDP, which enhances spectral cues, improved performances in the categorization tasks where some rhythmic information was added to the musical mode. This observation, together with the music experience through questionnaires, suggests that CI patients exploit not only rhythmical indications, but also spectral cues to enjoy music and that tests based on intervals, rhythm and melody recognition cannot fully comprehend these cues. Further work on these potential spectral cues will guide the development of next generation sound processing strategies.

Author Contributions: Conceptualization, G.L., E.B. and A.B.G.; methodology, A.B.G.; software, G.G. and E.B.; validation, E.B. and A.B.G.; formal analysis, A.B.G.; investigation, G.L. and G.G.; resources, E.B. and G.G.; data curation, G.L. ang G.G.; writing—original draft preparation, A.B.G. and C.G.; writing—review and editing, A.B.G. and C.G.; visualization, A.B.G.; supervision, A.B.G.; project administration, A.B.G.; Funding: A.B.G. All authors have read and agreed to the published version of the manuscript.

Funding: The authors acknowledge Oticon Medical for the financial assistance regarding publication fees.

Institutional Review Board Statement: The study was conducted in accordance with the Declaration of Helsinki and approved by the Institutional Review Board (or Ethics Committee) of CCP grand Est III.

Informed Consent Statement: All patients were clearly informed and provided their oral and written consent for this study.

Data Availability Statement: Not applicable.

Acknowledgments: The authors are grateful to Manuel Segovia Martinez, Michel Hoen, and Dan Gnansia from Oticon Medical for their technical assistance.

Conflicts of Interest: The authors declare no conflict of interest.

References

1. Musacchia, G.; Sams, M.; Skoe, E.; Kraus, N. Musicians have enhanced subcortical auditory and audiovisual processing of speech and music. *Proc. Natl. Acad. Sci. USA* **2007**, *104*, 15894–15898. [CrossRef] [PubMed]
2. Limb, C.J.; Rubinstein, J.T. Current research on music perception in cochlear implant users. *Otolaryngol. Clin. N. Am.* **2012**, *45*, 129–140. [CrossRef] [PubMed]
3. Lassaletta, L.; Castro, A.; Bastarrica, M.; Pérez-Mora, R.; Madero, R.; De Sarriá, J.; Gavilán, J. Does music perception have an impact on quality of life following cochlear implantation? *Acta Otolaryngol.* **2007**, *127*, 682–686. [CrossRef] [PubMed]
4. Mandikal Vasuki, P.R.; Sharma, M.; Ibrahim, R.; Arciuli, J. Statistical learning and auditory processing in children with music training: An ERP study. *Clin. Neurophysiol.* **2017**, *128*, 1270–1281. [CrossRef]
5. Patel, A.D. Why would Musical Training Benefit the Neural Encoding of Speech? The OPERA Hypothesis. *Front. Psychol.* **2011**, *2*, 142. [CrossRef]
6. Li, X.; Nie, K.; Imennov, N.S.; Won, J.H.; Drennan, W.R.; Rubinstein, J.T.; Atlas, L.E. Improved perception of speech in noise and Mandarin tones with acoustic simulations of harmonic coding for cochlear implants. *J. Acoust. Soc. Am.* **2012**, *132*, 3387–3398. [CrossRef]
7. Trehub, S.E.; Vongpaisal, T.; Nakata, T. Music in the lives of deaf children with cochlear implants. *Ann. N. Y. Acad. Sci.* **2009**, *1169*, 534–542. [CrossRef]
8. Gfeller, K.; Driscoll, V.; Kenworthy, M.; Van Voorst, T. Music Therapy for Preschool Cochlear Implant Recipients. *Music Ther. Perspect.* **2011**, *29*, 39–49. [CrossRef]
9. Gfeller, K.; Witt, S.; Woodworth, G.; Mehr, M.A.; Knutson, J. Effects of frequency, instrumental family, and cochlear implant type on timbre recognition and appraisal. *Ann. Otol. Rhinol. Laryngol.* **2002**, *111*, 349–356. [CrossRef]

10. Petersen, B.; Andersen, A.S.F.; Haumann, N.T.; Højlund, A.; Dietz, M.J.; Michel, F.; Riis, S.K.; Brattico, E.; Vuust, P. The CI MuMuFe—A New MMN Paradigm for Measuring Music Discrimination in Electric Hearing. *Front. Neurosci.* **2020**, *14*, 2. [CrossRef]
11. Hughes, S.; Llewellyn, C.; Miah, R. Let's Face the Music! Results of a Saturday Morning Music Group for Cochlear-Implanted Adults. *Cochlear Implant. Int.* **2010**, *11*, 69–73. [CrossRef]
12. Steel, M.M.; Polonenko, M.J.; Giannantonio, S.; Hopyan, T.; Papsin, B.C.; Gordon, K.A. Music Perception Testing Reveals Advantages and Continued Challenges for Children Using Bilateral Cochlear Implants. *Front. Psychol.* **2020**, *10*, 3015. [CrossRef]
13. Zhu, M.; Chen, B.; Galvin, J.J., 3rd; Fu, Q.-J. Influence of pitch, timbre and timing cues on melodic contour identification with a competing masker (L). *J. Acoust. Soc. Am.* **2011**, *130*, 3562–3565. [CrossRef]
14. Rubinstein, J.T.; Hong, R. Signal coding in cochlear implants: Exploiting stochastic effects of electrical stimulation. *Ann. Otol. Rhinol. Laryngol.* **2003**, *191*, 14–19. [CrossRef]
15. Hochmair, I.; Hochmair, E.; Nopp, P.; Waller, M.; Jolly, C. Deep electrode insertion and sound coding in cochlear implants. *Hear. Res.* **2015**, *322*, 14–23. [CrossRef]
16. Clark, G.M. The multiple-channel cochlear implant: The interface between sound and the central nervous system for hearing, speech, and language in deaf people-a personal perspective. *Philos. Trans. R. Soc. Lond. B Biol. Sci.* **2006**, *361*, 791–810. [CrossRef]
17. Pfingst, B.E.; Zhou, N.; Colesa, D.J.; Watts, M.M.; Strahl, S.B.; Garadat, S.N.; Schvartz-Leyzac, K.C.; Budenz, C.L.; Raphael, Y.; Zwolan, T.A. Importance of cochlear health for implant function. *Hear. Res.* **2015**, *322*, 77–88. [CrossRef]
18. Wang, S.; Chen, B.; Yu, Y.; Yang, H.; Cui, W.; Li, J.; Fan, G.G. Alterations of structural and functional connectivity in profound sensorineural hearing loss infants within an early sensitive period: A combined DTI and fMRI study. *Dev. Cogn. Neurosci.* **2019**, *38*, 100654. [CrossRef]
19. Mitani, C.; Nakata, T.; Trehub, S.E.; Kanda, Y.; Kumagami, H.; Takasaki, K.; Miyamoto, I.; Takahashi, H. Music recognition, music listening, and word recognition by deaf children with cochlear implants. *Ear Hear.* **2007**, *28*, 29S–33S. [CrossRef]
20. Cheng, X.; Liu, Y.; Shu, Y.; Tao, D.D.; Wang, B.; Yuan, Y.; Galvin, J.J., 3rd; Fu, Q.J.; Chen, B. Music Training Can Improve Music and Speech Perception in Pediatric Mandarin-Speaking Cochlear Implant Users. *Trends Hear.* **2018**, *22*, 2331216518759214. [CrossRef]
21. McDermott, H.J.; McKay, C.M.; Richardson, L.M.; Henshall, K.R. Application of loudness models to sound processing for cochlear implants. *J. Acoust. Soc. Am.* **2003**, *114*, 2190–2197. [CrossRef]
22. Riley, P.E.; Ruhl, D.S.; Camacho, M.; Tolisano, A.M. Music Appreciation after Cochlear Implantation in Adult Patients: A Systematic Review. *Otolaryngol. Head Neck Surg.* **2018**, *158*, 1002–1010. [CrossRef]
23. Irvine, D.R.F. Auditory perceptual learning and changes in the conceptualization of auditory cortex. *Hear. Res.* **2018**, *366*, 3–16. [CrossRef]
24. Galvin, J.J., 3rd; Fu, Q.J.; Oba, S. Effect of instrument timbre on melodic contour identification by cochlear implant users. *J. Acoust. Soc. Am.* **2008**, *124*, EL189–EL195. [CrossRef]
25. Moore, B.C. Coding of sounds in the auditory system and its relevance to signal processing and coding in cochlear implants. *Otol. Neurotol.* **2003**, *24*, 243–254. [CrossRef]
26. Suied, C.; Agus, T.R.; Thorpe, S.J.; Mesgarani, N.; Pressnitzer, D. Auditory gist: Recognition of very short sounds from timbre cues. *J. Acoust. Soc. Am.* **2014**, *135*, 1380–1391. [CrossRef]
27. Carlyon, R.P.; van Wieringen, A.; Long, C.J.; Deeks, J.M.; Wouters, J. Temporal pitch mechanisms in acoustic and electric hearing. *J. Acoust. Soc. Am.* **2002**, *112*, 621–633. [CrossRef]
28. Mistrík, P.; Jolly, C. Optimal electrode length to match patient specific cochlear anatomy. *Eur. Ann. Otorhinolaryngol. Head Neck Dis.* **2016**, *133*, S68–S71. [CrossRef] [PubMed]
29. Shannon, R.V.; Fu, Q.J.; Galvin, J.J., 3rd. The number of spectral channels required for speech recognition depends on the difficulty of the listening situation. *Acta Otolaryngol.* **2004**, *552*, 50–54. [CrossRef] [PubMed]
30. Luo, X.; Garrett, C. Dynamic current steering with phantom electrode in cochlear implants. *Hear. Res.* **2020**, *390*, 107949. [CrossRef] [PubMed]
31. Roy, A.T.; Carver, C.; Jiradejvong, P.; Limb, C.J. Musical Sound Quality in Cochlear Implant Users: A Comparison in Bass Frequency Perception Between Fine Structure Processing and High-Definition Continuous Interleaved Sampling Strategies. *Ear Hear.* **2015**, *36*, 582–590. [CrossRef]
32. Crew, J.D.; Iii, J.J.G.; Fu, Q.-J. Channel interaction limits melodic pitch perception in simulated cochlear implants. *J. Acoustic. Soc. Am.* **2012**, *132*, EL429–EL435. [CrossRef]
33. Tang, Q.; Benítez, R.; Zeng, F.-G. Spatial channel interactions in cochlear implants. *J. Neural Eng.* **2011**, *8*, 046029. [CrossRef]
34. James, C.J.; Blamey, P.J.; Martin, L.; Swanson, B.; Just, Y.; Macfarlane, D. Adaptive dynamic range optimization for cochlear implants: A preliminary study. *Ear Hear.* **2002**, *23*, 49S–58S. [CrossRef]
35. Blamey, P.J. Adaptive Dynamic Range Optimization (ADRO): A Digital Amplification Strategy for Hearing Aids and Cochlear Implants. *Trends Amplif.* **2005**, *9*, 77–98. [CrossRef]
36. Mao, Y.; Yang, J.; Hahn, E.; Xu, L. Auditory perceptual efficacy of nonlinear frequency compression used in hearing aids: A review. *J. Otol.* **2017**, *12*, 97–111. [CrossRef]
37. Vaisbuch, Y.; Santa Maria, P.L. Age-Related Hearing Loss: Innovations in Hearing Augmentation. *Otolaryngol. Clin. N. Am* **2018**, *51*, 705–723. [CrossRef]

38. Bozorg-Grayeli, A.; Guevara, N.; Bebear, J.P.; Ardoint, M.; Saaï, S.; Hoen, M.; Gnansia, D.; Romanet, P.; Lavieille, J.P. Clinical evaluation of the xDP output compression strategy for cochlear implants. *Eur. Arch. Otorhinolaryngol.* **2016**, *273*, 2363–2371. [CrossRef]
39. Dalla Bella, S.; Peretz, I.; Rousseau, L.; Gosselin, N. A developmental study of the affective value of tempo and mode in music. *Cognition* **2001**, *80*, B1–B10. [CrossRef]
40. Spitzer, E.R.; Landsberger, D.M.; Friedmann, D.R.; Galvin, J.J., 3rd. Pleasantness Ratings for Harmonic Intervals with Acoustic and Electric Hearing in Unilaterally Deaf Cochlear Implant Patients. *Front. Neurosci.* **2019**, *13*, 922. [CrossRef]
41. Di Lella, F.; Bacciu, A.; Pasanisi, E.; Vincenti, V.; Guida, M.; Bacciu, S. Main peak interleaved sampling (MPIS) strategy: Effect of stimulation rate variations on speech perception in adult cochlear implant recipients using the Digisonic SP cochlear implant. *Acta Otolaryngol.* **2010**, *130*, 102–107. [CrossRef] [PubMed]
42. Brockmeier, S.J.; Grasmeder, M.; Passow, S.; Mawmann, D.; Vischer, M.; Jappel, A.; Baumgartner, W.; Stark, T.; Müller, J.; Brill, S.; et al. Comparison of musical activities of cochlear implant users with different speech-coding strategies. *Ear Hear.* **2007**, *28*, 49S–51S. [CrossRef] [PubMed]
43. Bonett, D.G. Sample size requirements for testing and estimating coefficient alpha. *J. Educ. Behav. Stat.* **2002**, *27*, 335–340. [CrossRef]
44. Müllensiefen, D.; Gingras, B.; Musil, J.; Stewart, L. The Musicality of Non-Musicians: An Index for Assessing Musical Sophistication in the General Population. *PLoS ONE* **2014**, *9*, e89642. [CrossRef]
45. Kang, R.; Nimmons, G.L.; Drennan, W.; Longnion, J.; Ruffin, C.; Nie, K.; Won, J.H.; Worman, T.; Yueh, B.; Rubinstein, J. Development and validation of the University of Washington Clinical Assessment of Music Perception test. *Ear Hear.* **2009**, *30*, 411–418. [CrossRef]
46. Drennan, W.R.; Oleson, J.J.; Gfeller, K.; Crosson, J.; Driscoll, V.D.; Won, J.H.; Anderson, E.S.; Rubinstein, J.T. Clinical evaluation of music perception, appraisal and experience in cochlear implant users. *Int. J. Audiol.* **2015**, *54*, 114–123. [CrossRef]
47. Kohlberg, G.D.; Mancuso, D.M.; Chari, D.A.; Lalwani, A.K. Music Engineering as a Novel Strategy for Enhancing Music Enjoyment in the Cochlear Implant Recipient. *Behav. Neurol.* **2015**, *2015*, 829680. [CrossRef]
48. Hopyan, T.; Gordon, K.A.; Papsin, B.C. Identifying emotions in music through electrical hearing in deaf children using cochlear implants. *Cochlear Implants Int.* **2011**, *12*, 21–26. [CrossRef]
49. Hopyan, T.; Manno, F.A.M., 3rd; Papsin, B.C.; Gordon, K.A. Sad and happy emotion discrimination in music by children with cochlear implants. *Child Neuropsychol.* **2016**, *22*, 366–380. [CrossRef]
50. Levitin, D.J. What Does It Mean to Be Musical? *Neuron* **2012**, *73*, 633–637. [CrossRef]
51. Giannantonio, S.; Polonenko, M.J.; Papsin, B.C.; Paludetti, G.; Gordon, K.A. Experience Changes How Emotion in Music Is Judged: Evidence from Children Listening with Bilateral Cochlear Implants, Bimodal Devices, and Normal Hearing. *PLoS ONE* **2015**, *10*, e0136685. [CrossRef]
52. Bowling, D.L. A vocal basis for the affective character of musical mode in melody. *Front. Psychol.* **2013**, *4*, 464. [CrossRef]
53. Gfeller, K.; Lansing, C. Musical perception of cochlear implant users as measured by the Primary Measures of Music Audiation: An item analysis. *J. Music Ther.* **1992**, *29*, 18–39. [CrossRef]
54. Swanson, B.; Dawson, P.; McDermott, H. Investigating cochlear implant place-pitch perception with the Modified Melodies test. *Cochlear Implants Int.* **2009**, *10*, 100–104. [CrossRef]
55. Swanson, B.A.; Marimuthu, V.M.R.; Mannell, R.H. Place and Temporal Cues in Cochlear Implant Pitch and Melody Perception. *Front. Neurosci.* **2019**, *13*, 1266. [CrossRef]
56. Fu, Q.-J.; Nogaki, G. Noise susceptibility of cochlear implant users: The role of spectral resolution and smearing. *J. Assoc. Res. Otolaryngol.* **2005**, *6*, 19–27. [CrossRef]
57. Johnson-Laird, P.N.; Kang, O.E.; Leong, Y.C. On musical dissonance. *Music Percept.* **2012**, *30*, 19–35. [CrossRef]
58. Plomp, R.; Levelt, W.J. Tonal consonance and critical bandwidth. *J. Acoust. Soc. Am.* **1965**, *38*, 548–560. [CrossRef]
59. Cousineau, M.; McDermott, J.H.; Peretz, I. The basis of musical consonance as revealed by congenital amusia. *Proc. Natl. Acad. Sci. USA* **2012**, *109*, 19858–19863. [CrossRef]
60. Nemer, J.S.; Kohlberg, G.D.; Mancuso, D.M.; Griffin, B.M.; Certo, M.V.; Chen, S.Y.; Chun, M.B.; Spitzer, J.B.; Lalwani, A.K. Reduction of the Harmonic Series Influences Musical Enjoyment with Cochlear Implants. *Otol. Neurotol.* **2017**, *38*, 31–37. [CrossRef]
61. Bruns, L.; Mürbe, D.; Hahne, A. Understanding music with cochlear implants. *Sci. Rep.* **2016**, *6*, 32026. [CrossRef]
62. Vuust, P.; Witek, M.A. Rhythmic complexity and predictive coding: A novel approach to modeling rhythm and meter perception in music. *Front. Psychol.* **2014**, *5*, 1111. [CrossRef]
63. Huron, D. (Ed.) *Sweet Anticipation: Music and the Psychology of Expectation*; MIT Press: Cambridge, UK, 2006; p. 462.
64. Matthews, T.E.; Witek, M.A.G.; Heggli, O.A.; Penhune, V.B.; Vuust, P. The sensation of groove is affected by the interaction of rhythmic and harmonic complexity. *PLoS ONE* **2019**, *14*, e0204539. [CrossRef]
65. Gfeller, K.; Christ, A.; Knutson, J.; Witt, S.; Mehr, M. The effects of familiarity and complexity on appraisal of complex songs by cochlear implant recipients and normal hearing adults. *J. Music Ther.* **2003**, *40*, 78–112. [CrossRef]
66. Holden, L.K.; Finley, C.C.; Firszt, J.B.; Holden, T.A.; Brenner, C.; Potts, L.G.; Gotter, B.D.; Vanderhoof, S.S.; Mispagel, K.; Heydebrand, G.; et al. Factors affecting open-set word recognition in adults with Cochlear Implants. *Ear Hear.* **2013**, *34*, 342–360. [CrossRef]

67. Frederigue-Lopes, N.B.; Bevilacqua, M.C.; Costa, O.A. Munich Music Questionnaire: Adaptation into Brazilian Portuguese and application in cochlear implant users. *Codas* **2015**, *27*, 13–20. [CrossRef]
68. Zhou, Q.; Gu, X.; Liu, B. The music quality feeling and music perception of adult cochlear implant recipients. *Lin Chung Er Bi Yan Hou Tou Jing Wai Ke Za Zhi* **2019**, *33*, 47–51.
69. Falcón-González, J.C.; Borkoski-Barreiro, S.; Limiñana-Cañal, J.M.; Ramos-Macías, A. Recognition of music and melody in patients with cochlear implants, using a new programming approach for frequency assignment. *Acta Otorrinolaringol. Esp.* **2014**, *65*, 289–296. [CrossRef] [PubMed]
70. Belfi, A.M.; Kasdan, A.; Rowland, J.; Vessel, E.A.; Starr, G.G.; Poeppel, D. Rapid Timing of Musical Aesthetic Judgments. *J. Exp. Psychol. Gen.* **2018**, *147*, 1531–1543. [CrossRef] [PubMed]
71. Goehring, T.; Chapman, J.L.; Bleeck, S.; Monaghan, J.J.M. Tolerable delay for speech production and perception: Effects of hearing ability and experience with hearing aids. *Int. J. Audiol.* **2018**, *57*, 61–68. [CrossRef] [PubMed]

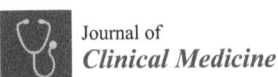

Article

Cochlear Implantation in Obliterated Cochlea: A Retrospective Analysis and Comparison between the IES Stiff Custom-Made Device and the Split-Array and Regular Electrodes

Julia Anna Christine Hoffmann [1,†], Athanasia Warnecke [1,2,†], Max Eike Timm [1,2], Eugen Kludt [1,2], Nils Kristian Prenzler [1,2], Lutz Gärtner [1,2], Thomas Lenarz [1,2] and Rolf Benedikt Salcher [1,2,*]

1. Department of Otorhinolaryngology, Head and Neck Surgery, Hannover Medial School, 30625 Hannover, Germany
2. Cluster of Excellence "Hearing4all", Hannover Medical School, 30625 Hannover, Germany
* Correspondence: salcher.rolf@mh-hannover.de
† These authors contributed equally to this work.

Abstract: Anatomical malformations, obliterations of the cochlea, or re-implantations pose particular challenges in cochlear implantation. Treatment methods rely on radiological and intraoperative findings and include incomplete insertion, the implantation of a double array, and radical cochleostomy. In addition, a stiff electrode array, e.g., the IE stiff (IES) custom-made device (CMD, MED-EL), was prescribed individually for those special cases and pre-inserted prior to facilitate cochlear implantation in challenging cases. Data on outcomes after implantation in obliterated cochleae are usually based on individual case reports since standardised procedures are lacking. A retrospective analysis was conducted to analyse our cases on obliterated cochleae treated with MED-EL devices in order to allow the different cases to be compared. Impedances and speech perception data of patients treated with the IES CMD and the double array were retrospectively compared to patients treated with a STANDARD or FLEX electrode array (the REGULAR group). Patients with a Split-Array CMD had a poor speech perception when compared to patients treated with the IES CMD device. Thus, the IES CMD can successfully be used in patients with obliterated cochleae who would otherwise be non-users, candidates for a Split-Array CMD, or candidates for partial insertion with insufficient cochlear coverage.

Keywords: inner ear; cochlear implant; obliteration of the inner ear; ossification; fibrous tissue growth; electrode impedance; insertion probe

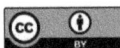

1. Introduction

Hearing loss and deafness are associated with severe consequences for the affected patients, such as insufficient speech development, anxiety, depression, as well as lower educational and career opportunities due to social isolation [1,2] and an increased risk for the development of dementia [3]. Thus, the early diagnosis and treatment of hearing loss has a high socio-economical value.

Patients with severe sensorineural hearing loss are treated with a cochlear implant (CI) [4]. The surgical technique and the insertion technique are largely standardised, and regular CI electrodes can be inserted in the majority of cases. Special cases, however, such as the implantation of patients with anatomical malformations, obliterations of the cochlea, or re-implantations pose a challenge in cochlear implantation and may require special devices. Obliteration of the cochlea, for example, occurs after meningitis, trauma, or infection which result in hearing loss and subsequent intracochlear tissue growth, such as connective tissue or bone formation. When the cochlea is obliterated or ossified to a particularly significant degree, the conventional insertion of the mechanically flexible electrode array may be impossible [5], and alternative surgical techniques, such as incomplete insertion, the implantation of double arrays [6], implantation into the scala vestibuli [7,8], or a radical cochleostomy, must be considered. All these methods are associated with some disadvantages, such as the poor performance of the implant. However, despite a significantly higher risk for injuring the facial nerve, the internal carotid artery, or the modiolus [9], such alternative procedures are recommended in cases of partial and complete ossification.

To enable insertion even in cases with abnormal cochlear anatomies, special electrode arrays have been developed. MED-EL (Innsbruck, Austria), for example, created a compressed array as well as a Split-Array CMD for special requirements. The compressed array features 12 pairs of electrodes with an active stimulation range (ASR) of 12.1 mm (standard array ASR 31 mm), allowing the array to be placed in close proximity to the neurons, especially in malformed or partially ossified cochleae [10]. The split electrode array (MED-EL) with a double-branch electrode array was designed for the severe ossification of the cochlea. It contains five and seven electrode pairs on separated arrays on an ASR of 4.4 and 6.6 mm, respectively, which can be inserted through two cochleostomies (one in the basal and the second in the medial part of the cochlea) to increase the number of completely inserted electrode contacts in the ossified cochlea. Nevertheless, it can be shown that the speech performance of patients treated with this type of electrode is in the lower range of the spectrum that can be achieved by patients with a regular cochlear anatomy implanted with MED-EL's STANDARD and FLEX electrodes [10,11].

Since August 2015, some of those challenging cases were also treated with a custom-made device (CMD, MED-EL) in our clinic. The CMD comprises a stiff insertion electrode (insertion electrode stiff, IES) and was prescribed in individual cases when the patients received a flexible lateral wall electrode array and there is an obstruction of the scala tympani (e.g., due to fibrosis or ossification). In such cases, the device is inserted prior to electrode insertion to dilate the cochlear lumen. This retrospective analysis evaluates speech performance data and impedance values as well as postoperative symptoms of patients treated with the IES CMD and compares them to the current available treatment options, a Split-Array CMD or a normal insertion.

2. Materials and Methods

2.1. Patients

A retrospective analysis of all patients treated between August 2015 and March 2019 with a MED-EL device revealed 33 patient ears which were treated with lateral wall CI electrodes using the IES CMD prior to electrode insertion (the IES group). Demographic and clinical data, impedance values, hearing results, and speech performance results of the patients were collected retrospectively. We also retrospectively identified patients treated with the STANDARD or FLEX electrode arrays to be included in our analysis as part of a comparative control group (the REGULAR group). The REGULAR group consisted of patients selected to match the patient's age (± 5 years), the patient's gender, the electrode carrier, and the type of implantation (first implantation or re-implantation) of the IES group. As an additional control, we identified and included patients treated with a Split-Array CMD (the SPLIT group). In these patients, implantation with regular electrode arrays was impossible. Due to the special electrode carrier, there were no suitable match patients for the SPLIT group to form a comparative collective.

2.2. Study Design

Based on the retrospective design of the study, ethical board approval was not required. The data for the present analysis were extracted from our cochlear implantation database. This database was established to routinely collect all clinical, audiological, radiological, and surgical data of the patients. We retrospectively identified patients, in whom either a IES CMD or a Aplit-Array CMD was used for cochlear implantation. In addition to the data obtained from the database, we also collected data retrospectively from the patients' surgical reports to determine the indication criteria used to determine the electrode type in individual cases. After identifying these patients, measurement protocols for impedances and hearing tests were evaluated, as well as clinical data collected from patient records to ensure a comprehensive evaluation. The REGULAR group served as a control group and included routinely treated patients without any cochlear abnormalities, as radiologically and intraoperatively determined.

2.3. The Fibrotic Obliteration Probe

The IE stiff CMD (IES, MED-EL, Innsbruck, Austria) (Figure 1) is a custom-made device which can be used individually when fibrotic tissue is present in the inner ear. It is used for the dilation of the cochlear lumen prior to electrode insertion. Thus, the IES consisted of an electrode dummy, which was used prior to electrode insertion as a surgical tool with no electrical function. The outer geometry was the same as the distal 50 mm of MED-EL's STANDARD electrode, with a diameter of 1.3 mm at the proximal end and 0.5 mm at the distal end of the array (Figure 1a,b). It was made of medical-grade silicone with multiple stiff metal wires incorporated into its matrix. The markings on the IES CMD array at 20, 24, and 28 mm indicate the possible insertion depths (Figure 1b).

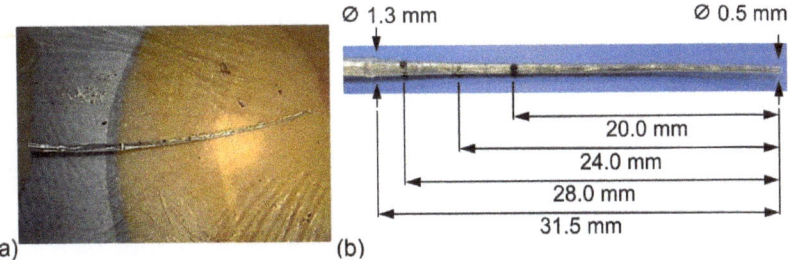

Figure 1. Dimensions of the IE stiff CMD. (**a**) Intraoperative; (**b**) markings on the IES CMD array. The IES CMD has a maximal insertion length of 31.5 mm.

2.4. The Surgical Procedure

Electrode insertion via the round window is the preferred approach in cochlear implantation. After opening the round window for insertion, the IES CMD was carefully inserted into the inner ear for the dilatation of obstructed scala tympani or for depth measurement prior to the actual insertion of the electrode array in the IES group. In any case, the electrode array was inserted slowly into the scala tympani up to the previously defined insertion depth. The insertion site was sealed with muscle fascia from the temporal muscle after electrode placement. The array was usually fixed in a 1 mm bony notch drilled in the chorda facial angle. At the end of the surgical intervention, cone beam computed tomography (CB-CT) was performed to assess the intracochlear position of the electrode array.

In cases of ossification of the round window region or of ossification commencing at the basal turn, cochleostomy was performed in order to insert the electrode array. Therefore, the opening of the membrane was extended in an antero-inferior direction with a bur.

In order to supply the severe ossification patients with a split electrode array, superior cochleostomy at the level of the second turn was performed for the full insertion of the apical array (the SPLIT group).

2.5. Impedance Measurement

The impedance values were measured with the MED-EL telemetry system (MAX interface box, clinical software Maestro), enabling an impedance field telemetry (IFT) on all 12 electrode contacts. The used stimuli were biphasic pulses (24.2 µs) with a nominal amplitude of 300 current units (cu), where 1 cu approximates 1 µA [12]. The measurements were carried out at defined points after surgery as follows. The first measurement was taken during surgery (intraoperatively, after electrode insertion). The second measurement was taken at the end of the first fitting (FF), usually 4–10 weeks after surgery, or sometimes longer in rare exceptional cases due to previous complications. The following measurements were performed 3, 6, and 12 months (±4 weeks) after the FF. Until the FF, the implant was not activated since there was no audio processor worn by the patient, meaning that there was no electrical stimulation. After the first fitting, the implant was activated and the cochlea was electrically stimulated on a daily basis.

2.6. Statistical Analysis

For the statistical analysis, the impedance values of all 12 electrode contacts of a patient were averaged at one time point to obtain a mean value. The one-way ANOVA and post-hoc Tukey HSD multiple-comparison tests were used to compare the means and calculate the p values using IBM SPSS Statistics 26.0. Differences were considered statistically significant for p values < 0.05. All data were visualized using GraphPad Prism Version 8.3.0 and Microsoft Excel.

2.7. Hearing Tests

In order to evaluate speech understanding after cochlear implantation, the Freiburg monosyllabic speech test (FMB) and the Hochmair–Desoyer–Schulz–Moser (HSM) sentence tests [13], both in quiet and in noise at 0° azimuth (S0N0) and at a 10 dB signal-to-noise ratio (SNR), were performed in our clinical routine and evaluated retrospectively. All speech tests were conducted in the free field or were directly coupled with sentences and monosyllables presented at 65 dB SPL [14]. The measurements were carried out at the same time points as the impedance measurements.

2.8. Clinical Data

Clinical data were collected from the patients' medical history and routine measurements retrospectively. For example, prior to and after implantation, patients were asked whether they suffered from vertigo, tinnitus, and facial stimulation.

2.9. Ethical Statement

This research is based on data collected from a retrospective analysis. Upon admission, all patients or their legal representatives signed an informed consent with regards to the anonymized use of their data for research purposes.

3. Results

3.1. Patients

Patients who underwent implantation with a MED-EL cochlear implant and who used the IES CMD prior to the insertion of the electrode array were included in the IES-group. Patients with different types of electrodes were included: FLEX 16 CMD ($n = 1$), FLEX 20 ($n = 3$), FLEX 24 ($n = 3$), FLEX 28 ($n = 21$), and STANDARD ($n = 5$).

Of these patients, twenty-seven were treated unilaterally and three were implanted bilaterally. In the following, each implanted ear is considered individually, yielding a dataset of 33 ears with nearly equal sex distribution (17 male and 16 female). Of the implantations, 20 (60.6%) were performed on the right side and 13 (39.4%) on the left side. At the time of implantation, the mean age was 37.6 years (range: 10 months–80 years).

The SPLIT group consisted of eight patients (five male and three female; mean age at the time of implantation 38.5 years; range: 1–74 years) who were implanted with a Split-Array CMD. In this group, the IES CMD was not used or its application was unsuccessful in the previous intervention ($n = 3$).

Both groups, the IES group and the SPLIT group, consisted of diverse and partly multimorbid patients. Table 1 provides an overview of the relevant comorbidities of the subjects as listed in their medical records.

Table 1. A summary of the occurrence of relevant concomitant diseases in subjects of the IES, SPLIT, and REGULAR groups.

relevant comorbidities; n (%)	IES Group n = 33	SPLIT Group n = 8	REGULAR Group n = 32
hypertension	10 (30.3)	4 (50.0)	8 (25.0)
meningitis	7 (21.2)	5 (62.5)	0 (0)
syndromes, genetic malformations	5 (15.2)	0 (0)	5 (15.6)
tumor in the head area	3 (9.1)	0 (0)	0 (0)
cardiac arrhythmia	2 (6.1)	2 (25.0)	1 (3.1)
diabetes mellitus (type I)	0 (0)	0 (0)	1 (3.1)
diabetes mellitus (type II)	2 (6.1)	2 (25.0)	4 (12.5)
coagulopathy	2 (6.1)	1 (12.5)	1 (3.1)
pulmonary diseases	2 (6.1)	3 (37.5)	4 (12.5)
epilepsy	1 (3.0)	1 (12.5)	0 (0)
apoplexy	1 (3.0)	1 (12.5)	1 (3.1)
hyperlipoproteinemia	1 (3.0)	0 (0)	1 (3.1)
osteoporosis	1 (3.0)	0 (0)	0 (0)
craniocerebral injury, fracture of temporal bone	1 (3.0)	2 (25.0)	1 (3.1)
facial nerve paresis	1 (3.0)	0 (0)	0 (0)
depression	1 (3.0)	2 (25.0)	1 (3.1)
sepsis	0 (0)	1 (12.5)	0 (0)

For better comparability with various CI patients, for whom no IES CMD application was necessary or indicated, the REGULAR group was included. The REGULAR group consisted of patients who were age- (± 5 years) and gender-matched (17 male and 15 female) to the subjects of the IES group. For the implanted patients of this group, the distribution of electrode variants was identical to the IES group. Only the implantation with a Flex 16 electrode array was excluded from the REGULAR group as no suitable comparison case was identified. This resulted in a dataset of 32 subjects for the REGULAR group. Table 1 shows the concomitant diseases of the REGULAR group to provide a complete survey.

3.2. Aetiology of Deafness

Regarding the aetiology of deafness in the IES group, seven patients (21.2%) suffered from meningitis, eight (24.2%) suffered from anatomical malformations in the inner ear, five (15.2%) suffered from other congenital hearing impairment, two (6.1%) suffered from sudden hearing loss, one (3.0%) suffered from trauma of the temporal bone, one (3.0%) suffered from otosclerosis, and the aetiology was unknown or not documented in nine other patients (27.3%).

In the SPLIT group, four patients (50%) suffered from meningitis, two (25%) suffered from trauma of the temporal bone, one (12.5%) suffered from sepsis due to pneumonia, and the cause was unknown or not documented for one other patient (12.5%).

3.3. Indication of the IES CMD

The IES CMD was used in our clinic for different indications. The possible applications included the penetration into a cochlea obstructed with fibrotic or ossified tissue, which could not be achieved by common electrodes due to their lack of stiffness and their inability to dilate the lumen. It was also used as an aid in re-implantations. Furthermore, the IES CMD was utilised as an instrument to estimate the depth of possible electrode insertion in the malformed cochleae.

Thus, the IES was deployed in the evaluated IES group to measure the depth of the cochlea prior to implantation ($n = 7$; 21.2%), due to intracochlear tissue which hampered the insertion of the electrode array ($n = 10$; 30.3%), as well as to ossify the basal turn or the round window region ($n = 9$; 27.3%). The IES was also used four times (12.1%) as a tool during device re-implantation to clear out fibrotic tissue. In three cases (9.1%), the reason for using the IES was to eliminate any resistance that occurred when trying to insert the stimulation electrode.

In the evaluation above, a variable was disregarded, depending on whether the surgical intervention was a first implantation or a re-implantation of a CI. In the IES group, 22 subjects (66.7%) underwent first implantation with an average duration of hearing loss of 8.57 years (range: 1 month–31 years). Eleven cases (33.3%) underwent re-implantation surgery due to soft failure or malfunction of the implant. The previous implant was in situ for a mean of 9.82 years (range: 6 month–31 years).

In the REGULAR group, patients were matched to the IES group (n = 22 first implantations and n = 11 re-implantations). An exact adjustment to the duration of hearing loss or the duration of the previous implant in situ was not possible due to the limited number of patients available.

In the SPLIT group, six cases (75%) were provided with a Split-Array CMD during the initial implantation procedure and showed an average duration of deafness of 5.04 years (range: 6 month–24 years). Two cases (25%) received a Split-Array CMD during a re-implantation procedure after 25 years in the first case and after 1 year in the second case.

3.4. Impedances

The course of impedances over time is depicted in Figure 2. Here, the median values of the overall impedances of all electrode contacts of the IES and SPLIT groups were plotted and compared to those of the REGULAR group (Figure 2). The median values were almost equal between the three groups immediately after the insertion at the intraoperative measurement. Thereafter, an increase in the impedance values up to the first fitting (FF; 4–6 weeks after implantation) was observed in all groups, but at slightly different levels. In the IES group, impedances continued to rise with a slight linear increase up to 12 months after the FF, while in the REGULAR group, a slight decrease was observed and finally constant impedance values were measured at a much lower level than the IES group. The values of the SPLIT group stayed relatively stable on all contacts up to 3 months. Thereafter, a strong increase in impedance values up to 12 months was observed that went far beyond the measured values of the IES group. Statistically significant differences could be observed at the FF between the IES and REGULAR groups ($p < 0.05$) and at M6 between the IES/CONTROL group ($p < 0.01$) and the IES-/SPLIT group ($p < 0.05$). At M12, all three groups showed a significant difference to each other (IES/REGULAR, $p < 0.001$; IES/SPLIT, $p < 0.05$; SPLIT/REGULAR, $p < 0.001$).

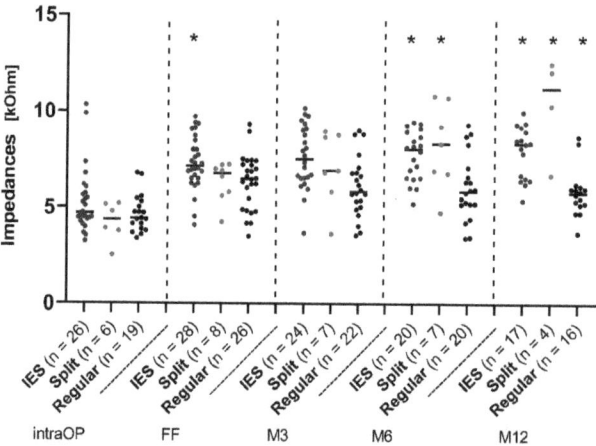

Figure 2. Change in impedances over time across the IES, SPLIT, and REGULAR groups. Median overall electrode contacts C1–C12. Since the number of patients varied over time, the existing patients were additionally marked as individual dots at each point in time. The red dots represent the IES patients, the blue dots represent the patients from the SPLIT group, and the black dots represent the patients from the REGULAR group. Asterisks mark the significant differences between groups.

3.4.1. Impedances at Different Indications of IES Use in the IES Group

In order to examine the diverse IES group in more detail, a retrospective subdivision into four subgroups, based on the indications for which the IES CMD was prescribed in the implanted ears and thus on the aetiology of the patients' deafness, was performed. Figure 3 shows the impedance data over time of the subgroup, where the IES CMD was applied due to an existing ossification in the inner ear (magenta dots, the O group, Figure 3), as well as the subgroup with IES CMD application due to fibrosis in the inner ear (red dots, the F group, Figure 3). The third subgroup indicates that IES CMD use after a resistance occurred during the actual implantation of the stimulation electrode (purple dots, the R group, Figure 3). In the fourth subgroup, the IES was used to determine the depth of the cochlea (light blue dots, the DM group, Figure 3). To facilitate a constant comparison, the REGULAR group was also depicted here with impedance data over time (black dots, Figure 3).

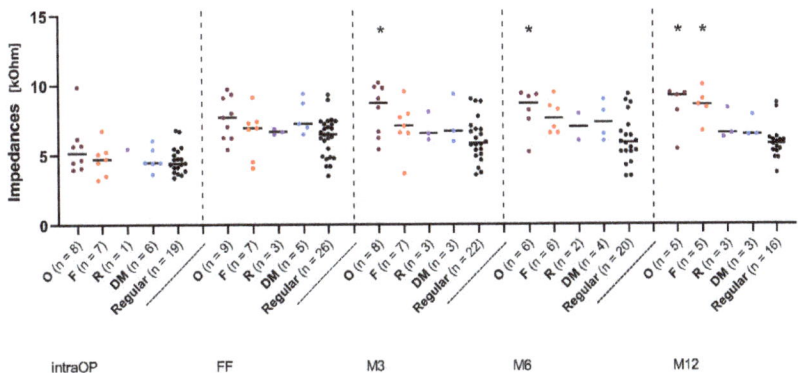

Figure 3. Change in impedances over time in subjects with different indications of IES use. Median overall electrode contacts C1–C12. The magenta dots represent patients with cochlear ossification (O), the red dots represent patients with fibrosis (F), the purple dots represent patients with occurring resistance (R), and the light blue dots represent patients for which the IES was used for cochlear depth measurement (DM). The black dots represent patients from the REGULAR group. Asterisks mark significant differences between groups.

Figure 3 shows the median impedance values over time over all electrode contacts. From the FF onwards, there was a slight drop in the impedance values and finally a constant lower level in the REGULAR group, while all other groups continued to show slight impedance increases. The O group showed the highest values over the whole time, followed by the F group. The R and DM groups, on the contrary, were at almost the same median level, but showed slightly higher values than the REGULAR group. From month 3 (M3) onwards, there was a statistically significant difference between the O group and the REGULAR group ($p < 0.05$). After 12 months, the F group also showed significantly higher impedance values than the REGULAR group ($p < 0.01$). All other groups showed no significant differences at any time.

3.4.2. Impedances Re-Implantation vs. First Implantation

In order to evaluate whether the re-implantation procedure and the usage of the IES CMD has an influence on impedance development, we distinguished between the cases of first implantation and the cases of re-implantation in both the IES group and the REGULAR group, as follows:

1. Re-implantation in the REGULAR group (RR): consists of 10 patients who received a re-implantation without using the IES;

2. Re-implantation in the IES group (RI): consists of 11 patients who were re-implanted using the IES;
3. First implantation in the IES group (FI): consists of 22 patients who were implanted for the first time using the IES;
4. First implantation in the REGULAR group (FR): consists of 22 patients who were implanted for the first time without the IES.

The course of median values over all electrode contacts over time is presented in Figure 4. Up to the FF, there was a similar increase in impedance values in all groups. In the further course, the median values of the RR, RI, and FI groups increased, while a decrease in the impedances could be observed in the FR group. Statistically significant differences between the FR and FI groups ($p < 0.05$), FR and RI groups ($p < 0.01$), and FR and RR groups ($p < 0.05$) could also be observed, which remained until month 6 (M6). After 12 months, there was no longer any significant difference between the FR and RR groups.

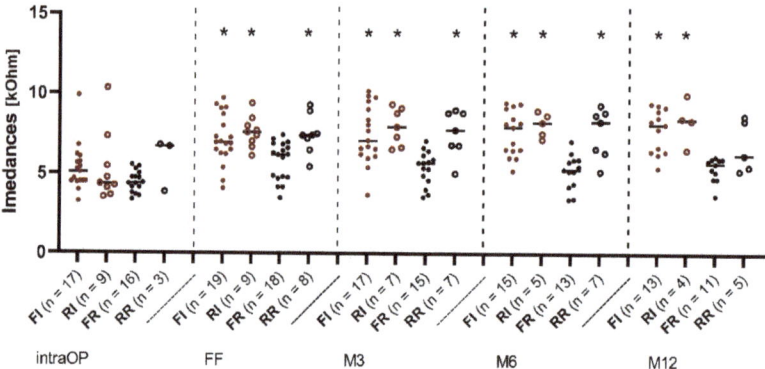

Figure 4. Change in impedances over time re-implantation vs. first implantation in the IES and REGULAR groups. Median over all electrode contacts C1–C12. The filled red dots represent the patients from the IES group who received first implantation (FI) and the hollow red dots represent the patients from the IES group who underwent re-implantation (RI). The filled black dots represent the patients with first implantation from the REGULAR group (FR) and the hollow black dots represent the patients who underwent re-implantation from the REGULAR group (RR). Asterisks mark significant differences between groups.

3.5. Speech Comprehension

Due to the retrospective analysis and the resulting limited availability of datasets, both patients whose speech tests were conducted in the free field as well as in direct coupling were included in the following speech data evaluation.

To avoid bilateral benefits, based on the results of the audiogram, an additional measurement in direct coupling was carried out if it was suspected that the non-test ear was influenced. Therefore, it can be assumed that the influence of the non-test ear was selected entirely from the speech results (Figure 5).

For the SPLIT group, only a few datasets were available since not every patient could complete each of the tests. As a consequence, the number of subjects varied between tests at measurement point after 6 months (M6). Furthermore, the results of a bilaterally implanted child in the SPLIT group were excluded from an evaluation of the speech data, as speech development was not possible due to child's age. The exclusion allowed an unbiased trend of hearing performance in patients implanted with a split-array CMD.

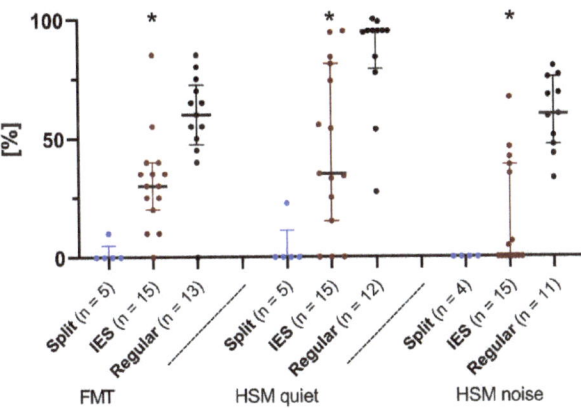

Figure 5. The Freiburg monosyllabic word test (FMT), and the HSM sentence test in quiet and in noise. Median scores (in % correct) after 6 months of device use. Comparing patients from the IES group (red dots), the REGULAR group (black dots), and the SPLIT group (blue dots). Asterisks mark significant differences between groups.

After 6 months of device use, for FMT, the subjects belonging to the IES group scored a median of 30%. The median was 60% after 6 months in the REGULAR group and 0% in the SPLIT group. There were significant differences between the IES and REGULAR groups (IES/REGULAR $p < 0.01$). Due to the small size of the test group, no statistical evaluation of the SPLIT group was carried out.

For the HSM test in quiet, the subjects of the IES group scored a median of 34.9% after 6 months of device use. In comparison, the median values of the REGULAR group were 95% after 6 months and 0% after 6 months in the SPLIT group. An intergroup comparison between the IES and REGULAR groups showed a significant difference in the results of the HSM test in quiet ($p < 0.01$).

For the HSM test in noise, patients of the IES and SPLIT groups achieved median values of 0% after 6 months of device use, as opposed to the REGULAR group (63.49%; $p < 0.001$).

3.6. Clinical Data

The clinical data presented here are based on a retrospective analysis of the patients' medical history before and after cochlear implantation. The numbers of patients suffering from tinnitus, vertigo, or facial stimulation at the respective times are shown in Table 2. Furthermore, seven patients in the IES group and two patients in the SPLIT group suffered from meningitis before surgery. None of the patients in the REGULAR group had a pre-existing meningitis in their medical history. After surgery, there was no evidence of postoperative meningitis in all three groups.

In order to alleviate facial stimulation in affected patients, triphasic pulses were utilized in four of the affected cases (Table 2), but were only temporarily sufficient for one of the cases. In the three remaining patients, individual electrode contacts had to be switched off and the stimulation level was lowered below the facial nerve stimulation (FNS) threshold in order to remedy the symptoms. The remaining two cases were not further documented because one patient was lost for follow-up (patient in the SPLIT group) or the other patient was currently no longer fitted with a CI (patient in the IES group).

Table 2. Clinical data.

Clinical Data; n^1 (%)	SPLIT Group	IES Group	REGULAR Group
vertigo			
preoperative	1 (12.5)	8 (24.2)	7 (25.0)
postoperative	1 (12.5)	7 (24.1)	4 (14.3)
tinnitus			
preoperative	5 (62.5)	12 (36.4)	9 (32.1)
postoperative	4 (50.0)	4 (13.8)	6 (21.4)
facial stimulation			
preoperative	0 (0.0)	2 (6.1)	0 (0.0)
postoperative	2 (25.0)	4 (13.8)	2 (7.1)
after triphasic pulses	2 (25.0)	1 (3.4)	1 (3.6)

[1] $n = 8$ patients were evaluated in the SPLIT group; $n = 28$ patients were evaluated in the REGULAR group; and $n = 33$ and $n = 29$ patients were preoperatively and postoperatively evaluated in the IES group, respectively.

4. Discussion

To our knowledge, this was the first comparative yet retrospective analysis to show that the IES CMD can facilitate the implantation of flexible lateral wall CI electrodes in patients with fibrotic, ossified, and malformed cochleae. Moreover, we showed that individual treatment with the IES CMD allowed a regular electrode array to be implanted without significantly impairing the performance of the patients.

Specifically, intraoperative impedance values of all three test groups were equally high and a presumed increase from insertion up to the FF was also evident in all three groups (Figure 2). At the timepoint M12, it can be stated that the median values of impedances of the IES and SPLIT groups were significantly higher than the median value of the REGULAR group. However, in relation to this, the median value of the SPLIT group was also significantly higher than the median value of the IES group.

In the REGULAR group, no significant increase in the median impedance values over time can be observed. Thus, based on the impedance values, an increased trauma due to the electrode insertion seemed unlikely here [15–17]. In contrast, there was an increase in impedances over time in the IES and SPLIT groups. A correlation between the level of fibrotic material and the impedance levels was found in preclinical cochlear implant models consisting of guinea pigs [18]. It could be possible that increased tissue formation due to insertion trauma may account for the increased impedance values observed in the IES and SPLIT patients. The increase in the IES group could be due to an increased amount of fibrous tissue growth around the electrode. However, it must be critically questioned whether this deviation, especially in comparison to the REGULAR group, is solely due to the use of the IES during surgery and the additional microtraumas that may have arisen. Patients in the IES group, unlike patients in the REGULAR group, already had increased cochlear damage (fibrosis, ossification, and malformation) before implantation and this damage may also explain the different impedance values. Another hypothesis therefore could be that the initial fibrotic tissue formation prior to implantation continues afterwards and leads to higher impedances. Furthermore, increased surgical trauma, such as cochlear drilling, as performed in some patients, could also trigger inflammation reaction with new tissue formation accounting for the increase in impedances [19]. In addition, it has not been evaluated whether other traumatic events, such as scalar shift, occurred after implantation, and whether they influenced the data. However, no scalar shift was described in the regular radiological evaluations of the postoperative CT images.

Further typical changes in electrode impedances occurred with the onset of electrical stimulation. It has been reported that the impedances of intracochlear electrodes are lower after stimulation compared to the levels before stimulation onset [20,21]. After implantation, a cell [22] and passivation [23] layer accumulated on the electrode surface of inactive electrode contacts. This layer was disrupted by the onset of electrical stimulation and resulted in a decrease in impedances, as clinically observed. Within 3 months after starting the electrical stimulation (after the FF), a decrease in impedances in all three groups, i.e., the IES group, the SPLIT group, and the REGULAR group, was observed in the present study. This decrease might corroborate studies showing that chronical electrical stimulation may lower electrode impedances [24–26].

As a result, it must be questioned whether patients in the SPLIT and IES groups have a shorter or more irregular wearing time of the implant processor to M12 and thus a non-regular electrical stimulation, thus contributing to an increase in impedances. However, this parameter was not recorded in our study.

Significantly increased impedance values 12 months after the FF were demonstrated in the groups with pre-damage of the cochlea (O and F groups) when compared to the REGULAR group (Figure 3). Pre-damage of the inner ear might have a significant influence on the further development of the electrode environment after implantation, leading to increased impedance values. No significant difference was found between patients who used the IES as a depth probe (the DM group) and patients in the REGULAR group, indicating that the IES is rather less traumatic when used in non-pre-damaged ears.

This assumption is contradicted by impedance values measured 12 months after implantation (M12), as depicted in Figure 4. While the impedances between all groups were still intraoperatively equal, the impedances of the IES group (FI and RI) were significantly increased from the FF onwards, as well as the values of the RR group. At M12, the values of the RR group dropped again. It is therefore assumed that without the use of the IES, the impedances will return to lower values over time. Thus, the IES could account for higher impedance values over time and should not be routinely used as a depth sensor, as the electrode environment appears to recover better without the use of the IES.

When interpreting the results, the usefulness of impedance values needs careful consideration. It is well accepted that electrode impedances may be a useful biomarker of inner ear pathology after cochlear implantation [27] and low impedances are desirable to minimize battery consumption. As such, impedances represent a non-invasive measuring method for obtaining information about the environment between electrodes and the respective neural interfaces [28]. It is believed that changes in the electrode impedances are related to the formation of a fibrous tissue matrix around the electrode array [18,22,29,30]. Foreign body immune responses may help to encapsulate the electrode array in fibrous tissue within the first few weeks of implantation [20,31]. Clinical studies on patients treated with cochlear implants show that, in the days and weeks following implantation, electrode impedances increase, forming a plateau after 4–6 weeks in situ [22,32].

Foggia et al. describes an inflammatory or fibrotic reaction as a response to the electrode array in the cochlea that occurs with every implantation [20]. Both the acute tissue response immediately after implantation (due to the insertion trauma) and the delayed response as a host-mediated foreign body response caused by nearly all biomaterials may help to explain the observed increase in impedance values [20]. Interestingly, a recent study has shown that impedances values do not correlate with speech understanding [33]. Considering the results of speech comprehension of the different groups 6 months after implantation, the patients of the REGULAR group achieved fairly good speech performance. The results obtained are consistent with those taken from other studies [34]. For the SPLIT group, poor results for speech perception were observed in our study, as corroborated by other studies [10]. Degeneration in spiral ganglion cells is particularly high in patients whose cause of deafness is bacterial meningitis [35]. Since many patients in the IES group had preoperative meningitis in their medical history, it can be assumed that a reduced number of spiral ganglion cells is one of the reasons for lower speech comprehension scores between the IES group and the REGULAR group. Therefore, as an important observation based on our results, it can be concluded that patients with implantation of a long lateral wall electrode using the IES CMD prior to insertion experience significant benefits in terms of speech understanding, as compared to those who were fitted with a Split-Array CMD (Figure 5). However, the case of a child implanted bilaterally with split arrays, which was excluded from our speech comprehension data, also shows that a long-term evaluation is indispensable in order to be able to make further statements. The child did not show any measurable scores at time M6 of the speech comprehension data evaluation as the tests were not age-appropriate; however, measurable speech understanding has developed in the meantime. To conclude, if conditions permit, normal implantation with the aid of the IES CMD should be favoured over the implantation of a Split-Array CMD. Speech recognition after cochlear implantation is further dependent on the degree of spiral ganglion cell preservation.

Since there are other stiff electrodes available for cochlear implantation, questions surrounding the use of delicate electrodes, such as the FLEX series from MED-EL, arise since the recipients presented with an obliteration of the cochlea with no residual hearing. The FLEX electrode array series includes atraumatic devices with variably sized lengths up to 28 mm. As such, this series allows the length of the electrode array to be correlated with the size of the patient's cochlea, thus adapting to variations in cochlear geometry. An advantage of flexible electrode arrays is the avoidance of pronounced trauma to the cochlea during electrode insertion. Since patients in the IES group have previous damage up to the anatomically complete obstruction of the cochlea, there is no residual hearing worth protecting. Thus, the use of flexible electrodes does not seem beneficial from this point of view. However, several studies, such as those by Buchmann et al. [36] or Büchner et al. [34], have shown that speech understanding after implantation significantly depends on the insertion depth of the electrode and that the insertion of longer electrodes allows better speech perception. With this in mind, the electrodes used represent a promising means of achieving better speech understanding in affected patients, not due to their flexibility, but because of their potential increased cochlear coverage. Moreover, the various malformations in the IES group that we evaluated are cases in which the insertion length can often only be determined intraoperatively. The ability to adjust the insertion length accordingly is essential.

Meningitis may occur more frequently in patients implanted with a CI either due to local infections or as a result of the actual surgical intervention. Other risk factors such as congenital or acquired anatomical defects, previous meningitis, or immunodeficiencies are described [37]. In the IES group, no postoperative meningitis occurred at the time of evaluation, although many of the risk factors apply to the evaluated group (Table 1). Furthermore, the IES CMD does not appear to increase the risk for meningitis. Vertigo and vestibular dysfunction may occur postoperatively after cochlear implantation [38]. Patients of the IES group already showed symptoms of this category preoperatively, and the number of affected patients slightly decreased postoperatively (Table 2). Here, it must be considered that the pre- and postoperatively affected patients do not necessarily correlate with one another. However, it seems that the use of the IES CMD does not result in a strongly increased trauma risk, since clinical symptoms and adverse events are to be regarded as indicators. Postoperative facial stimulation is observed in patients of all three groups. In the REGULAR and IES groups, facial stimulation could be controlled and improved by the use of triphasic pulses, while no change occurred in the SPLIT group (Table 2).

There are several limitations associated with the present study. First of all, the small number of patients included in this study limits the conclusions that can be drawn from the data. Additionally, the inhomogeneous patients, especially in the IES group, make it difficult to compare the data to the other study groups. Despite these limitations, we were able to demonstrate significant differences between groups and we could derive some important observations from our data.

5. Conclusions

In summary, this study shows that the IES CMD can successfully treat patients who would otherwise be non-users or would only be able to receive a split-array CMD or an insufficient number of inserted electrode contacts. The IES CMD offers a method to insert long flexible lateral-wall electrodes into the cochlea with a concomitant low risk of clinical complications.

The above evaluation also shows the broad applicability of the IES CMD, as it is a tool that can be used in almost all age groups and for a wide range of diseases. The IES CMD forms an important safe surgical aid for special cases, which does not greatly prolong surgical intervention and makes successful implantation possible.

Nevertheless, the IES CMD should not be applied as a standard instrument for cochlear implantation because its use leads to higher postoperative impedances, possibly due to a more invasive and traumatic implantation when compared to the FLEX arrays without the IES CMD. If possible, imaging techniques, or, more specifically, manufactured insertion electrodes, should be used to determine cochlear length, eliminating any negative influence on hearing results using the IES. In the future, it may be interesting to evaluate whether steroid administration via an inner ear catheter [15] can lead to a further reduction in impedances after implantation with the IES CMD. Furthermore, the IES CMD also provides a means of overcoming restrictions in the cochlea, allowing more electrode contacts to be inserted when only partial insertion would be possible without its use. The question around whether speech understanding can be improved also needs to be clarified further in future research endeavours.

Author Contributions: Conceptualization, A.W. and R.B.S.; data curation, J.A.C.H., A.W. and R.B.S.; formal analysis, J.A.C.H. and R.B.S.; funding acquisition, T.L.; investigation, J.A.C.H., A.W. and R.B.S.; methodology, J.A.C.H., A.W. and R.B.S.; project administration, A.W. and R.B.S.; resources, M.E.T., E.K., N.K.P., L.G. and T.L.; software, E.K. and L.G.; supervision, A.W., T.L. and R.B.S.; validation, E.K. and L.G.; visualization, J.A.C.H., A.W. and R.B.S.; writing—original draft, J.A.C.H.; writing—review and editing, J.A.C.H., A.W., M.E.T., E.K., N.K.P., L.G., T.L. and R.B.S. All authors have read and agreed to the published version of the manuscript.

Funding: This research received no external funding.

Institutional Review Board Statement: For the evaluation of anonymized intra-departmental and routine patient data, there was no obligation to submit the data to the Ethics Committee of Hannover Medical School in principle. Protocol code: 1897-2013. Date of approval: 9 July 2013. The study was conducted in accordance with the Declaration of Helsinki.

Informed Consent Statement: Informed consent was obtained from all subjects involved in the study.

Data Availability Statement: The data presented in this retrospective analysis are available on request from the corresponding author. The data are not publicly available as they contain personal and sensitive patient data. All data are stored on the servers of Hannover Medical School, Department of Otorhinolaryngology.

Acknowledgments: We are grateful to Cornelia Batsoulis and Max Fröhlich, both from the MED-EL Hannover Research Center, for their scientific support in this retrospective study.

Conflicts of Interest: The authors declare no conflict of interest.

References

1. Wallhagen, M.; Strawbridge, W.J.; Kaplan, W.A. 6-year impact of hearing impairment on psychosocial and physiologic functioning. *Nurse Pract.* **1996**, *21*, 11–14. [PubMed]
2. Dawes, P.; Emsley, R.; Cruickshanks, K.J.; Moore, D.R.; Fortnum, H.; Edmondson-Jones, M.; McCormack, A.; Munro, K.J. Hearing Loss and Cognition: The Role of Hearing Aids, Social Isolation and Depression. *PLoS ONE* **2015**, *10*, e0119616. [CrossRef] [PubMed]
3. Griffiths, T.D.; Lad, M.; Kumar, S.; Holmes, E.; McMurray, B.; Maguire, E.A.; Billig, A.J.; Sedley, W. How Can Hearing Loss Cause Dementia? *Neuron* **2020**, *108*, 401–412. [CrossRef] [PubMed]
4. Deutsche Gesellschaft für Hals-Nasen-Ohren-Heilkunde, Kopf- und Hals-Chirurgie. Leitlinie Cochlea-Implantat Versorgung und zentral-auditorischer Impantate 05/2012. AWMF Register-Nr. 017-071. Available online: https://www.awmf.org/leitlinien/detail/ii/017-071.html (accessed on 21 May 2019).
5. Lenarz, T. Cochlear implant—State of the art. *GMS Curr. Top. Otorhinolaryngol. Head Neck Surg.* **2018**, *16*, Doc04. [CrossRef] [PubMed]
6. Lenarz, T.; Lesinski-Schiedat, A.; Weber, B.P.; Issing, P.R.; Frohne, C.; Büchner, A.; Battmer, R.D.; Parker, J.; Von Wallenberg, E. The Nucleus Double Array Cochlear Implant: A New Concept for the Obliterated Cochlea. *Otol. Neurotol.* **2001**, *22*, 24–32. [CrossRef]

7. Steenerson, R.L.; Gary, L.B.; Wynens, M.S. Scala vestibuli cochlear implantation for labyrinthine ossification. *Am. J. Otol.* **1990**, *11*, 360–363.
8. Pijl, S.; Noel, F. The Nucleus Multichannel Cochlear Implant: Comparison of Scala Tympani vs. Scala Vestibuli Electrode Placement in a Single Patient. *Otolaryngol. Head Neck Surg.* **1992**, *107*, 472–474. [CrossRef]
9. Gantz, B.J.; McCabe, B.F.; Tyler, R.S. Use of Multichannel Cochlear Implants in Obstructed and Obliterated Cochleas. *Otolaryngol. Head Neck Surg.* **1988**, *98*, 72–81. [CrossRef]
10. Bauer, P.W.; Roland, P.S. Clinical Results with the Med-El Compressed and Split Arrays in the United States. *Laryngoscope* **2004**, *114*, 428–433. [CrossRef]
11. Bredberg, G.; Lindström, B.; Löppönen, H.; Skarżyński, H.; Hyodo, M.; Sato, H. Electrodes for ossified cochleas. *Am. J. Otol.* **1997**, *18*, S42–S43.
12. Zierhofer, C.M.; Hochmair, I.J.; Hochmair, E.S. The advanced Combi 40+ cochlear implant. *Am. J. Otol.* **1997**, *18*, S37–S38. [PubMed]
13. Lehnhardt, E. Sprachaudiometrie. In *Praxis der Audiometrie [in German]*; Lehnhardt, E., Laszig, R., Eds.; Georg Thieme-Verlag: Stuttgart, Germany, 2001; pp. 173–196.
14. Hochmair-Desoyer, I.; Schulz, E.; Moser, L.; Schmidt, M. The HSM sentence test as a tool for evaluating the speech understanding in noise of cochlear implant users. *Am. J. Otol.* **1997**, *18*, S83. [PubMed]
15. Prenzler, N.K.; Salcher, R.; Timm, M.; Gaertner, L.; Lenarz, T.; Warnecke, A. Intracochlear administration of steroids with a catheter during human cochlear implantation: A safety and feasibility study. *Drug Deliv. Transl. Res.* **2018**, *8*, 1191–1199. [CrossRef] [PubMed]
16. Prenzler, N.K.; Kappelmann, C.; Steffens, M.; Lesinski-Schiedat, A.; Lenarz, T.; Warnecke, A. Single Intravenous High Dose Administration of Prednisolone Has No Influence on Postoperative Impedances in the Majority of Cochlear Implant Patients. *Otol. Neurotol.* **2018**, *39*, e1002–e1009. [CrossRef]
17. Prenzler, N.K.; Salcher, R.; Lenarz, T.; Gaertner, L.; Warnecke, A. Dose-Dependent Transient Decrease of Impedances by Deep Intracochlear Injection of Triamcinolone with a Cochlear Catheter Prior to Cochlear Implantation–1 Year Data. *Front. Neurol.* **2020**, *11*, 258. [CrossRef]
18. Wilk, M.; Hessler, R.; Mugridge, K.; Jolly, C.; Fehr, M.; Lenarz, T.; Scheper, V. Impedance Changes and Fibrous Tissue Growth after Cochlear Implantation Are Correlated and Can Be Reduced Using a Dexamethasone Eluting Electrode. *PLoS ONE* **2016**, *11*, e0147552. [CrossRef]
19. Burghard, A.; Lenarz, T.; Kral, A.; Paasche, G. Insertion site and sealing technique affect residual hearing and tissue formation after cochlear implantation. *Hear. Res.* **2014**, *312*, 21–27. [CrossRef]
20. Fuggia, M.J.; Quevedo, R.V.; Hansen, M.R. Intracochlear fibrosis and the foreign body response to cochlear implant biomaterials. *Laryngoscope Investig Otolaryngol.* **2019**, *4*, 678–683. [CrossRef]
21. de Sauvage, R.C.; da Costa, D.L.; Erre, J.-P.; Aran, J.-M. Electrical and physiological changes during short-term and chronic electrical stimulation of the normal cochlea. *Hear. Res.* **1997**, *110*, 119–134. [CrossRef]
22. Newbold, C.; Richardson, R.; Huang, C.Q.; Milojevic, D.; Cowan, R.; Shepherd, R. An in vitro model for investigating impedance changes with cell growth and electrical stimulation: Implications for cochlear implants. *J. Neural Eng.* **2004**, *1*, 218–227. [CrossRef]
23. Topalov, A.A.; Cherevko, S.; Zeradjanin, A.R.; Meier, J.C.; Katsounaros, I.; Mayrhofer, K.J.J. Towards a comprehensive understanding of platinum dissolution in acidic media. *Chem. Sci.* **2014**, *5*, 631–638. [CrossRef]
24. Saunders, E.; Cohen, L.; Aschendorff, A.; Shapiro, W.; Knight, M.; Stecker, M.; Richter, B.; Waltzman, S.; Tykocinski, M.; Roland, T.; et al. Threshold, Comfortable Level and Impedance Changes as a Function of Electrode-Modiolar Distance. *Ear Hear.* **2002**, *23*, 28S–40S. [CrossRef] [PubMed]
25. Newbold, C.; Mergen, S.; Richardson, R.; Seligman, P.; Millard, R.; Cowan, R.; Shepherd, R. Impedance changes in chronically implanted and stimulated cochlear implant electrodes. *Cochlear Implant. Int.* **2014**, *15*, 191–199. [CrossRef]
26. Newbold, C.; Risi, F.; Hollow, R.; Yusof, Y.; Dowell, R. Long-term electrode impedance changes and failure prevalence in cochlear implants. *Int. J. Audiol.* **2015**, *54*, 453–460. [CrossRef]
27. Choi, J.; Payne, M.R.; Campbell, L.J.; Bester, C.W.; Newbold, C.; Eastwood, H.; O'Leary, S.J. Electrode Impedance Fluctuations as a Biomarker for Inner Ear Pathology After Cochlear Implantation. *Otol. Neurotol.* **2017**, *38*, 1433–1439. [CrossRef] [PubMed]
28. Needham, K.; Stathopoulos, D.; Newbold, C.; Leavens, J.; Risi, F.; Manouchehri, S.; Durmo, I.; Cowan, R. Electrode impedance changes after implantation of a dexamethasone-eluting intracochlear array. *Cochlear Implant. Int.* **2020**, *21*, 98–109. [CrossRef] [PubMed]
29. Newbold, C.; Richardson, R.; Millard, R.; Huang, C.; Milojevic, D.; Shepherd, R.; Cowan, R. Changes in biphasic electrode impedance with protein adsorption and cell growth. *J. Neural Eng.* **2010**, *7*, 056011. [CrossRef] [PubMed]
30. Newbold, C.; Richardson, R.; Millard, R.; Seligman, P.; Cowan, R.; Shepherd, R. Electrical stimulation causes rapid changes in electrode impedance of cell-covered electrodes. *J. Neural Eng.* **2011**, *8*, 036029. [CrossRef]
31. Xu, J.; Shepherd, R.K.; Millard, R.E.; Clark, G.M. Chronic electrical stimulation of the auditory nerve at high stimulus rates: A physiological and histopathological study. *Hear. Res.* **1997**, *105*, 1–29. [CrossRef]
32. Tykocinski, M.; Cohen, L.T.; Cowan, R.S. Measurement and Analysis of Access Resistance and Polarization Impedance in Cochlear Implant Recipients. *Otol. Neurotol.* **2005**, *26*, 948–956. [CrossRef]

33. Prenzler, N.K.; Weller, T.; Steffens, M.; Lesinski-Schiedat, A.; Büchner, A.; Lenarz, T.; Warnecke, A. Impedance Values Do Not Correlate With Speech Understanding in Cochlear Implant Recipients. *Otol. Neurotol.* **2020**, *41*, e1029–e1034. [CrossRef] [PubMed]
34. Büchner, A.; Illg, A.; Majdani, O.; Lenarz, T. Investigation of the effect of cochlear implant electrode length on speech comprehension in quiet and noise compared with the results with users of electro-acoustic-stimulation, a retrospective analysis. *PLoS ONE* **2017**, *12*, e0174900. [CrossRef] [PubMed]
35. Nadol, J.B., Jr. Patterns of neural degeneration in the human cochlea and auditory nerve: Implications for cochlear implantation. *Otolaryngol. Neck Surg.* **1997**, *117*, 220–228. [CrossRef]
36. Buchman, C.A.; Dillon, M.T.; King, E.R.; Adunka, M.C.; Adunka, O.F.; Pillsbury, H.C. Influence of Cochlear Implant Insertion Depth on Performance: A prospective randomized trial. *Otol. Neurotol.* **2014**, *35*, 1773–1779. [CrossRef] [PubMed]
37. Wooltorton, E. Cochlear implant recipients at risk for meningitis. *Can. Med. Assoc. J.* **2002**, *167*, 670.
38. Fina, M.; Skinner, M.; Goebel, J.A.; Piccirillo, J.F.; Neely, J.G. Vestibular Dysfunction after Cochlear Implantation. *Otol. Neurotol.* **2003**, *24*, 234–242. [CrossRef]

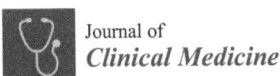

Article

Development of Sound Localization in Infants and Young Children with Cochlear Implants

Filip Asp [1,2,*], Eva Karltorp [1,2] and Erik Berninger [1,3]

[1] Department of Clinical Science, Intervention and Technology, Karolinska Institutet, 17177 Stockholm, Sweden
[2] Hearing Implant Unit, Department of ENT, Karolinska University Hospital, 14186 Stockholm, Sweden
[3] Department of Audiology and Neurotology, Karolinska University Hospital, 14186 Stockholm, Sweden
* Correspondence: filip.asp@ki.se

Abstract: Cochlear implantation as a treatment for severe-to-profound hearing loss allows children to develop hearing, speech, and language in many cases. However, cochlear implants are generally provided beyond the infant period and outcomes are assessed after years of implant use, making comparison with normal development difficult. The aim was to study whether the rate of improvement of horizontal localization accuracy in children with bilateral implants is similar to children with normal hearing. A convenience sample of 20 children with a median age at simultaneous bilateral implantation = 0.58 years (0.42–2.3 years) participated in this cohort study. Longitudinal follow-up of sound localization accuracy for an average of ≈1 year generated 42 observations at a mean age = 1.5 years (0.58–3.6 years). The rate of development was compared to historical control groups including children with normal hearing and with relatively late bilateral implantation (≈4 years of age). There was a significant main effect of time with bilateral implants on localization accuracy (slope = 0.21/year, R^2 = 0.25, F = 13.6, $p < 0.001$, $n = 42$). No differences between slopes (F = 0.30, $p = 0.58$) or correlation coefficients (Cohen's q = 0.28, $p = 0.45$) existed when comparing children with implants and normal hearing (slope = 0.16/year since birth, $p = 0.015$, $n = 12$). The rate of development was identical to children implanted late. Results suggest that early bilateral implantation in children with severe-to-profound hearing loss allows development of sound localization at a similar age to children with normal hearing. Similar rates in children with early and late implantation and normal hearing suggest an intrinsic mechanism for the development of horizontal sound localization abilities.

Keywords: sound localization; infants; bilateral cochlear implants; development

Citation: Asp, F.; Karltorp, E.; Berninger, E. Development of Sound Localization in Infants and Young Children with Cochlear Implants. *J. Clin. Med.* 2022, 11, 6758. https://doi.org/10.3390/jcm11226758

Academic Editor: Nicolas Guevara

Received: 25 October 2022
Accepted: 14 November 2022
Published: 15 November 2022

Publisher's Note: MDPI stays neutral with regard to jurisdictional claims in published maps and institutional affiliations.

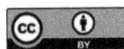

Copyright: © 2022 by the authors. Licensee MDPI, Basel, Switzerland. This article is an open access article distributed under the terms and conditions of the Creative Commons Attribution (CC BY) license (https://creativecommons.org/licenses/by/4.0/).

1. Introduction

Humans can identify the source of a sound with high accuracy [1]. Interaural differences in time and level are analyzed in the central auditory system and associated with events or locations in our environment. Even though both animals [2,3] and humans [4] can localize sound just after birth, accuracy refines with experience from such associations [5,6]. In barn owls, an extensively studied species, the visual system plays a key role for the brain to learn and build an auditory space map based on these associations [7,8]. Occlusion of one ear [9] or displacement of the visual field [10] in the barn owl have shown corrections of sound localization behavior in response to these manipulations. These corrections in localization behavior are experience-driven and demonstrated using various experimental manipulations of sensory input in many species. Experience gained early in life is demonstrated to be most important for the formation and refinement of a subcortical auditory space map [11–13], but capability of adaptation to altered cues is shown behaviorally in adult humans [6,14,15] and ferrets [16]. Plasticity in the neural circuitry underlying sound localization, thus, exists across species and age (see [16] for an overview).

Children with congenital bilateral severe-to-profound hearing loss represent an opportunity for the study of plasticity in the human auditory system. For these children, cochlear implantation is a clinically well-established treatment resulting in an ability to recognize speech and development of speech and language in many cases [17–20]. To promote normal speech and language development, implantation preferably should occur no later than 12 months of age [21,22] and family centered early intervention is important. However, horizontal sound localization, an important and early obtainable auditory ability dependent on bilateral implantation [17], develops systematically despite relatively late sequential bilateral cochlear implantation ($\approx$4 years of age) following long periods of unilateral hearing ($\approx$2 years) [23]. Once bilateral stimulation is provided, development of sound localization accuracy occurs over several years [23], with subsequent persistent abilities [24], albeit, worse than normal [17,24]. Accordingly, the age at which implants are provided does not seem to determine development of sound localization [23], consistent with findings that adult humans can adapt to altered localization cues [6,25].

While a number of large centers perform cochlear implantation early, implants are generally provided beyond the infant period [26,27] and the US Food and Drug administration grants implantation no earlier than 0.75 years (for one of three major manufacturers). Relatively late implantation in combination with assessment of behavioral outcomes after years of implant use makes comparison with normal developmental trajectories difficult.

Here, we study development of horizontal sound localization in infants and young children listening through bilateral cochlear implants (BiCI) since $\approx$0.6 years of age, and contrast the results with previous findings from children with normal hearing [28], and children with late cochlear implantation [23]. We asked whether early bilateral cochlear implantation allows experience-driven improvement of horizontal localization accuracy and if the rate of improvement was similar to children with normal hearing.

2. Materials and Methods

2.1. Study Design

This was a longitudinal clinical study with an inclusion period between March 2019 and February 2021. The study was approved by the regional ethical review board in Stockholm, Sweden (permit number 2012/189-31/3 and 2013/2248-32). To be included, children were required to have received bilateral cochlear implantation in a simultaneous procedure and be available and willing to participate in the study during regular clinical follow-up. Within 3 months after surgery, parents were asked for their child's participation at a visit to the clinic. At clinical follow-ups (initial fitting of external parts of the cochlear implant system about 3 weeks after surgery, and then approximately 1, 3, 6, 12, 18 and 24 months after initial fitting), children participated in a 3 min horizontal sound localization task adapted to children from about 6 months of age [28]. The rate of development of sound localization accuracy was compared to children with normal hearing and older children using cochlear implants.

2.2. Subjects

Twenty children were included in the study at a median age of 0.87 years (0.58–2.53 years, 8 females) (Table 1). Parental informed consent was obtained for all children. Children were implanted bilaterally at a median age of 0.58 years (0.42–2.3 years) with devices from Cochlear (Cochlear Corporation, Sydney, Australia) or Med-El (Med-El GmbH, Innsbruck, Austria).

Thirteen children who met the inclusion criteria were not asked to participate due to limited time during regular clinical follow-up. Another two children declined participation. These 15 children were implanted at the same median age as the included subjects.

Table 1. Background data on the children who participated in the study. Children are sorted in ascending age order. Two of twenty included children did not cooperate to sound localization testing and are not shown.

Age at Implantation (Years)	Cochlear Implant Model	Sound Processor	Sex	Etiology
0.42	CI522	CP1000	M	Connexin 26
0.45	CI522	CP1000	M	Genetic testing performed; no mutation found
0.45	Synchrony 2 Flex 28	Sonnet 2	M	Cause not investigated
0.47	CI612	CP1000	F	Cause not investigated
0.48	CI532	CP1000	F	Genetic testing performed; no mutation found
0.51	Synchrony 2 Flex 28	Sonnet 2	F	Unknown; no positive cCMV infection found
0.51	CI612	CP1000	M	Connexin 26
0.55	CI522	CP1000	F	Connexin 26
0.56	Synchrony 2 Flex 28	Sonnet 2	F	Connexin 26
0.58	CI522	CP1000	F	cCMV
0.58	CI512	CP1000	M	cCMV
0.65	CI612	CP1000	M	Cause not investigated
0.76	Synchrony 2 Flex 28	Sonnet 2	F	Genetic testing performed; uncertain causative gene mutation
0.91	CI612	CP1000	M	Genetic testing performed; no mutation found
1.0	Synchrony 2 Flex 28	Sonnet 2	M	Connexin 26
1.6	CI612	CP1000	M	Cause not investigated
1.8	CI522	CP1000	M	Unknown; no positive cCMV infection found
2.3	CI612	CP1000	F	Cause not investigated

CI522, CI512, CI532, and CI612; cochlear implants manufactured by Cochlear Corporation, Sydney, Australia. Synchrony 2 Flex28; cochlear implant manufactured by Med-El GmbH, Innsbruck, Austria. CP1000; sound processor manufactured by Cochlear Corporation, Sydney, Australia. Sonnet 2; sound processor manufactured by Med-El GmbH, Innsbruck, Austria. M; Male. F; Female. cCMV; congenital cytomegalovirus.

2.3. Setup, Stimulus and Test Procedure

The setup, stimulus, test procedure and acquisition of behavioral responses is described in detail previously [28]. Children were seated in the lap of a parent in front of 12 active loudspeakers (ARGON 7340A; Argon Audio, Sweden) spanning a 110-degree arc in the frontal horizontal plane (Figure 1) in an audiometric test room. Loudspeakers were at ear level and spaced 10 degrees, resulting in loudspeaker positions at ± 55, ± 45, ± 35, ± 25, ± 15, and ± 5 degrees azimuth with respect to the subject. A 7-inch thin film transistor (TFT) display was mounted below each loudspeaker, resulting in 12 loudspeaker/display (LD)-pairs. An eye-tracking system (Smart Eye Pro; Smart Eye AB, Gothenburg, Sweden) was used for objective positioning of children's pupil positions relative to the LD-pairs.

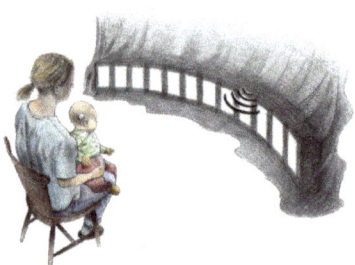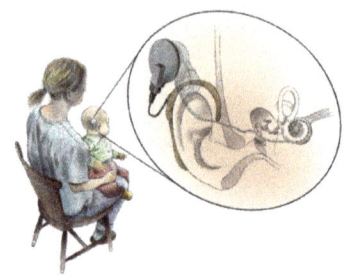

Figure 1. Experimental setup for determination of horizontal sound localization accuracy in infants and young children listening through bilateral cochlear implants. The left panel illustrates the position of the child relative to an array of loudspeaker/display-pairs. Loudspeakers were covered in black cloth to attract the child's gaze to the visual displays. A continuous auditory-visual stimulus was presented from a loudspeaker/display-pair and randomly shifted in azimuth. Simultaneously with an azimuthal shift, the visual part of the stimulus was stopped for 1.6 s and eye-gaze patterns in response to the auditory stimulus were recorded before the visual part of the stimulus returned. The right panel illustrates the implanted and external parts of a cochlear implant system. An array of electrode contacts resides in the cochlea, stimulating the auditory nerve. The electronics of the cochlear implant are driven by an external sound processor behind the ear. Illustration by Mats Ceder.

A sound localization test consisted of 24 azimuthal shifts of an ongoing auditory-visual stimulus (a colorful cartoon movie playing a continuous melody with a long-term frequency spectrum similar to female speech) presented at 63 dBA. In each azimuthal shift, the sound was changed to another randomly assigned loudspeaker on average every 7th second (5–9 s) with a simultaneous stop of the visual stimulus. The visual stimulus was reintroduced on the visual display corresponding to the sounding loudspeaker 1.6 s after the azimuthal sound shift. The procedure allowed acquisition of gaze behavior during 1.6 s in response to a spatial change of the sound. A test lasted ≈3 min.

Localization accuracy was quantified by an Error Index [29,30]. An EI = 0 corresponds to perfect performance. An EI = 1 corresponds to average random performance. A Monte Carlo simulation showed that the 95% confidence interval (C.I.) for random performance using the current procedure was [0.72, 1.28].

Children were not given any instructions before or during testing. The parent having the child on their knee was instructed to remain seated and unmoving and to not talk to the child.

2.4. Analyses

To analyze cross-sectional data, linear regression analyses of the first sound localization test (n = 18; two children were not possible to assess) were performed with EI (range = 0.31–1.0) as dependent variable and time since activation of BiCI (i.e., auditory experience, range = 0.03–1.7 years) as the independent variable. To account for between- and within-subject variability despite missing data points, a linear mixed model was constructed, with the EI as dependent variable and time since activation of BiCI, age at implantation, and the number of obtained responses in a localization test as fixed effects. A random intercept for subjects was included in the model and interaction terms between fixed effects and random intercepts were evaluated. Selection of a final model was guided by minimizing the Aikaike information criterion. The slope of the regression line was statistically compared to slopes obtained in children with normal hearing [28] by an analysis of covariance, and qualitatively to older children with cochlear implants [23]. Statistical analyses were performed using Statistica version 13 (Statsoft, Inc., Tulsa, OK, USA) and R Version 3.4.2 (R Foundation for Statistical Computing, Austria)

Test reliability was computed by dividing each test into two parts and comparing the EI between part 1 (test) and part 2 (retest) [28]. The statistical reliability of the localization test was then quantified by analysis of the variability in test–retest differences and by estimation of the variance in EI for a single SLA measurement (see Equation (10) in [28] for the variance estimate).

3. Results

Longitudinal follow-up generated 42 sound localization measurements (1 to 5 measurements per child) in 18 children (2 of 20 children were not willing to cooperate to testing). The average time since activation of BiCI was 0.9 years (0.09 years–1.7 years, n = 42) with a mean age at test = 1.5 years (0.58 years–3.6 years, n = 42).

3.1. Development of Sound Localization Accuracy Is Driven by Time since Activation of Bilateral Implants

Simple linear regression analyses of cross-sectional data (first test, n = 18) indicated that increasing time since activation of BiCI was associated with increasing sound localization accuracy (EI = 0.83–0.19 time since BiCI, r = -0.47, p = 0.05). A linear mixed model for the entire longitudinal dataset (n = 42) showed a significant main effect of time since BiCI on the EI, whereas no effect of random intercept (i.e., of subject) or interaction with number of trials existed. The final linear model, thus, included time since activation of BiCI, which explained 25% of the variance in the EI (R^2 = 0.25, F = 13.6, n = 42, p = 0.0007) (Figure 2). According to the model equation, which was similar to the linear fit from the cross-sectional analysis, the EI decreased by 0.21/year with an intercept of 0.82.

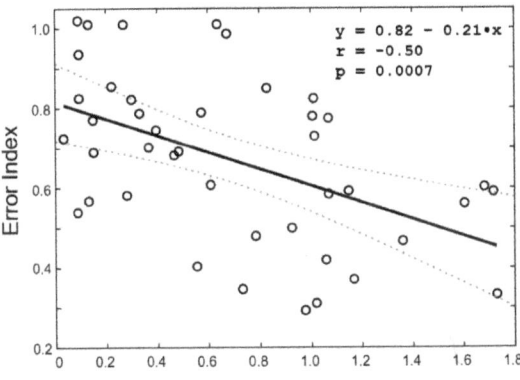

Figure 2. Children with congenital severe-to-profound hearing loss develop horizontal sound localization abilities with increasing time since activation of bilateral cochlear implants. The black open circles depict localization accuracy (Error Index) for 18 infants measured at 1 to 5 occasions (n = 42, mean follow-up time = 0.9 years (0.09 years–1.7 years); mean age at test = 1.5 years (0.58 years–3.6 years). Localization accuracy increased as a function of time since activation of bilateral cochlear implants (R^2 = 0.25, F = 13.6, n = 42, p = 0.0007, linear mixed model). The black solid line is the linear fit from a linear mixed model analysis, and the dotted lines depict the 95% confidence interval of the fit.

Individual perceived versus presented azimuths were plotted for the child with the longest time since activation of BiCI (Figure 3), to visualize development of behavioral response patterns. With increasing time since activation of BiCI (4 measurements over 1.4 years follow-up), perceived azimuths were approaching target azimuths.

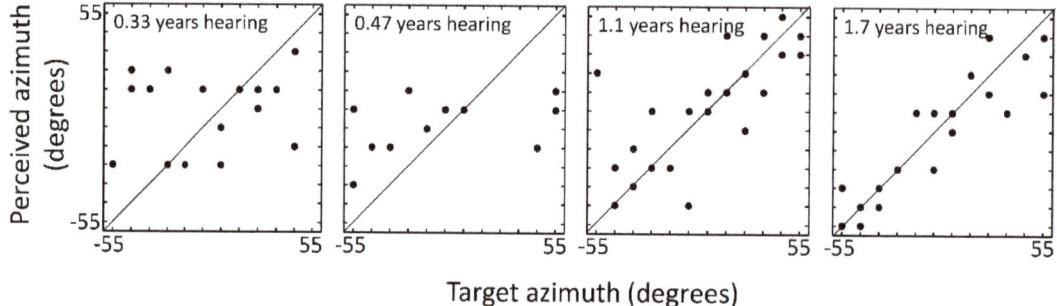

Figure 3. Perceived as a function of target sound-source azimuth at 4 occurrences (one per panel) for an individual child. In the left panel, this child had bilateral cochlear implants activated for 0.33 years. As experience with bilateral cochlear implants increases (from left to right), datapoints approach the line of equality corresponding to perfect sound localization accuracy in this task.

3.2. Comparison between Children with Early Bilateral Cochlear Implantation and Young Children with Normal Hearing

To study whether implanted children develop sound localization accuracy similar to children with normal hearing, data were compared with previously reported cross-sectional results from 12 children (median age = 1.0 years) with normal hearing tested with the same technique [28]. Figure 4, panel A, illustrates that children with implants (black open circles) overlap in their performance with children with normal hearing (filled blue circles).

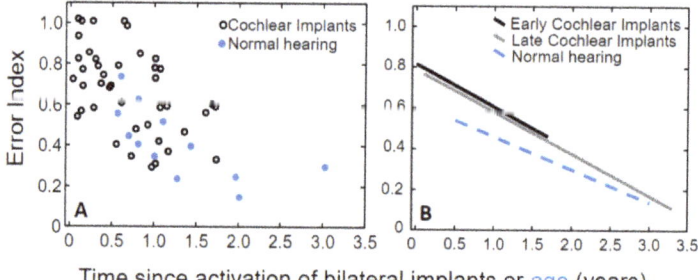

Figure 4. (**A**): The black open circles depict localization accuracy in children with bilateral cochlear implants, and the blue filled circles depict localization accuracy in children with normal hearing from Asp et al. (2016) [28]. (**B**): The lines show linear fits based on data from the present study in infants (black) and previous data from children with normal hearing (blue, Asp et al. (2016) [28]) and children with relatively late sequential bilateral implantation (grey, Asp et al. (2011) [23]).

The slopes of the regression lines for each group were similar (Normal hearing: 0.16/year, $p = 0.015$); Cochlear implant: 0.21/year, $p = 0.0007$) (Figure 4, panel B), with no difference between correlation coefficients (Cohen's q = 0.28, $p = 0.45$). An analysis of covariance with group as categorical factors (cochlear implants versus normal hearing) and time since bilateral hearing onset/age as a covariate, showed no statistically significant interaction (F = 0.30, $p = 0.58$), that is, no significant difference between developmental rates. In addition, no significant difference in localization accuracy existed between children with implants and normal hearing (F = 3.0, $p = 0.09$).

3.3. Comparison between Children with Early Bilateral Cochlear Implantation and Relatively Late Sequential Bilateral Cochlear Implantation

To study the effect of age at implantation on development of sound localization accuracy, data were further compared to results from children with relatively late sequential bilateral cochlear implantation (median age first CI = 1.9 years, median age second CI = 4.1 years, $n = 66$) [23]. These children, implanted and tested at the same tertiary referral center as the subjects in the present study, were assessed at a median age of 5.6 years (range = 2.8–17.3 years), i.e., they were substantially older than the children in the present study. Despite methodological and procedural differences (i.e., number of sound-sources, spatial range and resolution of the test, spectral and temporal characteristics of the auditory stimulus, and quantification of behavioral responses), a striking resemblance in development of localization between early (this study) and late bilateral implantation existed (Figure 4, panel B). The rate of development was identical, whereas intercepts differed slightly (late cochlear implants: slope = 0.21/year, intercept = 0.79; early cochlear implants: slope = 0.21/year, intercept = 0.82).

3.4. Reliability of Sound Localization Measurements

The 95% C.I. of the test–retest differences (−0.098 to 0.037) included 0, reflecting that no significant learning effect occurred. The 95% C.I. for the EI for a single measurement was ±0.11 ($n = 42$). The test–retest differences did not depend on the number of obtained responses during a test (r = 0.13, $p = 0.40$).

4. Discussion

We found that infants with bilateral severe-to-profound congenital hearing loss develop horizontal sound localization abilities after bilateral cochlear implantation. When contrasting data from the current study with previous data from infants with normal hearing, we found that the developmental rates in these groups were similar. While it seems unlikely that localization will reach the same accuracy as in normal hearing based on CI studies in adults [31], the rate of improvement emphasizes the need of early provision of hearing in both ears for children with severe-to-profound hearing loss to allow development of spatial hearing near ages for which development normally occurs. In addition to being a safety matter in for example traffic, adults with hearing loss report that difficulties in localization of sounds are associated with loss of concentration, confusion of sounds, and a wish to escape settings in which this occurs [32]. Additionally, accurate localization is likely to improve communication since audiovisual cues are important for speech understanding when hearing loss is present [33]. Less is known about how impaired sound localization during infancy affects learning and interaction in daily life and should be targeted in future research. For children with unilateral hearing loss, a condition that typically is associated with impaired localization [34], it is 10 times more common having to repeat at least one year in school [35].

When contrasting the current data with previous data from children with relatively late cochlear implantation, we found a striking resemblance between infants and children in early school-age in the rate of development following implantation. This demonstrates that a sensitive period for human spatial hearing is not restricted to early development, corroborating findings in adult humans [6] and ferrets [16] who adapt their behavior to altered spatial cues. Results differ from barn owls [36] and mice [37], for which age limits sensitive periods for development of sound localization or the binaural cues it is based on. In children implanted bilaterally after 5 years of age, localization performance is poor one year after implantation [38], but data on long-term localization performance for late bilateral implantation is unknown. It is noteworthy that the high similarity in the rate of development and between-subject variability of sound localization abilities found in the present study between younger and older children with cochlear implants occurred despite methodological differences in how localization accuracy was measured. Infants' responses in the present study were obtained through eye-gaze, whereas older children with implants [23] pointed at or verbally indicated the perceived sound-source azimuth. In addition, children in the present study listened to a continuous sound, whereas older children listened to sounds of relatively short duration. For both groups, between-subject variability in localization accuracy was high and time since activation of BiCI explained the same amount of variance in localization accuracy (25%). The underlying causes for variability in binaural hearing in individuals with implants have been targeted in recent years [39–43], revealing etiology of the hearing loss, duration of hearing loss, and surgical procedures and subsequent bilateral fitting of sound processors as variables that may affect results. Importantly, while current and previous data presented together here show that the developmental rate of localization accuracy is comparable for children with normal hearing and cochlear implants, localization performance after prolonged cochlear implant use does not reach that of individuals with normal hearing [17,44,45]. One reason for less accurate localization despite many years of cochlear implant stimulation is that thresholds for important cues underlying accurate localization (interaural level and time differences) typically are substantially worse for listeners with cochlear implants compared to normal hearing [46], owing to technical and surgical limitations (see, e.g., ref. [47] for a discussion). Future studies including long-term follow up of children who received bilateral cochlear implants as infants may reveal if localization performance plateaus at higher accuracy than later implanted children, and if early localization abilities have implications for, e.g., learning, language and social interaction. Factors of interest in such future studies should be to determine underlying causes for between-subject variability through genetic testing (≈50% of congenital sensorineural hearing loss are genetic in origin [48,49]) and radiological investigation of bilateral cochlear implant electrode placement to assess the impact of interaural frequency mismatch which negatively affects binaural hearing [39].

A limitation of the comparison between data collected in the current study and data from children with NH from previous work is that previous data are cross-sectional and based on a relatively small sample. However, the data from children with NH should be representative given previously performed analyses [28] of localization accuracy in larger samples of children with NH aged 0.5 to 1.5 years ($n = 80$) showing a rate of improvement similar to what was found in our smaller sample [28,50].

Data presented here suggest an intrinsic mechanism for the development of horizontal sound localization abilities. Our study improves on previous work on spatial hearing in children with cochlear implants [17,23,51,52] due to its inclusion of children at a very young age and its longitudinal follow-up before school-age. As long as cochlear implantation may be performed safely in infants, our findings suggest that implantation should occur as early as possible to allow development of spatial hearing near ages for which development normally occurs.

Author Contributions: Conceptualization, F.A. and E.B.; methodology, F.A. and E.B.; software, F.A.; validation, F.A., E.K. and E.B.; formal analysis, F.A. and E.B.; investigation, F.A.; resources, F.A.; data curation, F.A.; writing—original draft preparation, F.A.; writing—review and editing, F.A., E.K. and E.B.; visualization, F.A. and E.B.; supervision, F.A. and E.B.; project administration, F.A. and E.K.; funding acquisition, F.A., E.K. and E.B. All authors have read and agreed to the published version of the manuscript.

Funding: This research was funded by the Tysta Skolan Foundation (FB16-0023) and the Foundation for promotion and development of clinical research at Karolinska Institutet. The project was also supported by the regional agreement on medical training and clinical research (ALF) between Stockholm County Council and Karolinska Institutet, and the foundation of the Swedish Order of Freemasons (Konung Gustaf VI Adolfs frimurarefond, 2022).

Institutional Review Board Statement: The study was conducted in accordance with the Declaration of Helsinki, and approved by the regional ethical review board in Stockholm, Sweden (permit number 2012/189-31/3 and 2013/2248-32) for studies involving humans.

Informed Consent Statement: Parental informed consent was obtained for all subjects involved in the study. Written informed consent has been obtained from the parents to the children to publish this paper.

Data Availability Statement: The data presented in this study are available on request from the corresponding author. The data are not publicly available due to ethical, legal and privacy issues.

Acknowledgments: We wish to extend our appreciation to the children and parents that participated in this study. The authors are grateful for the continued support of Scientific Center for Advanced Pediatric Audiology at Karolinska Institute, to Åke Olofsson for technical assistance, and to Mats Ceder for illustrating the setup used for sound localization measurements in Figure 1.

Conflicts of Interest: The authors declare no conflict of interest.

References

1. Middlebrooks, J.C.; Green, D.M. Sound localization by human listeners. *Annu. Rev. Psychol.* **1991**, *42*, 135–159. [CrossRef] [PubMed]
2. Ashmead, D.H.; Clifton, R.K.; Reese, E.P. Development of auditory localization in dogs: Single source and precedence effect sounds. *Dev. Psychobiol.* **1986**, *19*, 91–103. [CrossRef] [PubMed]
3. Olmstead, C.E.; Villablanca, J.R. Development of behavioral audition in the kitten. *Physiol. Behav.* **1980**, *24*, 705–712. [CrossRef]
4. Field, J.; Muir, D.; Pilon, R.; Sinclair, M.; Dodwell, P. Infants' orientation to lateral sounds from birth to three months. *Child Dev.* **1980**, *51*, 295–298. [CrossRef] [PubMed]
5. Knudsen, E.I. Instructed learning in the auditory localization pathway of the barn owl. *Nature* **2002**, *417*, 322–328. [CrossRef]
6. Hofman, P.M.; Van Riswick, J.G.; Van Opstal, A.J. Relearning sound localization with new ears. *Nat. Neurosci.* **1998**, *1*, 417–421. [CrossRef]
7. Knudsen, E.I.; Knudsen, P.F. Vision calibrates sound localization in developing barn owls. *J. Neurosci.* **1989**, *9*, 3306–3313. [CrossRef]
8. Knudsen, E.I.; Knudsen, P.F. Vision guides the adjustment of auditory localization in young barn owls. *Science* **1985**, *230*, 545–548.
9. Knudsen, E.I.; Esterly, S.D.; Knudsen, P.F. Monaural occlusion alters sound localization during a sensitive period in the barn owl. *J. Neurosci.* **1984**, *4*, 1001–1011. [CrossRef]
10. Brainard, M.S.; Knudsen, E.I. Sensitive periods for visual calibration of the auditory space map in the barn owl optic tectum. *J. Neurosci.* **1998**, *18*, 3929–3942. [CrossRef]
11. Brainard, M.S.; Knudsen, E.I. Experience-dependent plasticity in the inferior colliculus: A site for visual calibration of the neural representation of auditory space in the barn owl. *J. Neurosci.* **1993**, *13*, 4589–4608. [CrossRef]
12. King, A.J.; Hutchings, M.E.; Moore, D.R.; Blakemore, C. Developmental plasticity in the visual and auditory representations in the mammalian superior colliculus. *Nature* **1988**, *332*, 73–76. [CrossRef]
13. Withington-Wray, D.J.; Binns, K.E.; Dhanjal, S.S.; Brickley, S.G.; Keating, M.J. The Maturation of the Superior Collicular Map of Auditory Space in the Guinea Pig is Disrupted by Developmental Auditory Deprivation. *Eur. J. Neurosci.* **1990**, *2*, 693–703. [CrossRef]
14. Kumpik, D.P.; Kacelnik, O.; King, A.J. Adaptive reweighting of auditory localization cues in response to chronic unilateral earplugging in humans. *J. Neurosci.* **2010**, *30*, 4883–4894. [CrossRef]
15. Zwiers, M.P.; Van Opstal, A.J.; Paige, G.D. Plasticity in human sound localization induced by compressed spatial vision. *Nat. Neurosci.* **2003**, *6*, 175–181. [CrossRef]
16. King, A.J.; Parsons, C.H.; Moore, D.R. Plasticity in the neural coding of auditory space in the mammalian brain. *Proc. Natl. Acad. Sci. USA* **2000**, *97*, 11821–11828. [CrossRef]
17. Asp, F.; Maki-Torkko, E.; Karltorp, E.; Harder, H.; Hergils, L.; Eskilsson, G.; Stenfelt, S. Bilateral versus unilateral cochlear implants in children: Speech recognition, sound localization, and parental reports. *Int. J. Audiol.* **2012**, *51*, 817–832. [CrossRef]
18. Dunn, C.C.; Walker, E.A.; Oleson, J.; Kenworthy, M.; Van Voorst, T.; Tomblin, J.B.; Ji, H.; Kirk, K.I.; McMurray, B.; Hanson, M.; et al. Longitudinal speech perception and language performance in pediatric cochlear implant users: The effect of age at implantation. *Ear Hear.* **2014**, *35*, 148–160. [CrossRef]
19. Houston, D.M.; Miyamoto, R.T. Effects of early auditory experience on word learning and speech perception in deaf children with cochlear implants: Implications for sensitive periods of language development. *Otol. Neurotol.* **2010**, *31*, 1248–1253. [CrossRef]
20. Leigh, J.; Dettman, S.; Dowell, R.; Sarant, J. Evidence-Based Approach for Making Cochlear Implant Recommendations for Infants With Residual Hearing. *Ear Hear.* **2011**, *32*, 313–322. [CrossRef]
21. Karltorp, E.; Eklof, M.; Ostlund, E.; Asp, F.; Tideholm, B.; Lofkvist, U. Cochlear implants before 9 months of age led to more natural spoken language development without increased surgical risks. *Acta Paediatr.* **2020**, *109*, 332–341. [CrossRef]
22. Dettman, S.J.; Dowell, R.C.; Choo, D.; Arnott, W.; Abrahams, Y.; Davis, A.; Dornan, D.; Leigh, J.; Constantinescu, G.; Cowan, R.; et al. Long-term Communication Outcomes for Children Receiving Cochlear Implants Younger Than 12 Months: A Multicenter Study. *Otol. Neurotol.* **2016**, *37*, e82–e95. [CrossRef] [PubMed]
23. Asp, F.; Eskilsson, G.; Berninger, E. Horizontal sound localization in children with bilateral cochlear implants: Effects of auditory experience and age at implantation. *Otol. Neurotol.* **2011**, *32*, 558–564. [CrossRef] [PubMed]
24. Asp, F.; Maki-Torkko, E.; Karltorp, E.; Harder, H.; Hergils, L.; Eskilsson, G.; Stenfelt, S. A longitudinal study of the bilateral benefit in children with bilateral cochlear implants. *Int. J. Audiol.* **2015**, *54*, 77–88. [CrossRef] [PubMed]
25. Mendonca, C.; Campos, G.; Dias, P.; Santos, J.A. Learning auditory space: Generalization and long-term effects. *PLoS ONE* **2013**, *8*, e77900. [CrossRef]

26. Bruijnzeel, H.; Bezdjian, A.; Lesinski-Schiedat, A.; Illg, A.; Tzifa, K.; Monteiro, L.; Volpe, A.D.; Grolman, W.; Topsakal, V. Evaluation of pediatric cochlear implant care throughout Europe: Is European pediatric cochlear implant care performed according to guidelines? *Cochlear Implant. Int.* **2017**, *18*, 287–296. [CrossRef]
27. Armstrong, M.; Maresh, A.; Buxton, C.; Craun, P.; Wowroski, L.; Reilly, B.; Preciado, D. Barriers to early pediatric cochlear implantation. *Int. J. Pediatr. Otorhinolaryngol.* **2013**, *77*, 1869–1872. [CrossRef]
28. Asp, F.; Olofsson, A.; Berninger, E. Corneal-Reflection Eye-Tracking Technique for the Assessment of Horizontal Sound Localization Accuracy from 6 Months of Age. *Ear Hear.* **2016**, *37*, e104–e118. [CrossRef]
29. Asp, F.; Reinfeldt, S. Horizontal sound localisation accuracy in individuals with conductive hearing loss: Effect of the bone conduction implant. *Int. J. Audiol.* **2018**, *57*, 657–664. [CrossRef]
30. Gardner, M.B.; Gardner, R.S. Problem of localization in the median plane: Effect of pinnae cavity occlusion. *J. Acoust. Soc. Am.* **1973**, *53*, 400–408. [CrossRef]
31. van Hoesel, R.J. Exploring the benefits of bilateral cochlear implants. *Audiol. Neurootol.* **2004**, *9*, 234–246. [CrossRef]
32. Noble, W.; Ter-Horst, K.; Byrne, D. Disabilities and handicaps associated with impaired auditory localization. *J. Am. Acad. Audiol.* **1995**, *6*, 129–140.
33. Lachs, L.; Pisoni, D.B.; Kirk, K.I. Use of audiovisual information in speech perception by prelingually deaf children with cochlear implants: A first report. *Ear Hear.* **2001**, *22*, 236–251. [CrossRef]
34. Bess, F.H.; Tharpe, A.M.; Gibler, A.M. Auditory performance of children with unilateral sensorineural hearing loss. *Ear Hear.* **1986**, *7*, 20–26. [CrossRef]
35. Tharpe, A.M. Unilateral and mild bilateral hearing loss in children: Past and current perspectives. *Trends Amplif.* **2008**, *12*, 7–15. [CrossRef]
36. Knudsen, E.I.; Knudsen, P.F. The sensitive period for auditory localization in barn owls is limited by age, not by experience. *J. Neurosci.* **1986**, *6*, 1918–1924. [CrossRef]
37. Polley, D.B.; Thompson, J.H.; Guo, W. Brief hearing loss disrupts binaural integration during two early critical periods of auditory cortex development. *Nat. Commun.* **2013**, *4*, 2547. [CrossRef]
38. Galvin, K.L.; Mok, M.; Dowell, R.C.; Briggs, R.J. 12-month post-operative results for older children using sequential bilateral implants. *Ear Hear.* **2007**, *28*, 19S–21S. [CrossRef]
39. Goupell, M.J.; Stoelb, C.A.; Kan, A.; Litovsky, R.Y. The Effect of Simulated Interaural Frequency Mismatch on Speech Understanding and Spatial Release From Masking. *Ear Hear.* **2018**, *39*, 895–905. [CrossRef]
40. Kan, A.; Litovsky, R.Y.; Goupell, M.J. Effects of interaural pitch matching and auditory image centering on binaural sensitivity in cochlear implant users. *Ear Hear.* **2015**, *36*, e62–e68. [CrossRef]
41. Kan, A.; Goupell, M.J.; Litovsky, R.Y. Effect of channel separation and interaural mismatch on fusion and lateralization in normal-hearing and cochlear-implant listeners. *J. Acoust. Soc. Am.* **2019**, *146*, 1448. [CrossRef] [PubMed]
42. Kan, A.; Stoelb, C.; Litovsky, R.Y.; Goupell, M.J. Effect of mismatched place-of-stimulation on binaural fusion and lateralization in bilateral cochlear-implant users. *J. Acoust. Soc. Am.* **2013**, *134*, 2923–2936. [CrossRef] [PubMed]
43. Goupell, M.J.; Stoelb, C.; Kan, A.; Litovsky, R.Y. Effect of mismatched place-of-stimulation on the salience of binaural cues in conditions that simulate bilateral cochlear-implant listening. *J. Acoust. Soc. Am.* **2013**, *133*, 2272–2287. [CrossRef] [PubMed]
44. Murphy, J.; Summerfield, A.Q.; O'Donoghue, G.M.; Moore, D.R. Spatial hearing of normally hearing and cochlear implanted children. *Int. J. Pediatr. Otorhinolaryngol.* **2011**, *75*, 489–494. [CrossRef] [PubMed]
45. Dorman, M.F.; Loiselle, L.H.; Cook, S.J.; Yost, W.A.; Gifford, R.H. Sound Source Localization by Normal-Hearing Listeners, Hearing-Impaired Listeners and Cochlear Implant Listeners. *Audiol. Neurootol.* **2016**, *21*, 127–131. [CrossRef]
46. Laback, B.; Egger, K.; Majdak, P. Perception and coding of interaural time differences with bilateral cochlear implants. *Hear. Res.* **2015**, *322*, 138–150. [CrossRef]
47. Loiselle, L.H.; Dorman, M.F.; Yost, W.A.; Cook, S.J.; Gifford, R.H. Using ILD or ITD Cues for Sound Source Localization and Speech Understanding in a Complex Listening Environment by Listeners with Bilateral and with Hearing-Preservation Cochlear Implants. *J. Speech Lang. Hear. Res.* **2016**, *59*, 810–818. [CrossRef]
48. Morton, C.C.; Nance, W.E. Newborn Hearing Screening—A Silent Revolution. *N. Engl. J. Med.* **2006**, *354*, 2151–2164. [CrossRef]
49. Smith, R.J.H.; Bale, J.F.; White, K.R. Sensorineural hearing loss in children. *Lancet* **2005**, *365*, 879–890. [CrossRef]
50. Morrongiello, B.A.; Rocca, P.T. Infants' localization of sounds in the horizontal plane: Effects of auditory and visual cues. *Child Dev.* **1987**, *58*, 918–927. [CrossRef]
51. Bennett, E.E.; Litovsky, R.Y. Sound Localization in Toddlers with Normal Hearing and with Bilateral Cochlear Implants Revealed through a Novel "Reaching for Sound" Task. *J. Am. Acad. Audiol.* **2020**, *31*, 195–208. [CrossRef]
52. Grieco-Calub, T.M.; Litovsky, R.Y. Sound localization skills in children who use bilateral cochlear implants and in children with normal acoustic hearing. *Ear Hear.* **2010**, *31*, 645–656. [CrossRef]

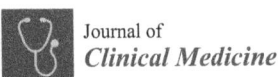

Article

Robot-Assisted Electrode Insertion in Cochlear Implantation Controlled by Intraoperative Electrocochleography— A Pilot Study

Wojciech Gawęcki [1,2,*], Andrzej Balcerowiak [2], Paulina Podlawska [2], Patrycja Borowska [2], Renata Gibasiewicz [2], Witold Szyfter [2] and Małgorzata Wierzbicka [2,3]

1 Department of Otolaryngology and Laryngological Oncology, Poznan University of Medical Sciences, 60-355 Poznan, Poland
2 Department of Otolaryngology and Laryngological Oncology, Heliodor Swiecicki Clinical Hospital, 60-355 Poznan, Poland
3 Institute of Human Genetics, Polish Academy of Sciences, 60-479 Poznan, Poland
* Correspondence: wojgaw@interia.pl; Tel.: +48-61-8691-387

Abstract: Robotics in otology has been developing in many directions for more than two decades. Current clinical trials focus on more accurate stapes surgery, minimally invasive access to the cochlea and less traumatic insertion of cochlear implant (CI) electrode arrays. In this study we evaluated the use of the RobOtol® (Collin, Bagneux, France) otologic robot to insert CI electrodes into the inner ear with intraoperative ECochG analysis. This prospective, pilot study included two adult patients implanted with Advanced Bionics (Westinghouse PI, CA, USA) cochlear implant, with HiFocus™ Mid-Scala electrode array. The standard surgical approach was used. For both subjects, who had residual hearing in the implanted ear, intraoperative and postoperative ECochG was performed with the AIM™ system. The surgeries were uneventful. A credible ECochG response was obtained after complete electrode insertion in both cases. Preoperative BC thresholds compared to intraoperative estimated ECochG thresholds and 2-day postoperative BC thresholds had similar values at frequencies where all thresholds were measurable. The results of the ECochG performed one month after the surgery showed that in both patients the hearing residues were preserved for the selected frequencies. The RobOtol® surgical robot allows for the correct, safe and gentle insertion of the cochlear implant electrode inside the cochlea. The use of electrocochleography measurements during robotic cochlear implantation offers an additional opportunity to evaluate and modify the electrode array insertion on an ongoing basis, which may contribute to the preservation of residual hearing.

Keywords: cochlear implant; robot; residual hearing; electrocochleography

1. Introduction

Robotics in otology has overtaken other fields of head and neck surgery and has been developing in many directions for more than two decades. Robots for otology can be classified as collaborative when intervention is constrained by the robot but the surgeon directly actuates the end-effector, teleoperated when a remotely controlled robot enables the tremor reduction, or autonomous when the surgeon monitors the robot performing a task [1–3]. Current clinical trials focus on more accurate stapes surgery, minimally invasive access to the cochlea and less traumatic insertion of cochlear implant (CI) electrode arrays. A robot-based holder may combine the benefits of endoscopic exposure with a two-handed technique. Robot-assisted endoscopy is a safe and trustworthy tool for several categories of middle ear procedures, such as myringoplasty, partial ossiculoplasty and total ossiculoplasty [4,5]. Robot-assisted manipulation of the ossicular chain in cadaveric temporal bones using a robotic arm (RobOtol®) was described as reliable [6]. Otosclerosis surgery with robotic assistance enhances the precise amplitude of motion and the surgeon's dexterity and rapidly reduces the learning curve [7]. Moreover, the surgical simulator has been developed to plan new procedures that exploit the robot's capacities, enhancing gesture accuracy and allowing exploration of new procedures for middle ear surgery [8].

Robot-assisted cochlear implantation is the result of over a decade of research & development work but is still in its childhood era [9,10]. Successful hearing rehabilitation with a CI is a complex, multi-stage process. "Clinical Practice Guidelines" are widely accepted for the standardization of such processes; however, there is still room for refining the diagnostic and technical steps for optimal results, which is where robotic surgery comes in [11]. As the first device to obtain European certification for clinical use (CE mark), the RobOtol® system has been used in France and China since 2019 for robotic-assisted CI in profoundly deaf adults and children [5,6,12]. The beginning of research dates back to 2005, the commercial launch of RobOtol® on the market in 2018 and soon after, in 2019, the first robotic cochlear implantation at the APHP Pitié-Salpêtrière Department took place. Recently the robotic system has been implemented in clinical practice [6,12–14] and the assumption was optimization of the electrode array insertion into the scala tympani (ST). The subject of discussion and the key question is how to compare and how to measure the superiority of a robotic electrode insertion over a manual one. This was performed based on the analysis of retrospective (manual insertion) and prospective (robotic) pair-matched patients based on imaging studies and on the results of speech rehabilitation [12–14].

One method of accurately assessment of electrode array placement in the cochlea is intracochlear electrocochleography (ECochG) [15,16]. Intracochlear ECochG is also a promising method for pre-curved electrodes [17]. In general, ECochG is a measurement technique based on recording electrical potentials generated by the inner ear and auditory nerve in response to acoustically evoked stimulation [18]. Contrary to the well-known and described standard extracochlear ECochG measurement techniques that require the use of surface electrodes, trans-tympanic or extra-tympanic electrodes, in intracochlear ECochG measurement application, the CI electrode array is used as the measuring electrode [17]. The ECochG response to low-frequency tone burst stimulus is mainly composed of the cochlear microphonic (CM) and the auditory nerve neurophonic (ANN) [19]. The CM is derived from the stereocilia of the outer hearing cells and follows the stimulus waveform [20]. The ANN is the electric potential correlate of phase-locking in the auditory nerve [19]. Therefore, monitoring of extracted CM electrical potentials allows indirect insight into the inner ear's micromechanical activity and provides data for assessing electrode insertion trauma during the electrode array insertion and after cochlear implantation at subsequent follow-ups. Previous work has also demonstrated that ECochG recordings correlate with postoperative pure-tone thresholds in subjects with sensorineural hearing loss [21]. Additionally, CI recipients who show preserved residual hearing perform better than those without postoperative hearing [22].

Thus, we evaluated the use of the RobOtol® otologic robot to insert CI electrodes into the inner ear with intraoperative ECochG (iECochG) analysis. The objective of the study was to clarify how the iECochG can improve the robotic cochlear electrode array insertion.

2. Materials and Methods

2.1. Study Design and Patients

This prospective, pilot study included two adult patients (females, aged 57 and 61 years) who underwent cochlear implantation in a tertiary referral center. Robot-assisted cochlear implantations were performed on 12–13 July 2022. The surgeries were preceded by surgical training on an artificial temporal bone (Figure 1). The patients had passed the typical procedure for qualifying for a cochlear implant at our center before surgery. Both patients had residual hearing in the implanted ear (Figure 2). The preoperative CT of the temporal bone (Siemens, Somatom Definition Edge, Munich, Germany) showed normal anatomy of the ear qualified for cochlear implantation in the both cases (case 1–right ear, case 2–left ear) (Figure 3). The patients provided informed, written consent for their participation in the study and the publication of its findings. The study was approved by the local Bioethics Committee (decision number 1033/19).

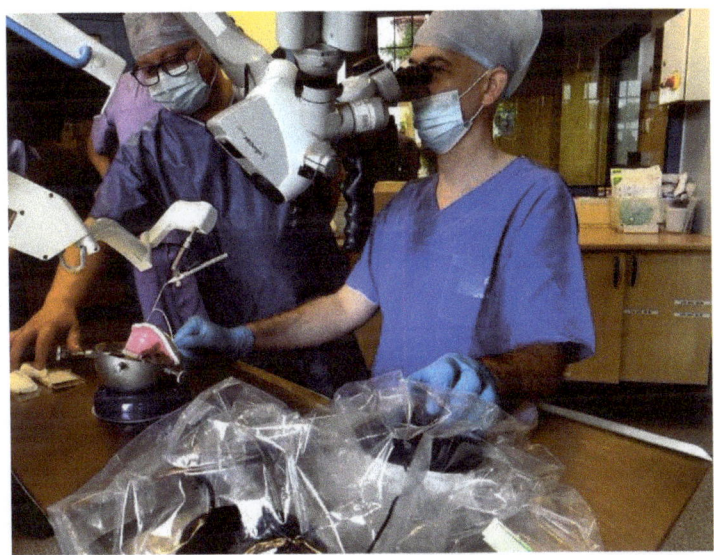

Figure 1. Surgical training with RobOtol® on artificial temporal bone.

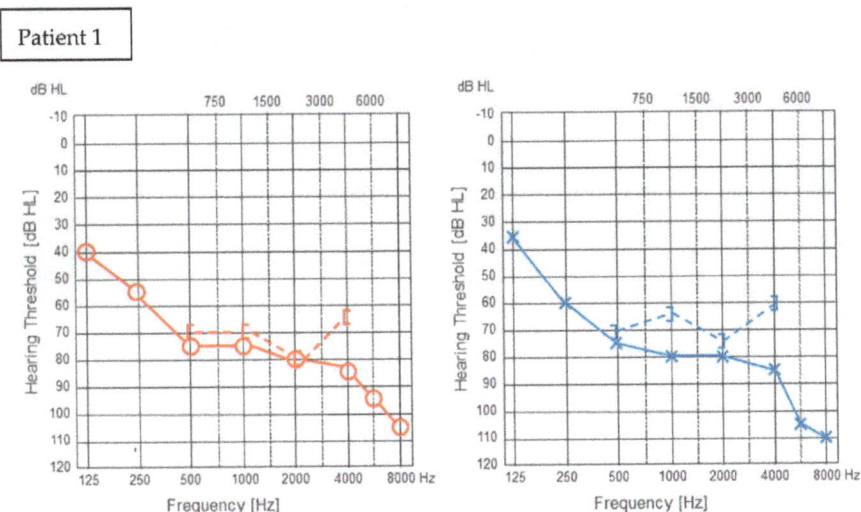

Figure 2. *Cont.*

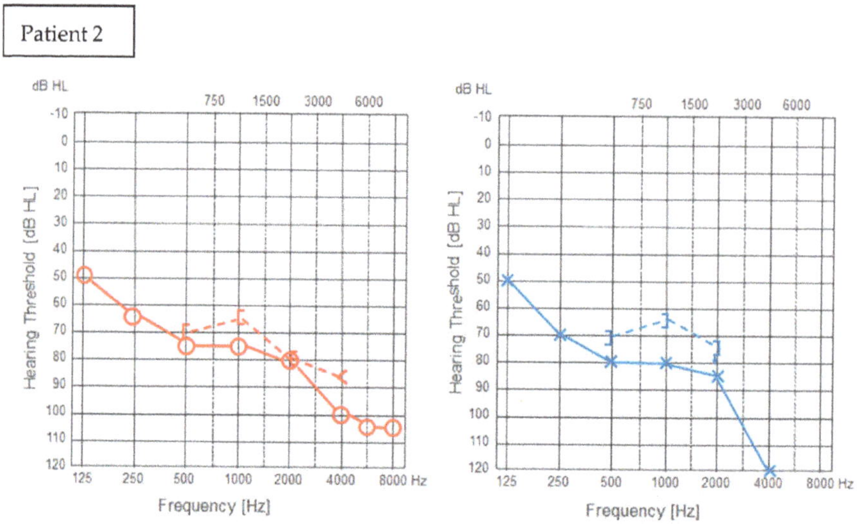

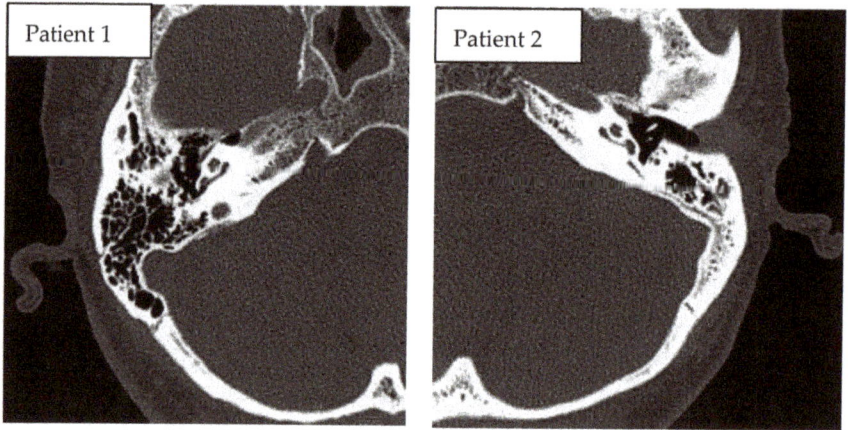

Figure 2. Preoperative audiograms of the patients.

Figure 3. Preoperative CT of temporal bones of the patients, both cases with normal anatomy of the temporal bone.

2.2. Types of Device and Electrode Arrays

Both patients had chosen the Advanced Bionics cochlear implant and the same type of electrode array was inserted: HiFocus™ Mid-Scala electrode array. This pre-curved electrode array has an active length of 15.5 mm and 16 electrodes.

2.3. Robot-Assisted Electrode Array Insertion

The surgeries were performed with the use of RobOtol® (Collin, Bagneux, France). The RobOtol® arm was controlled by the surgeon using a SpaceMouse® (3DConnexion, Waltham, MA, USA). The speed of the robotic arm could be switched between three gears (high speed: 10 mm/s; medium speed: 2 mm/s; low speed: 0.1–1 mm/s). Before the robot-assisted procedure, RobOtol® was sterile covered, moved into the optimal surgical position and then the Boglock sterilized connector (Collin, Bagneux, France; AB Mid-Scala: RBT-0406) was set on the arm. The internal coil of CI was inserted into the subperiosteal pocket and the transducer was positioned in the bone bed and fixed with surgical thread. Then Mid-Scala array was positioned on the insertion tool previously attached to the dedicated connector and the prepared set was coupled to the robot arm by Boglock.

2.4. Surgical Technique

The cochlear implantations were performed by the senior otologist (WG). The same standard surgical approach was used in both cases (via mastoidectomy and posterior tympanotomy). The electrode array was inserted through the round window in the first patient and through the cochleostomy in the second (due to the poorly visible round window).

2.5. Cochlear Implant System Activation

The cochlear implant system's initial activation was carried out one month after the CI surgery.

2.6. Electrophysiological Measurements

Typical electrophysiological measurements were performed during surgery (impedances of the electrodes and neural response telemetry) and at initial system activation (impedances of the electrodes). Additionally, intraoperative and postoperative monitoring of CM electrical potentials (ECochG) was performed.

2.7. ECochG Measurement

Intraoperative and postoperative ECochG measurements were performed with the Advanced Bionics Active Insertion Monitoring AIM^{TM} system. The system consists of the AIM System tablet, Naida CI Q90 sound processor, headpiece, cables, insert earphone and sterile inserts with an acoustic tube. Surgical preparation for the measurement was performed according to the AIM^{TM} system Intra-Operative Guide. During electrode array insertion, a 50 ms tone burst stimulus (500 Hz) of alternating polarity was delivered at 115 dB SPL via the external ear canal with sterile inserts and an acoustic tube. The ECochG responses were recorded with the apical-most electrode contact. The acoustic feedback on changes in ECochG magnitude during the electrode array insertion was automatically provided to the surgeon. The AIM system schematic block system diagram is presented in Figure 4.

After full electrode array insertion, the ECochG responses were recorded with selected active electrode contacts to assess estimated pure-tone thresholds at audiometric frequencies in the 125–4000 Hz range. For this purpose, implemented in the device, an automatic algorithm of the ECochG signal detection and associated gradually decreasing tone burst stimulus were used (subsequently referred to in the text as the estimated audiogram measurement). The same procedure was repeated during the initial system activation.

2.8. Imaging

CT of the temporal bone (Siemens, Somatom Definition Edge, Munich, Germany) was performed the day after surgery to confirm the proper position of the electrode.

2.9. Pure-Tone Audiometry

The pure-tone audiometry measurements (Interacoustics AC40) were performed preoperatively and postoperatively to assess air conduction (AC) and bone conduction (BC) thresholds in line with ISO 8253–1:2010 standards in selected periods, no earlier than one month before surgery (AC and BC thresholds), two days after the surgery (BC thresholds only), and 1-month after the surgery (AC and BC thresholds).

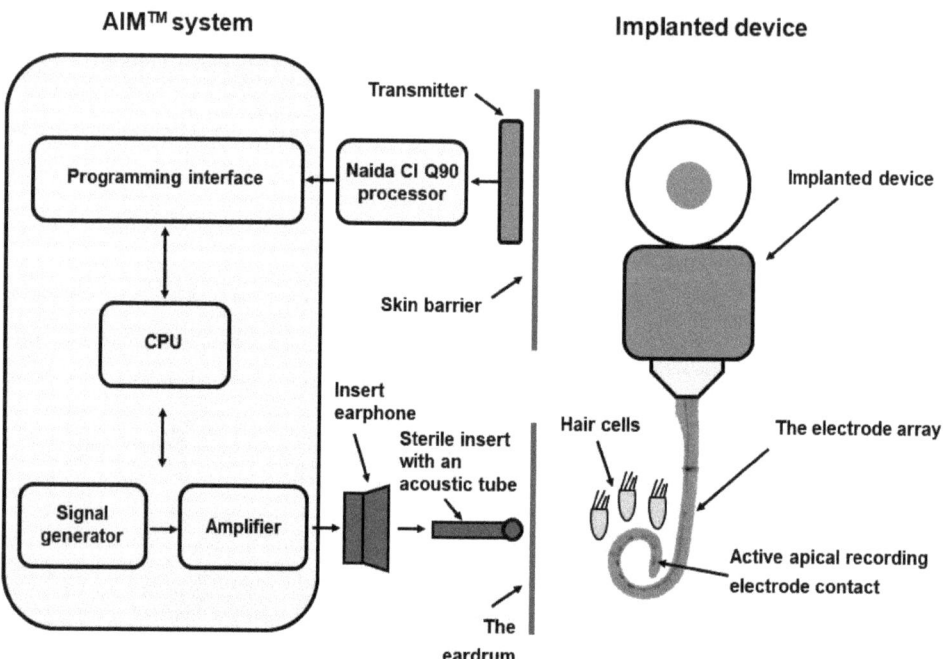

Figure 4. The AIM system schematic block diagram.

3. Results

3.1. Intraoperative Course

The surgery was uneventful for both patients. The approach to the cochlea was typically completed-by antro-mastoidectomy and posterior tympanotomy. The bone bed for the transducer was drilled. The cochlea was opened by the round window in the first patient and by performing cochleostomy (due to poor visibility of the round window) in the second. The internal coil of CI was inserted into the subperiosteal pocket and the transducer was positioned in the bone bed and fixed with surgical thread. Then the insertion tool was connected to a dedicated connector and coupled for a moment to the robot arm by Boglock (Collin, Bagneux, France; AB Mid-Scala: RBT-0406) to confirm the optimal position of the robot arm (Figure 5), and then decoupled. In the next stage, the Mid-Scala array was positioned on the insertion tool and connected to the robot (Figure 6). The electrode was moved directly to the cochlear opening and slowly inserted to the first blue marker using a robot (Figure 7). Further insertion was carried out by hand with a slider on the insertion tool. However, the stable position of the tool allowed for a very slow and gentle insertion. Moreover, it was possible to stop the electrode insertion and keep it in one position for a few or even several seconds if the ECochG potential decreased. What is more, the insertion axis of the electrode array was slightly modified when iECochG potentials decreased in case one, which improved the iECochG results. The full insertion (till the second blue marker) was carried out in both cases. Then the intraoperative measurements were completed. The connecting cable to the electrode was positioned in the antro-mastoidectomy and the wound was typically closed.

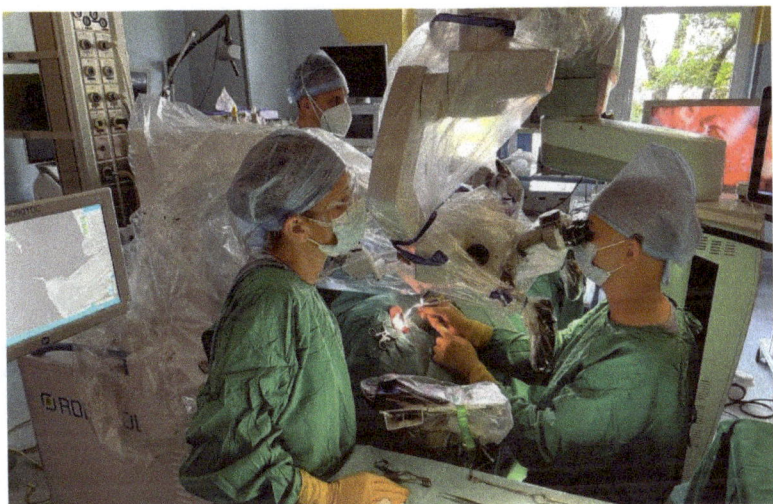

Figure 5. The RobOtol® system is ready to use. The insertion tool is attached to a dedicated connector and coupled to the robot arm by Boglock to confirm the optimal position of the robot arm.

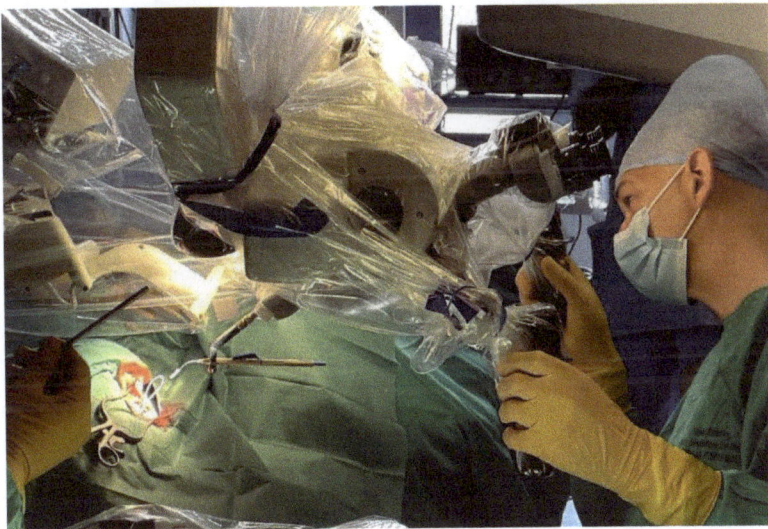

Figure 6. The Mid-Scala array is positioned on the insertion tool and connected to the robot. The system is ready for electrode array insertion.

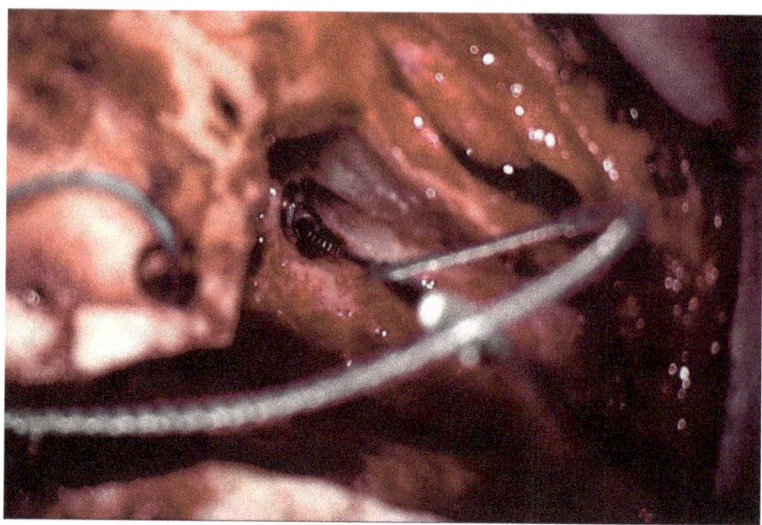

Figure 7. The electrode array insertion via typical (antromastoidectomy and facial recess) approach with a RobOtol® (case 1).

3.2. Intraoperative Electrocochleography

The results of intraoperative ECochG measurements are presented in Figure 8. The ECochG responses reflected the electro-mechanical activity of the inner ear on acoustic stimulation during the insertion of the electrode array into the cochlea. Ideally, the signal amplitude is expected to increase to some extent as the electrode array's most apical electrode contacts approach the cochlea's signal source. After bypassing the hair cells, which are probably responsible for the generated signal, the amplitude should gradually decrease with distance from this site. In fact, every movement of the electrode array can cause substantial disturbance in the micromechanical characteristic of the inner ear. Figure 8 shows the ECochG signal waveforms recorded for the two subjects who underwent CI surgery supported with the AIM system measurement. The observed changes in the amplitude of the ECochG signal are presumably results of electrode movement toward the cochlea, unintentional and unpredictable physical contact of the basilar membrane with the electrode array, slight movement of the robotic arm and surgeon's hand, as well as the implemented measurement technique. The maximum value of the recorded signal may vary for each subject. A credible ECochG response is considered to exceed 3 µV (internal noise of the implantable system does not exceed around 1 µV). The ECochG response was above the mentioned value after complete electrode insertion in both cases.

3.3. Imaging

The post-operative CT confirmed the intracochlear position of the electrode arrays (with the tip of the electrode array in the medial turn of the cochlea) in both patients (Figure 9).

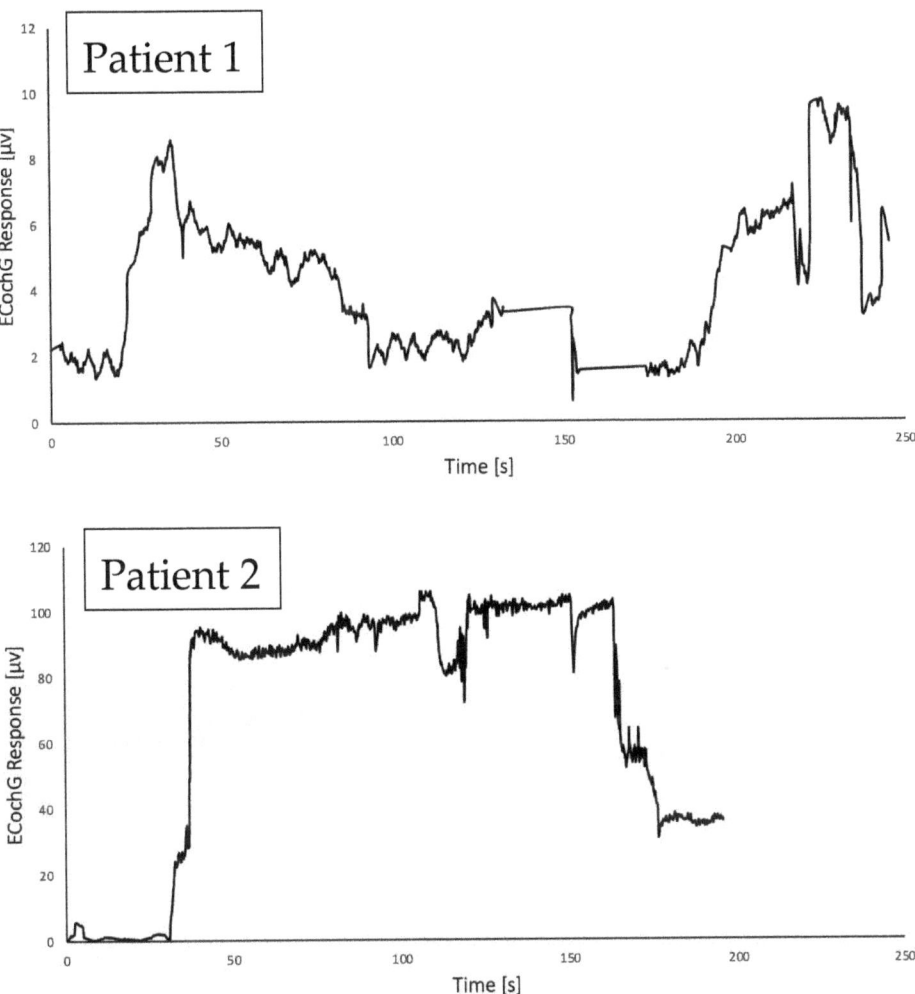

Figure 8. The intraoperative ECochG response measurements for patient 1 and patient 2.

3.4. Pure Tone Audiometry and the Estimated Audiogram

The results of pure tone audiometry and the estimated audiograms are presented in Figure 10. Preoperative BC thresholds compared to intraoperative estimated ECochG thresholds and 2-day postoperative BC thresholds had similar values at frequencies where all thresholds were measurable. However, for patient 1 the estimated threshold for 250 Hz seems an outlier (80 dB HL vs. 55 and 50 dB HL). The results of the ECochG performed one month after the surgery showed that in both patients the hearing residues were preserved for the selected frequencies. Moreover, in patient 2, the pure-tone audiometry results confirmed the maintenance of postoperative auditory thresholds for most frequencies.

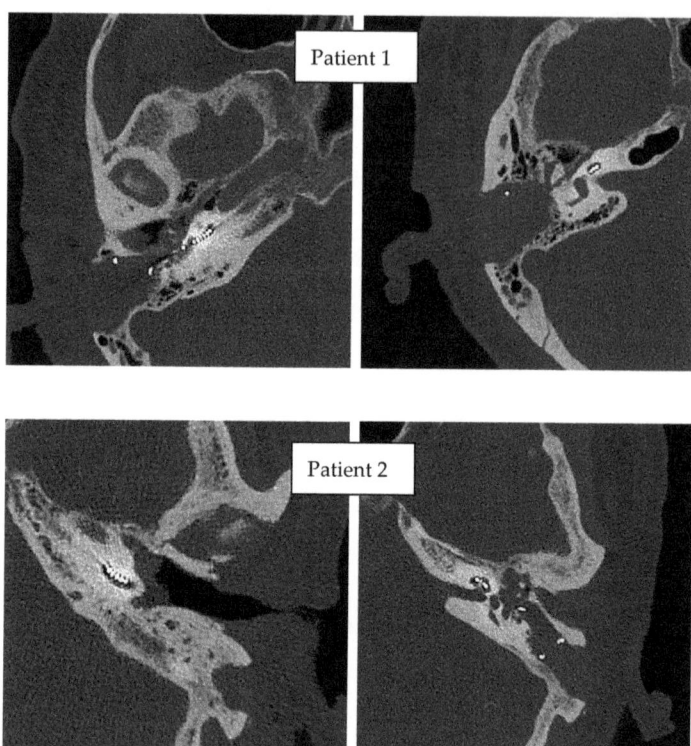

Figure 9. Postoperative CT scans of operated patients.

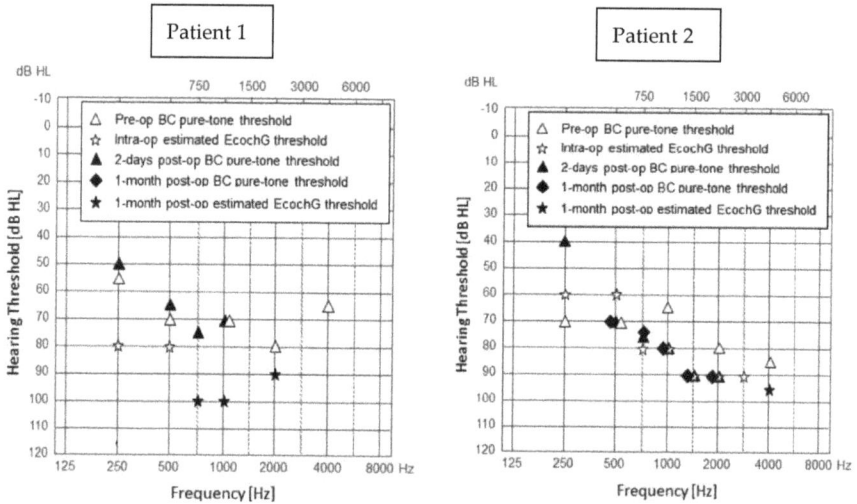

Figure 10. The patients' preoperative BC thresholds (triangles), intraoperative estimated ECochG thresholds (asterisks), 1-month postoperative estimated ECochG threshold (solid asterisks), postoperative BC thresholds after 2 days (solid triangles) and 1 month (solid diamonds).

4. Discussion

Cochlear implantation can benefit from robotic assistance in several steps of the surgical procedure: (i) the approach to the middle ear by automated mastoidectomy and posterior tympanotomy or through a tunnel from the postauricular skin to the middle ear (i.e., direct cochlear access); (ii) a minimally invasive cochleostomy by a robot-assisted drilling tool; (iii) alignment of the correct insertion axis on the basal cochlear turn; (iv) insertion of the electrode array with a motorized insertion tool [10]. Currently, there are four systems for clinical robotic cochlear implantation available. Three of them, Microtable® (Vanderbilt), HEARO® (Bern) and ROSA® (Amiens), are used for direct cochlear access but the number of cases implanted with these devices is still very limited [10,23–26]. The fourth system (RobOtol®) is not intended for drilling, but for robotic alignment of the electrode array and its insertion into the scala tympani. This system is clinically used in many European countries, mainly France and in China. More than 250 cochlear implantations with this system have been performed, both in adults and children [10,27–29].

The primary assumption of introducing RobOtol® was to optimize the electrode array insertion into the scala tympani and preserve the anatomical structures of the cochlea, which can have many benefits, mainly in patients with residual hearing. It was supposed to have an effect in better hearing if damage to the basilar membrane is avoided and residual hearing preservation is possible [30]. Currently, the RobOtol® can be used with many straight electrodes: SlimJ (Advanced Bionics), 522 and 622 (Cochlear), Flex (Medel), Evo (Oticon) and with one perimodiolar electrode–MidScala (Advanced Bionics) [5,6,9,13,14,28]. The system shows its advantage in eliminating human involuntary tremors and augmenting accuracy during micromanipulation. It can safely assist cochlear implantation to realize minimally invasive and full tympanic scala insertion of the electrode array and to ensure the preservation of the fine intracochlear structure [12]. Despite the promising results in laboratory tests in terms of minimal invasiveness, reduced trauma and better hearing preservation, so far, no clinical benefits on residual hearing preservation or better speech performance have been demonstrated [10]. It is emphasized that new robotic insertion tools should be provided with loop feedback systems capable of modifying the insertion parameters based on both insertion forces and ECochG responses. A preliminary study in vivo sheep model tested the feasibility of an ECochG-guided robotics-assisted CI insertion system [31].

The main goal of our study was to show the application of robotic electrode insertion with simultaneous iECochG measurements, which constituted intraoperative control. We wanted to clarify how the iECochG can improve the robotic cochlear electrode array insertion. To the best of our knowledge, the association between an innovative method of supporting CI surgery and an equally current method of tracking the intraoperative effect has not been published so far. During the electrode insertion with a RobOtol® in our patients with residual hearing, the continuous measurements of ECochG responses were recorded and the insertion speed and axis were constantly modified. For example, electrode insertion was slowed down or interrupted and the insertion axis of the electrode array was modified as the ECochG potential decreased. Perhaps thanks to this, we have managed to partially preserve residual hearing, confirmed by estimated audiograms at the end of the surgeries and during the system's activation and by measuring bone conduction thresholds by pure tone audiometry. However, our patients require longer follow-ups and subsequent measurements to explain the differences between obtained results and long-term effects.

Study Limitations

In this work, we wanted to show the possibilities of combining robotic surgery of cochlear implants with electrocochleographic measurement. However, we are aware of the limitations of our work, i.e., a small number of patients and a short observation time.

5. Conclusions

The RobOtol® surgical robot allows for the correct, safe and gentle insertion of the cochlear implant electrode inside the cochlea. The use of electrocochleography measurements during robotic cochlear implantation offers an additional opportunity to evaluate and modify the electrode array insertion on an ongoing basis, which may contribute to the preservation of residual hearing.

Author Contributions: Conceptualization, W.G. and M.W.; methodology, W.G. and A.B.; formal analysis, W.G., P.P. and P.B.; investigation, W.G., A.B., P.B. and R.G.; data curation, W.G., P.P. and P.B.; writing—original draft preparation, W.G., P.P. and M.W.; writing—review and editing, W.G., A.B., R.G. and M.W.; visualization, A.B. and P.B.; supervision, W.S. and M.W.; project administration, W.S. and M.W. All authors have read and agreed to the published version of the manuscript.

Funding: This research received no external funding.

Institutional Review Board Statement: The study was conducted in accordance with the Declaration of Helsinki and approved by the local Ethics Committee of Poznan University of Medical Sciences (decision number 1033/19, date of approval 7 November 2019).

Informed Consent Statement: Informed consent was obtained from all subjects involved in the study.

Data Availability Statement: The data presented in this study are available on request from the corresponding author.

Acknowledgments: We would like to thank Łukasz Olszewski (affiliated at Advanced Bionics, Poland) for his invaluable input to the present study. His contribution included support for electrocochleography measurements and preparation of several figures.

Conflicts of Interest: The authors declare no conflict of interest.

References

1. Bell, B.; Gerber, N.; Williamson, T.; Gavaghan, K.; Wimmer, W.; Caversaccio, M.; Weber, S. In vitro accuracy evaluation of image-guided robot system for direct cochlear access. *Otol. Neurotol.* **2013**, *34*, 1284–1290. [CrossRef] [PubMed]
2. Kratchman, L.B.; Blachon, G.S.; Withrow, T.J.; Balachandran, R.; Labadie, R.F.; Webster, R.J., 3rd. Design of a bone attached parallel robot for percutaneous cochlear implantation. *IEEE Trans. Biomed. Eng.* **2011**, *58*, 2904–2910. [CrossRef]
3. Riojas, K.E.; Labadie, R.F. Robotic Ear Surgery. *Otolaryngol. Clin. N. Am.* **2020**, *53*, 1065–1075. [CrossRef] [PubMed]
4. Veleur, M.; Lahlou, G.; Torres, R.; Daoudi, H.; Mosnier, I.; Ferrary, E.; Sterkers, O.; Nguyen, Y. Robot-Assisted Middle Ear Endoscopic Surgery: Preliminary Results on 37 Patients. *Front. Surg.* **2021**, *8*, 740935. [CrossRef] [PubMed]
5. Vittoria, S.; Lahlou, G.; Torres, R.; Daoudi, H.; Mosnier, I.; Mazalaigue, S.; Ferrary, E.; Nguyen, Y.; Sterkers, O. Robot-based assistance in middle ear surgery and cochlear implantation: First clinical report. *Eur. Arch. Oto-Rhino-Laryngol.* **2021**, *278*, 77–85. [CrossRef]
6. Daoudi, H.; Torres, R.; Mazalaigue, S.; Sterkers, O.; Ferrary, E.; Nguyen, Y. Analysis of forces during robot-assisted and manual manipulations of mobile and fixed footplate in temporal bone specimens. *Eur. Arch. Oto-Rhino-Laryngol.* **2021**, *278*, 4269–4277. [CrossRef]
7. Nguyen, Y.; Bernardeschi, D.; Sterkers, O. Potential of Robot-Based Surgery for Otosclerosis Surgery. *Otolaryngol. Clin. N. Am* **2018**, *51*, 475–485. [CrossRef]
8. Kazmitcheff, G.; Nguyen, Y.; Miroir, M.; Péan, F.; Ferrary, E.; Cotin, S.; Sterkers, O.; Duriez, C. Middle-ear microsurgery simulation to improve new robotic procedures. *BioMed Res. Int.* **2014**, *2014*, 891742. [CrossRef]
9. Panara, K.; Shahal, D.; Mittal, R.; Eshraghi, A.A. Robotics for Cochlear Implantation Surgery: Challenges and Opportunities. *Otol. Neurotol.* **2021**, *42*, e825–e835. [CrossRef]
10. De Seta, D.; Daoudi, H.; Torres, R.; Ferrary, E.; Sterkers, O.; Nguyen, Y. Robotics, automation, active electrode arrays, and new devices for cochlear implantation: A contemporary review. *Hear. Res.* **2022**, *414*, 108425. [CrossRef]
11. Loth, A.; Vazzana, C.; Leinung, M.; Guderian, D.; Issing, C.; Baumann, U.; Stöver, T. Quality control in cochlear implant therapy: Clinical practice guidelines and registries in European countries. *Eur. Arch. Oto-Rhino-Laryngol.* **2022**, *279*, 4779–4786. [CrossRef] [PubMed]
12. Jia, H.; Pan, J.X.; Li, Y.; Zhang, Z.H.; Tan, H.Y.; Wang, Z.Y.; Wu, H. Preliminary application of robot-assisted electrode insertion in cochlear implantation. *Zhonghua Er Bi Yan Hou Tou Jing Wai Ke Za Zhi Chin. J. Otorhinolaryngol. Head Neck Surg.* **2020**, *55*, 952–956. (In Chinese) [CrossRef]
13. Torres, R.; Daoudi, H.; Lahlou, G.; Sterkers, O.; Ferrary, E.; Mosnier, I.; Nguyen, Y. Restoration of High Frequency Auditory Perception After Robot-Assisted or Manual Cochlear Implantation in Profoundly Deaf Adults Improves Speech Recognition. *Front. Surg.* **2021**, *8*, 729736. [CrossRef] [PubMed]

14. Torres, R.; Hochet, B.; Daoudi, H.; Carré, F.; Mosnier, I.; Sterkers, O.; Ferrary, E.; Nguyen, Y. Atraumatic Insertion of a Cochlear Implant Pre-Curved Electrode Array by a Robot-Automated Alignment with the Coiling Direction of the Scala Tympani. *Audiol. Neurootol.* **2022**, *27*, 148–155. [CrossRef] [PubMed]
15. Giardina, C.K.; Brown, K.D.; Adunka, O.F.; Buchman, C.A.; Hutson, K.A.; Pillsbury, H.C.; Fitzpatrick, D.C. Intracochlear Electrocochleography: Response Patterns During Cochlear Implantation and Hearing Preservation. *Ear Hear.* **2019**, *40*, 833–848. [CrossRef]
16. Buechner, A.; Bardt, M.; Haumann, S.; Geissler, G.; Salcher, R.; Lenarz, T. Clinical experiences with intraoperative electrocochleography in cochlear implant recipients and its potential to reduce insertion trauma and improve postoperative hearing preservation. *PLoS ONE* **2022**, *17*, e0266077. [CrossRef] [PubMed]
17. Koka, K.; Riggs, W.J.; Dwyer, R.; Holder, J.T.; Noble, J.H.; Dawant, B.M.; Ortmann, A.; Valenzuela, C.V.; Mattingly, J.K.; Harris, M.M.; et al. Intra-Cochlear Electrocochleography During Cochear Implant Electrode Insertion Is Predictive of Final Scalar Location. *Otol. Neurotol.* **2018**, *39*, e654–e659. [CrossRef] [PubMed]
18. Pienkowski, M.; Adunka, O.F.; Lichtenhan, J.T. Editorial: New Advances in Electrocochleography for Clinical and Basic Investigation. *Front. Neurosci.* **2018**, *12*, 310. [CrossRef] [PubMed]
19. Riggs, W.J.; Roche, J.P.; Giardina, C.K.; Harris, M.S.; Bastian, Z.J.; Fontenot, T.E.; Buchman, C.A.; Brown, K.D.; Adunka, O.F.; Fitzpatrick, D.C. Intraoperative Electrocochleographic Characteristics of Auditory Neuropathy Spectrum Disorder in Cochlear Implant Subjects. *Front. Neurosci.* **2017**, *11*, 416. [CrossRef] [PubMed]
20. Harris, M.S.; Riggs, W.J.; Giardina, C.K.; O'Connell, B.P.; Holder, J.T.; Dwyer, R.T.; Koka, K.; Labadie, R.F.; Fitzpatrick, D.C.; Adunka, O.F. Patterns Seen During Electrode Insertion Using Intracochlear Electrocochleography Obtained Directly Through a Cochlear Implant. *Otol. Neurotol.* **2017**, *38*, 1415–1420. [CrossRef] [PubMed]
21. Attias, J.; Ulanovski, D.; Hilly, O.; Greenstein, T.; Sokolov, M.; HabibAllah, S.; Mormer, H.; Raveh, E. Postoperative Intracochlear Electrocochleography in Pediatric Cochlear Implant Recipients: Association to Audiometric Thresholds and Auditory Performance. *Ear Hear.* **2020**, *41*, 1135–1143. [CrossRef] [PubMed]
22. O'Connell, B.P.; Holder, J.T.; Dwyer, R.T.; Gifford, R.H.; Noble, J.H.; Bennett, M.L.; Rivas, A.; Wanna, G.B.; Haynes, D.S.; Labadie, R.F. Intra- and Postoperative Electrocochleography May Be Predictive of Final Electrode Position and Postoperative Hearing Preservation. *Front. Neurosci.* **2017**, *11*, 291. [CrossRef] [PubMed]
23. Caversaccio, M.; Wimmer, W.; Anso, J.; Mantoukoudis, G.; Gerber, N.; Rathgeb, C.; Schneider, D.; Hermann, J.; Wagner, F.; Scheidegger, O.; et al. Robotic middle ear access for cochlear implantation: First in man. *PLoS ONE* **2019**, *14*, e0220543. [CrossRef] [PubMed]
24. Labadie, R.F.; Balachandran, R.; Noble, J.H.; Blachon, G.S.; Mitchell, J.E.; Reda, F.A.; Dawant, B.M.; Fitzpatrick, J.M. Minimally invasive image-guided cochlear implantation surgery: First report of clinical implementation. *Laryngoscope* **2014**, *124*, 1915–1922. [CrossRef]
25. Labadie, R.F.; Riojas, K.; Von Wahlde, K.; Mitchell, J.; Bruns, T.; Webster, R., 3rd; Dawant, B.; Fitzpatrick, J.M.; Noble, J. Clinical Implementation of Second-generation Minimally Invasive Image-guided Cochlear Implantation Surgery. *Otol. Neurotol.* **2021**, *42*, 702–705. [CrossRef]
26. Klopp-Dutote, N.; Lefranc, M.; Strunski, V.; Page, C. Minimally invasive fully ROBOT-assisted cochlear implantation in humans: Preliminary results in five consecutive patients. *Clin. Otolaryngol.* **2021**, *46*, 1326–1330. [CrossRef]
27. Daoudi, H.; Lahlou, G.; Torres, R.; Sterkers, O.; Lefeuvre, V.; Ferrary, E.; Mosnier, I.; Nguyen, Y. Robot-assisted cochlear implant electrode array insertion in adults: A comparative study with manual insertion. *Otol. Neurotol.* **2021**, *42*, 438–444. [CrossRef]
28. Barriat, S.; Peigneux, N.; Duran, U.; Camby, S.; Lefebvre, P.P. The Use of a Robot to Insert an Electrode Array of Cochlear Implants in the Cochlea: A Feasibility Study and Preliminary Results. *Audiol. Neurootol.* **2021**, *26*, 361–367. [CrossRef]
29. Jia, H.; Pan, J.; Gu, W.; Tan, H.; Chen, Y.; Zhang, Z.; Jiang, M.; Li, Y.; Sterkers, O.; Wu, H. Robot-Assisted Electrode Array Insertion Becomes Available in Pediatric Cochlear Implant Recipients: First Report and an Intra-Individual Study. *Front. Surg.* **2021**, *8*, 695728. [CrossRef]
30. Gifford, R.H.; Dorman, M.F.; Skarzynski, H.; Lorens, A.; Polak, M.; Driscoll, C.L.W.; Peter Roland, P.; Buchman, C.A. Cochlear implantation with hearing preservation yields significant benefit for speech recognition in complex listening environments. *Ear Hear.* **2013**, *34*, 413–425. [CrossRef]
31. Henslee, A.M.; Kaufmann, C.R.; Andrick, M.D.; Reineke, P.T.; Tejani, V.D.; Hansen, M.R. Development and Characterization of an Electrocochleography-Guided Robotics-Assisted Cochlear Implant Array Insertion System. *Otolaryngol. Head Neck Surg.* **2022**, *167*, 334–340. [CrossRef] [PubMed]

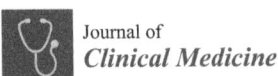

Article

Cochlear Implant Stimulation Parameters Play a Key Role in Reducing Facial Nerve Stimulation

Lutz Gärtner [1], Bradford C. Backus [2], Nicolas Le Goff [2], Anika Morgenstern [1], Thomas Lenarz [1,3] and Andreas Büchner [1,3,*]

1. Department of Otolaryngology, Hannover Medical School, 30625 Hannover, Germany; gaertner.lutz@mh-hannover.de (L.G.); morgenstern.anika@mh-hannover.de (A.M.); lenarz.thomas@mh-hannover.de (T.L.)
2. Oticon Medical, 06220 Vallauris, France; brba@oticonmedical.com (B.C.B.); nile@oticonmedical.com (N.L.G.)
3. Cluster of Excellence "Hearing4all", 30625 Hannover, Germany
* Correspondence: buechner.andreas@mh-hannover.de; Tel.: +49-511-5328589

Abstract: A percentage (i.e., 5.6%) of Cochlear Implant (CI) users reportedly experience unwanted facial nerve stimulation (FNS). For some, the effort to control this problem results in changing stimulation parameters, thereby reducing their hearing performance. For others, the only viable solution is to deactivate the CI completely. A growing body of evidence in the form of case reports suggests that undesired FNS can be effectively addressed through re-implantation with an Oticon Medical (OM) Neuro-Zti implant. However, the root of this benefit is still unknown: is it due to surgical adjustments, such as varied array geometries and/or positioning, or does it stem from differences in stimulation parameters and/or grounding? The OM device exhibits two distinct features: (1) unique stimulation parameters, including anodic leading pulses and loudness controlled by pulse duration—not current—resulting in lower overall current amplitudes; and (2) unconventional grounding, including both passive (capacitive) discharge, which creates a pseudo-monophasic pulse shape, and a 'distributed-all-polar' (DAP) grounding scheme, which is thought to reduce current spread. Unfortunately, case reports alone cannot distinguish between surgical factors and these implant-related ones. In this paper, we present a novel follow-up study of two CI subjects who previously experienced FNS before re-implantation with Neuro-Zti implants. We used the Oticon Medical Research Platform (OMRP) to stimulate a single electrode in each subject in two ways: (1) with traditional monopolar biphasic cathodic-first pulses, and (2) with distinct OM clinical stimulation. We progressively increased the stimulation intensity until FNS occurred or the sound became excessively loud. Non-auditory/FNS sensations were observed with the traditional stimulation but not with the OM clinical one. This provides the first direct evidence demonstrating that stimulation parameters and/or grounding—not surgical factors—play a key role in mitigating FNS.

Keywords: FNS; facial nerve; CI; cochlear implant; electrode; stimulation parameters; OMRP; Oticon Medical Research Platform

Citation: Gärtner, L.; Backus, B.C.; Le Goff, N.; Morgenstern, A.; Lenarz, T.; Büchner, A. Cochlear Implant Stimulation Parameters Play a Key Role in Reducing Facial Nerve Stimulation. *J. Clin. Med.* **2023**, *12*, 6194. https://doi.org/10.3390/jcm12196194

Academic Editor: Christof Röösli

Received: 26 August 2023
Revised: 18 September 2023
Accepted: 21 September 2023
Published: 25 September 2023

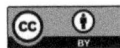

Copyright: © 2023 by the authors. Licensee MDPI, Basel, Switzerland. This article is an open access article distributed under the terms and conditions of the Creative Commons Attribution (CC BY) license (https://creativecommons.org/licenses/by/4.0/).

1. Introduction

Cochlear implants (CIs) are the most successful sensory prosthetic devices developed to date and have revolutionized the world of audiology, offering hope to individuals with severe to profound hearing loss [1–3]. However, while CIs significantly improve auditory perception for many, the technology is not without its challenges. One such issue is the unwanted stimulation of the facial nerve (FNS), a side effect reported in an estimated 5.6% of CI users [4]. FNS can lead to involuntary facial twitching, vertigo, or indistinct pain and thereby impact quality of life. To unlock the benefits of CIs for these individuals, we need to gain a better understanding of the contributing factors that lead to FNS and circumvent them.

Traditionally, FNS in CI users has been managed through the adjustment of stimulation parameters by the audiologist. The most common type of stimulation for cochlear implants consists of biphasic pulses with a leading cathodic phase—a method derived from animal studies, which suggested its superior effectiveness [5,6]. These biphasic pulses are then amplitude modulated based on the time-varying envelope output from the filter linked to the corresponding electrode. The majority of CI manufacturers employ this paradigm. For a more comprehensive overview of CI functionality, readers are directed to [3]. To prevent unpleasant facial nerve stimulation, clinicians often lower the pulse current (and expand the pulse duration) or deactivate troublesome electrodes altogether. However, these methods do not always work, and even when they do, they can compromise CI performance. In severe cases, the CI becomes unusable.

Some CI manufacturers, such as MED-EL (Innsbruck, Austria), offer a 'triphasic' stimulation mode. In this mode, there are 3 pulse phases: (1) a leading cathodic pulse phase; (2) an intermediate anodic phase presented with twice the phase duration; and (3) a final repeated cathodic phase. While this method has shown effectiveness in reducing unwanted FNS for some CI patients [5,6], it does not always work and usually results in reduced battery life.

Emerging evidence from case reports suggests a promising treatment for severe cases is re-implantation with the Oticon Medical (OM) (Smørumnedre, Denmark) Neuro-Zti implant. Re-implantation with this device has been shown to effectively address FNS. However, the reason for this is not yet fully understood. While surgical adjustments such as varying array geometries and positioning may play a role, there are also distinct implant-related attributes to consider. These include the unique stimulation parameters used by OM devices, such as anodic leading pulses, passive capacitive charge return, and their unconventional distributed all-polar (DAP) grounding scheme [7]. Both elements are distinct from other CI systems. Moreover, in the OM device, loudness is not coded by pulse current but rather by pulse duration. Understanding whether the reduced FNS seen in the literature stems from surgical factors or from these implant-related ones will provide valuable insight to further improve CI technology and enhance patient outcomes and quality of life for those suffering from FNS.

This analysis presents a novel follow-up study on two CI subjects who experienced FNS prior to re-implantation with OM Neuro-Zti implants [8] and reveals the reasons why this intervention helped them.

2. Materials and Methods

2.1. Subjects

Two subjects who had previously suffered from FNS during CI stimulation and had been re-implanted with Oticon Medical Neuro-Zti devices [8] were further investigated during a clinical follow-up visit. One of these patients was initially fitted with Advanced Bionics (Valencia, CA, USA) HiRes Ultra 3D implants and a mid-scala electrode in both ears. The other patient had originally been fitted with a MED-EL SYNCHRONY implant with a FLEX28 electrode in one ear.

Our goal was to gain deeper insight into the subjects' behavioral perceptions of different stimuli, with the ultimate aim of further improving their clinical outcomes.

2.2. Stimuli

We used the Oticon Medical Research Platform (OMRP) [9] to directly stimulate single electrodes on the Neuro-Zti Implant in two ways: (1) using stimulus parameters designed to replicate those of their prior CI, and (2) using the parameters of their current clinical CI mode. With Subject S2, we also investigated reversing the polarity of these pulses for a total of 4 stimulus types (Table 1 and Figure 1). All stimuli were presented in a pulse train with a 50% duty cycle (500 ms on and 500 ms off) using pulses presented at a rate of 500 Hz.

Table 1. Stimulus parameters that were used during this study.

Parameter	A− (Clinical)	A+	B+ (Clinical)	B−
charge return	active	active	passive	passive
leading phase	cathodic	anodic	anodic	cathodic
pulse shape	biphasic	biphasic	pseudo-monophasic	pseudo-monophasic
grounding	MP	MP	DAP [2]	DAP [2]
loudness coding	current/duration [1]	current/duration [1]	duration	duration

[1] Subject S1 used duration coding for stimuli A− and B+ (current = 0.6 mA). Subject S2 used duration coding for stimuli B−/B+ (current = 0.4 mA) and current coding for stimuli A+/A− (duration = 30 µs). Note: We improved the software between S1 and S2 to allow current coding. [2] Distributed-all-polar (DAP) [7] indicates that current returns via the case electrode, like MP (monopolar) grounding, and simultaneously to all non-stimulating intra-cochlear electrodes, sometimes called 'common ground' (CG) (Figure 1).

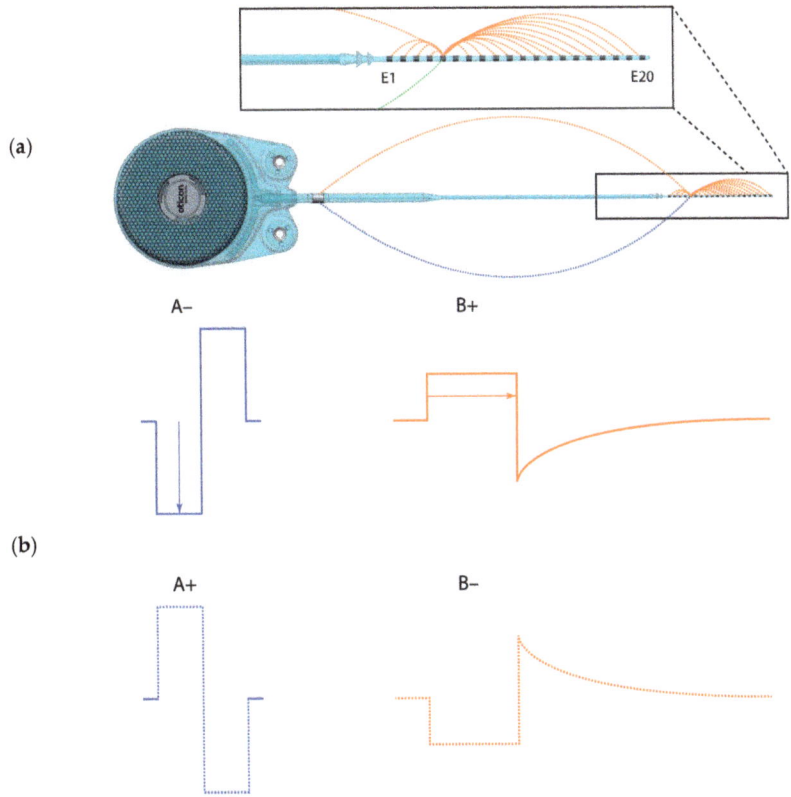

Figure 1. Panel (a) shows a diagram of the Neuro-Zti implant illustrating current paths (dotted lines) for monopolar (MP) grounding used for stimuli A− and A+ (blue) vs. distributed-all-polar (DAP) grounding used for B+ and B− (orange). It also shows the electrode positions and numbering. Panel (b) shows sketches of the pulse shapes used in the experiment for MP grounding (blue) and DAP grounding (orange). The first row shows the clinical pulses in each case, with arrows denoting clinical loudness coding; the second row shows the reversed polarity pulses used with Subject S2.

In each trial, we gradually increased the stimulation charge (i.e., pulse duration or amplitude) until either (1) the sound was too loud or (2) non-auditory sensations became too intense for the subject.

2.3. Procedure

Testing was conducted during a scheduled clinical fitting session. The session was divided into three parts, each lasting about 30 min, interspersed with 5-min breaks. The total testing time was approximately 2 h.

In the first session, we selected suitable electrodes for the experiment from the regions where subjects had previously reported strong FNS responses (Figure 2). We conducted a search to determine which electrode to use for each subject utilizing the 'A−' stimulus (Table 1). This was chosen to mimic their previous cochlear implant and thereby give a good chance of eliciting an FNS response. For the search, we incrementally increased the pulse charge until either the subject reported a non-auditory sensation or the loudness reached an uncomfortable level. Not all electrodes that previously caused FNS (Figure 2) induced FNS responses with the Oticon Medical implant. Those that did, did so at different charge levels than previously reported (higher ones for subject S1, and lower ones for subject S2). In the end, we selected the electrode that elicited the most substantial FNS response to study in detail.

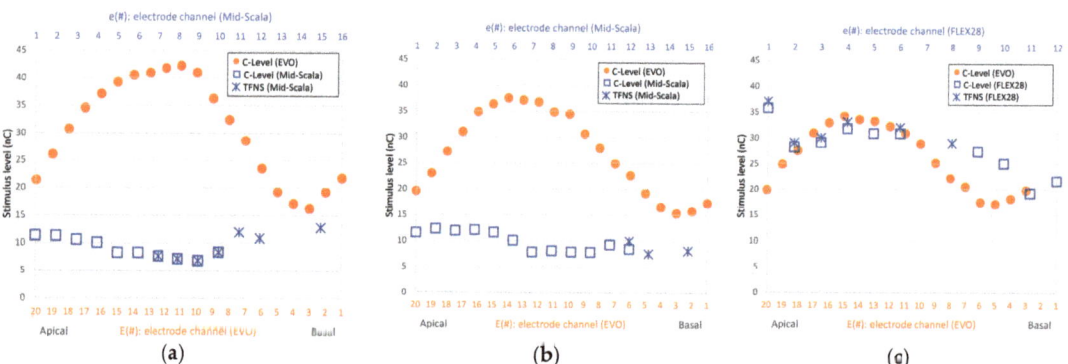

Figure 2. Selected results from case reports presented in [8]. C-level before and about half a year after re-implantation with Oticon Medical Neuro Zti EVO. Asterisks refer to the FNS thresholds with the previously implanted electrode. The upper x-axis refers to the channel number (#) of the previously implanted electrode; the lower x-axis refers to those of the EVO electrode. (**a**) Subject S1, right; (**b**) Subject S1, left; (**c**) Subject S2, right.

In the two following sessions, we stimulated the chosen electrode using either (1) the current clinical mode of their Oticon Medical CI (stimulus B+) or (2) a non-clinical mode designed to mimic their previous CI (stimulus A−). This allowed us to directly compare the in-situ effect of these stimulation modes while keeping implant hardware and subject factors consistent. For each stimulation mode, we gradually increased the intensity. At each charge level, we asked the subjects to: (1) rate the loudness on a scale from 0 (inaudible) to 10 (very loud); (2) describe any non-auditory sensations qualitatively; and (3) indicate whether they were comfortable enough to continue. Due to time constraints, we did not interleave testing modes; this would have necessitated reconfiguring the implant between presentations.

For subject S1, only stimuli of type A− and B+ were explored as described above, because it took some time until we found an electrode that exhibited strong non-auditory side effects. For all stimuli presented to subject S1, charge was increased using pulse duration due to a software limitation (Table 1). Fortunately, for subject S2, the software limitation was overcome, and we then used current coding for stimuli A−/A+ and duration coding for stimuli B−/B+ as would have been carried out clinically. We also had time to explore the effect of reversing pulse polarity for subject S2 in session 3 (Figure 1).

3. Results

The results of the main single electrode experiments for both subjects across all stimulus types are shown in Figure 3 as loudness growth curves. Reported non-auditory/FNS sensations are overlayed as separate symbols. For both subjects, the charge required to reach equivalent loudness levels was higher for stimulus B+ than for A− by more than a factor of 2. However, the growth in loudness was very different between the two. Subject S1 exhibited a rightward shift (~20 nC) and a slower loudness growth for the B+ stimulus, while Subject S2 only exhibited the rightward shift.

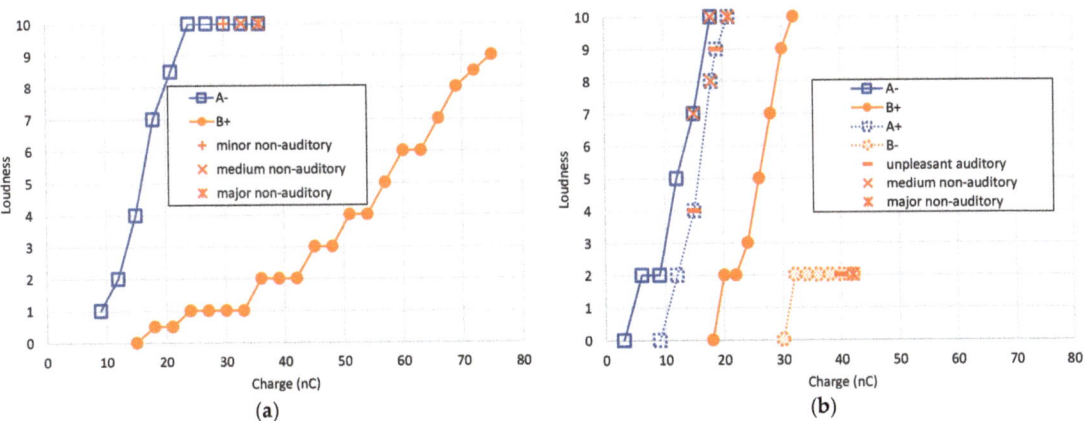

Figure 3. (a) Subject-reported loudness vs. individual pulse charge delivered for subject S1 (left electrode E5) showed faster loudness growth with stimulus A− than with B+. Stimulus A− also elicited non-auditory FNS sensations. (b) Subject S2 (right electrode E18) reported similar slopes but rightward-shifted loudness growth functions between A− and B+. Non-auditory sensations on both panels show how stimulus A− led to FNS stimulation at lower charge levels than for other stimulus types and how non-auditory sensations were affected in a markedly different way from the loudness percepts. Using stimulus B−, we were unable to achieve sufficient loudness. Instead, pronounced side effects were observed.

Reversing the polarity highlighted how non-auditory sensations were affected in a markedly different way than the loudness percept. More detailed results for each subject are presented individually below.

3.1. Subject S1

Using stimulus type A−, first the right ear was tested for side effects. On electrodes E3 and E7, the patient felt some vibration in the outer ear at very loud auditory perception (loudness 10, charge level 36 nC (E3) and 27 nC (E7)). On electrode E11, no non-auditory sensation was reported up to a charge level of 33 nC (loudness = 10). These three electrodes correspond approximately to electrodes e14, e11, and e8 of the previous CI (see Figure 2a), where severe FNS had previously been perceived at soft loudness levels. Thereafter, measurements were performed on the left side on electrodes E7 and E16, again without any non-auditory sensation (loudness 10, charge level 27 nC (E7) and 33 nC (E16). These electrodes matched approximately electrodes e11 and e4 of the previous CI (see Figure 2b).

Finally, measurements on electrode E5 (left) unveiled certain non-auditory side effects. Specifically, a peculiar sensation was reported at a charge level of 30 nC (perceived loudness level at 10). When the charge was increased to 33 nC, the subject described feeling a vibration in the outer ear (see Table 2 for a summary of these findings). Further, at a charge level of 36 nC, this sensation was accompanied by a facial tingle. At this point, a stapedial reflex was objectively confirmed using tympanometry, and we discovered that the reflex was elicited at charge levels from 30 nC upwards, matching the subject's reported perceptions. We selected this E5 electrode for our further investigation.

Table 2. Results of the search for electrodes with side effects. FNS thresholds taken from subject S1's prior implantation (left and right) are compared with observations using the re-implanted OM device and a similar stimulation type (A−). The OM device exhibited higher FNS thresholds for this subject during the acute testing.

Prior Implant (Stimulus A−)		Neuro-Zti Implant (Stimulus A−)			
electrode number	FNS Threshold (nC)	Electrode number	Charge (nC)	Loudness	Observation
e14 (R)	14	E3 (R)	36	10	outer ear vibration
e11 (R)	12	E7 (R)	27	10	outer ear vibration
e8 (R)	8	E11 (R)	33	10	none
e11 (L)	10	E7 (L)	27	10	none
e4 (L)	N/A	E16 (L)	33	10	none
e13 (L)	8	E5 (L)	36	10	facial tingle

While the type A− stimulus presented a rather rapid increase in loudness perception, type B+ exhibited a shallower growth and did not induce any non-auditory side effects (Figure 3a and Table 3). With the use of type B+ stimulation, the loudness level did not exceed 9, and even at charge levels of 75 nC—the maximum possible in our setup—the stapedial reflex was not elicited.

Table 3. Current and duration parameters used while testing subject S1 left ear electrode E5 using either stimulation style A− or B+ (Table 1) and the reported loudness (0 = unheard, 10 = very loud) perceptions for each of these. Comments and observations from the subject concerning any non-auditory sensations are highlighted with footnotes.

Stimulation	A−	B+
(fixed parameter)	(0.6 mA)	(0.6 mA)
Charge (nC)	Loudness	Loudness
9 *	1	
12	2	
15	4	
18	7	0
21	8.5	0.5
24	10	0.5
27	10	1
30	10 [1]	1
33	10 [2]	1
36	10 [3]	2
39		2
42		2
45		3
48		3
51		4
54		4
57		5
60		6
63		6
66		7
69		8
72		8.5
75		9

* The lowest possible value. [1] The subject reported 'feeling' something. [2] The subject reported an 'outer ear vibration'. [3] The subject reported stronger 'outer ear vibration' and a facial tingle.

3.2. Subject S2

The search for electrodes with side effects began with electrode E18, which was approximately equivalent to electrode e2 of the previous implant. This was where a comfortably loud stimulation level had previously evoked FNS (refer to Figure 2c). Using the A− stimulus, the patient experienced vertigo at 15 nC with a loudness level of 7. When the charge was increased to 18 nC, the patient reacted and described a mild but discomforting sensation akin to 'pain in the head' and a loudness level of 10 (Table 4). We selected this E18 electrode for our further investigation.

Table 4. Results of the search for electrodes with side effects. FNS thresholds taken from subject S2's prior implantation (right) are compared with observations using the re-implanted OM device and a similar stimulation type (A−). For this subject, the OM device exhibited non-auditory thresholds at slightly lower charge levels during acute testing.

Prior Implant (Stimulus A−)		Neuro-Zti Implant (Stimulus A−)			
Electrode number	FNS Threshold (nC)	Electrode number	Charge (nC)	Loudness	Observation
e2	28	E18	15	7	vertigo
		E18	18	10	mild pain in the head

With the anodic-leading, passive-discharge B+ stimulus, the patient reported no non-auditory side effects, even up to a charge level of 32 nC (loudness 10). When testing with the reversed polarity using stimulus A+, the patient described an unpleasant buzzing sensation at 15 nC (perceived loudness at level 4). By 18 nC, the subject experienced a sensation akin to 'a force pulling on the head' and rated the loudness at level 8. The buzzing persisted at 19 nC with a loudness perception of level 9. By the time stimulation reached 21 nC (loudness level 10), nystagmus was observed—indicative of an activation of the vestibular system due to the electrical stimulation.

In contrast, with cathodic-leading passive-discharge stimulation (B−), there was only a modest rise in perceived loudness, saturating at a level 2 perception between 32 and 42 nC with no additional growth. At 40 nC, the subject described a deterioration in auditory quality. By 42 nC, the sensations reported were uncomfortably familiar to those previously experienced with her prior cochlear implant, characterized by a blend of vague pain and dizziness. All loudness growth functions for subject S2 are shown in Figure 3b, and corresponding data is listed in Table 5.

Table 5. Current and duration parameters used while testing subject S2 right ear electrode E18 using stimulation styles A−, A+, B−, or B+ (Table 1) and the associated reported loudness (0 = unheard and 10 = very loud) for each of these. Comments and observations from the subject concerning any non-auditory sensations are highlighted with footnotes.

Stimulation (fixed parameter)	A− (30 μs)	A+ (30 μs)	B+ (0.4 mA)	B− (0.4 mA)
Charge (nC)	Loudness	Loudness	Loudness	Loudness
3	0			
6	2			
9	2	0		
12	5	2		
15	7 [1]	4 [3]		
18	10 [2]	8 [4]	0	
19		9 [5]		
20			2	

Table 5. Cont.

Stimulation	A−	A+	B+	B−
21		10 [6]		
22			2	
24			3	
26			5	
28			7	
30			9	0
32			10	2
34				2
36				2
38				2
40				2 [7]
42				2 [8]

[1] The subject reported that the sound was 'not unpleasantly loud' but that it came with vertigo. [2] The subject winced and reported an unpleasant but mild 'pain in the head'. [3,5] The subject reported an unpleasant buzzing sound. [4] The subject experienced a feeling similar to 'a force pulling on her head'. [6] Observed nystagmus (involuntary eyes moving), a vestibular effect. [7] The subject reported deterioration of sound quality. [8] Unpleasant non-auditory sensations. The subject reported that this is 'super unpleasant' but still auditorily soft; the sensation reminded her of her previous CI.

4. Discussion

Approximately 5.6% of all cochlear implant users report experiencing aberrant facial nerve stimulation (FNS) as a side effect of their CI implantation [4]. For users presenting with FNS, audiologists may first attempt to control the problem by re-programming the device to produce lower currents, followed by turning off offending electrodes—both of which can reduce speech comprehension [4]. If these solutions fail, clinics have observed that re-implantation with an Oticon Medical Neuro Zti implant can resolve FNS issues [8,10–13]. Indeed, for our two subjects, re-implantation with the Oticon Medical device not only completely resolved FNS but also improved speech recognition [8].

The mechanisms that underlie this improvement are not yet well understood. However, we can reasonably expect that factors that affect the local electrical fields near neural activation points for the auditory and facial nerves—combined with how those nerves respond to these fields—are involved. These factors include: (1) electrode proximity; (2) factors that affect current spread (e.g., grounding and pulse duration and shape); and (3) polarity. In the subsequent four sections, we explore these factors and discuss the distinct characteristics of the Oticon Medical device in these areas. It is important to clarify that our intention is to shed light on these differences and not to imply that these distinctions inherently make the Oticon Medical device superior to others.

4.1. Electrode Proximity

The proximity between the stimulating electrodes and the neural activation sites of the auditory nerve fibers (ANF) is influenced by the type of electrode array used. Common understanding suggests that modiolus-hugging or mid-scala arrays might offer advantages in minimizing FNS over the lateral wall array design, used—among others—in the Oticon Medical electrode array. Case studies, such as Battmer et al. [14], indicate that electrodes positioned closer to the ANF require less current for excitation. This reduced current potentially leads to limited current spread, decreasing the likelihood of stimulating more distant non-auditory neural structures. Indeed, when looking across the literature, electrode array type does emerge as a statistically significant factor [4]. However, other case studies—including those of the two subjects in this manuscript—demonstrate that the Oticon Medical device is effective in alleviating unwanted FNS. Consequently, as we've previously argued [8], stimulation-related factors likely have a larger impact.

4.2. Grounding

Beyond geometry, other factors determining the current spread are also relevant when considering the activation of more distant, non-auditory neural structures. A notable distinction between the OM devices and others lies in their DAP grounding scheme (see Figure 1). With DAP, approximately 80% of the current returns to intra-cochlear electrodes and the remaining 20% to an extra-cochlear electrode [7]. By contrast, conventional MP-grounding returns all the current through the extra-cochlear electrode. This MP grounding mechanism theoretically results in a broader dispersion of the overall electrical field, making it more likely to intersect with the facial nerve.

In addition to DAP and MP, 'bipolar' and 'common ground' schemes are also in clinical use, with the latter commonly observed in older Cochlear® (Cochlear Limited, Sydney, Australia) devices. Both return current via intracochlear electrodes. A study investigating the effects of different grounding strategies on FNS efficacy, conducted using 204 electrically evoked compound action potential (eCAP) input/output functions recorded from 33 ears of 26 guinea pigs, revealed that—for biphasic pulses—the broad-MP grounding was associated with a high occurrence of FNS (65%), while bipolar and an experimental tripolar configuration (expected to be the most focused) generated only 20% and 2% of FNS occurrences, respectively [15].

4.3. Pulse Duration and Shape

Altering the grounding scheme modifies the spatial distribution of current. While certain configurations might reduce this spread, predicting current pathways in individual anatomies is challenging. Specific grounding configurations, like bipolar or multipolar schemes—which are presumed to be more focused—typically require higher charge levels to reach equivalent loudness percepts vs. MP grounding [12]. This could, in turn, lead to a broader current spread again.

OM differs from most CI manufacturers in its encoding of loudness; it uses pulse duration rather than current amplitude. Consequently, the current is consistently set at a relatively low level, even for intense sounds. It has been shown that this approach can lead to a more focused area of excitation, especially at higher stimulation levels [16].

The OM pulse shape is also different than the standard biphasic one. It begins with an active rectangular phase, but rather than being followed by a symmetric shape, the charge return is via passive (capacitive) discharge, leading to an exponential decay (Figure 1). This unique pulse waveform requires only half the stimulation power needed for generating symmetric biphasic pulses. While the amplitude of the second phase varies based on the duration and current of the initial active phase, it is typically much smaller, creating a pulse shape akin to a pseudo-monophasic one. Such pseudo-monophasic (or asymmetric) pulses are known to be charge-efficient, activating nerve fibers with lower charge levels than symmetric biphasic pulses [17,18]. Mathematical modeling by Frijns et al. [19] also suggests that asymmetric pulses like these might act to reduce current spread to some extent compared to their symmetric counterparts.

In essence, employing pulse duration coding and pseudo-monophasic pulse shapes appears to limit current spread within the cochlea, potentially decreasing the likelihood of FNS.

4.4. Pulse Polarity

Not only does the OM device have a unique grounding scheme and pulse shape, but it also has opposite polarity to the standard clinical biphasic pulses. The majority of CI manufacturers initiate their biphasic pulses with a cathodic phase, while OM devices begin with an anodic phase. This alternative polarity, combined with the pseudo-monophasic pulse shape, seems to significantly impact the occurrence of FNS, as observed in our two subjects. Specifically, when using the OM's clinical pulses, both subjects experienced no side effects. However, when traditional biphasic active stimuli with MP grounding were applied, side effects were evident. To better understand the effect of the polarity alone, we inverted the polarity of the stimuli in the OM stimulation mode for subject S2. We found that those pseudo-monophasic cathodic-leading pulses (using DAP grounding) did induce FNS, even at low loudness levels and in the absence of any auditory loudness growth.

Notably, when using the clinical anodic leading pulses, the subject reached her maximum tolerable loudness (level 10) at a charge of 32 nC without any side effects. However, when cathodic-leading pulses of the same type were used, reported loudness plateaued at level 2, while side effects continued to escalate as charge levels were increased. This striking contrast between these two conditions suggests that, for this subject, anodic stimulation primarily excited auditory nerve structures, while cathodic stimulation was effective at activating other neural structures, such as the facial nerve.

4.5. Summary and Further Considerations

For our two subjects utilizing the OM Neuro ZTI implant, we observed that traditional symmetric biphasic cathodic-leading pulses in monopolar stimulation mode could elicit FNS. However, when using pseudo-monophasic anodic-leading pulses in DAP grounding mode—the clinical standard setting of the ZTI implant—it was impossible to trigger FNS even when raising charge levels at the subjects' maximum tolerable loudness.

Conversely, and of significant note, we found that pseudo-monophasic cathodic-leading pulses in all-polar grounding mode could induce FNS at lower charge levels, while provoking auditory sensations required much higher charge, and even then, the auditory sensations were only soft. This striking contrast between these two conditions strongly suggests that anodic stimulation is primarily effective at exciting auditory nerve structures, while cathodic stimulation appears to predominantly activate other neural structures, such as the facial nerve.

Our findings, though just from two subjects, lend further support to an expanding body of research suggesting that the auditory and facial nerves exhibit differential sensitivity to electrical stimulation based on polarity [20–24]. However, unlike previous studies, which have primarily relied on action potential recordings in CI subjects elicited with active biphasic pulses, our study provides novel evidence from direct subjective feedback obtained from two human subjects using pseudo-monophasic pulses. We demonstrate that anodic currents are markedly more effective in selectively stimulating the neural structures associated with the auditory nerve while minimizing activation of the facial and other non-auditory neural structures. The hypothesis that the auditory nerve may be more sensitive to anodic stimulation while the facial nerve is more responsive to cathodic stimulation could also partially explain the reduced FNS symptoms observed with triphasic stimulation in the MED-EL device, which also uses a longer and presumably dominant anodic phase. Using an anodic-leading (or anodic dominant) pulse could, in theory, allow for more targeted stimulation of the auditory nerve, potentially reducing unwanted activation of other nerves like the facial nerve [25].

5. Conclusions

We conclude that CI stimulus parameters and grounding rather than surgical or electrode array changes were key factors in reducing FNS for our two subjects, and we suggest that this may hold true more generally. Our data indicates that the active anodic phase of the stimulus predominantly activates the auditory nerve fibers. In contrast, the cathodic phase seems more inclined to stimulate other neural structures, such as the facial nerve, leading to undesired side effects. Further untangling the relative contributions of polarity, pulse shape, pulse current vs. duration, and grounding to FNS will be a rich area for future investigations.

Author Contributions: Conceptualization, L.G., A.B., B.C.B. and N.L.G.; methodology, A.B., A.M. and B.C.B.; software, B.C.B.; validation, B.C.B. and L.G.; investigation, A.B., A.M., B.C.B., L.G. and N.L.G.; resources, T.L. and A.B.; data curation, B.C.B., N.L.G., L.G., A.M. and A.B.; writing—original draft preparation, A.B., A.M., B.C.B., L.G. and N.L.G.; writing—review and editing, A.B., A.M., B.C.B., L.G., N.L.G. and T.L.; visualization, B.C.B. and L.G.; supervision, A.B., T.L. and N.L.G.; project administration, A.B., B.C.B., T.L. and N.L.G. All authors have read and agreed to the published version of the manuscript.

Funding: This research received no external funding.

Institutional Review Board Statement: The study was conducted in accordance with the Declaration of Helsinki, conducted during the normal clinical fitting routine, and approved by the ethics board of the Hannover Medical School (No. 1897-2013).

Informed Consent Statement: Subjects gave their written informed consent for taking part in these additional diagnostic measurements and for publishing the data.

Data Availability Statement: Data tables are included within the manuscript.

Conflicts of Interest: Authors L.G., A.M., T.L. and A.B. declare no conflict of interests. The other authors of this study declare competing interests: B.B. and N.L. are paid employees of Oticon Medical (Vallauris, France; https://www.oticonmedical.com/, accessed on 15 August 2023). They had roles in conceptualization, methodology, software, validation, investigation, data curation, writing—original draft preparation, writing—review and editing, visualization, supervision, and project administration. The specific roles of the authors employed by Oticon Medical are articulated in the 'author contributions' section. There are no patents, products in development, or marketed products associated with this research to declare.

References

1. World Health Organization. *World Report on Hearing*; World Health Organization: Geneva, Switzerland, 2021.
2. Wilson, B.S.; Dorman, M.F. Cochlear implants: A remarkable past and a brilliant future. *Hear. Res.* **2008**, *242*, 3–21. [CrossRef]
3. Niparko, J.K. (Ed.) *Cochlear Implants: Principles & Practices*; Lippincott Williams & Wilkins: Philadelphia, PA, USA, 2009.
4. Van Horn, A.; Hayden, C.; Mahairas, A.D.; Leader, P.; Bush, M.L. Factors Influencing Aberrant Facial Nerve Stimulation Following Cochlear Implantation: A Systematic Review and Meta-analysis. *Otol. Neurotol.* **2020**, *41*, 1050–1059. [CrossRef]
5. Braun, K.; Walker, K.; Sürth, W.; Löwenheim, H.; Tropitzsch, A. Triphasic Pulses in Cochlear Implant Patients with Facial Nerve Stimulation. *Otol. Neurotol.* **2019**, *40*, 1268–1277. [CrossRef]
6. Bahmer, A.; Baumann, U. The underlying mechanism of preventing facial nerve stimulation by triphasic pulse stimulation in cochlear implant users assessed with objective measure. *Otol. Neurotol.* **2016**, *37*, 1231–1237. [CrossRef] [PubMed]
7. Stahl, P.; Dang, K.; Vandersteen, C.; Guevara, N.; Clerc, M.; Gnansia, D. Current distribution of distributed all-polar cochlear implant stimulation mode measured in-situ. *PLoS ONE* **2022**, *17*, e0275961. [CrossRef]
8. Gärtner, L.; Lenarz, T.; Ivanauskaite, J.; Büchner, A. Facial nerve stimulation in cochlear implant users—A matter of stimulus parameters? *Cochlear Implant. Int.* **2022**, *23*, 165–172. [CrossRef]
9. Backus, B.; Adiloğlu, K.; Herzke, T. A Binaural CI Research Platform for Oticon Medical SP/XP Implants Enabling ITD/ILD and Variable Rate Processing. *Trends Hear.* **2015**, *19*, 2331216515618655. [CrossRef]
10. Zellhuber, N.; Helbig, R.; James, P.; Bloching, M.; Lyutenski, S. Multi-mode grounding and monophasic passive discharge stimulation avoid aberrant facial nerve stimulation following cochlear implantation. *Clin. Case Rep.* **2022**, *10*, e05360. [CrossRef]
11. Hyppolito, M.A.; Barbosa Reis, A.C.M.; Danieli, F.; Hussain, R.; Le Goff, N. Cochlear re-implantation with the use of multi-mode grounding associated with anodic monophasic pulses to manage abnormal facial nerve stimulation. *Cochlear Implant. Int.* **2023**, *24*, 55–64. [CrossRef]
12. Eitutis, S.T.; Carlyon, R.P.; Tam, Y.C.; Salorio-Corbetto, M.; Vanat, Z.; Tebbutt, K.; Bardsley, R.; Powell, H.R.; Tysome, J.R.; Bance, M.L.; et al. Management of Severe Facial Nerve Cross Stimulation by Cochlear Implant Replacement to Change Pulse Shape and Grounding Configuration: A Case-series. *Otol. Neurotol.* **2022**, *43*, 452–459. [CrossRef]
13. Danieli, F.; Hyppolito, M.A.; Hussain, R.; Hoen, M.; Karoui, C.; Reis, A.C.M.B. The Effects of Multi-Mode Monophasic Stimulation with Capacitive Discharge on the Facial Nerve Stimulation Reduction in Young Children with Cochlear Implants: Intraoperative Recordings. *J. Clin. Med.* **2023**, *12*, 534. [CrossRef] [PubMed]
14. Battmer, R.; Pesch, J.; Stöver, T.; Lesinski-Schiedat, A.; Lenarz, M.; Lenarz, T. Elimination of facial nerve stimulation by reimplantation in cochlear implant subjects. *Otol. Neurotol.* **2006**, *27*, 918–922. [CrossRef] [PubMed]
15. Konerding, W.S.; Baumhoff, P.; Kral, A. Anodic Polarity Minimizes Facial Nerve Stimulation as a Side Effect of Cochlear Implantation. *J. Assoc. Res. Otolaryngol.* **2023**, *24*, 31–46. [CrossRef] [PubMed]
16. Quass, G.L.; Baumhoff, P.; Gnansia, D.; Stahl, P.; Kral, A. Level coding by phase duration and asymmetric pulse shape reduce channel interactions in cochlear implants. *Hear. Res.* **2020**, *396*, 108070. [CrossRef]

17. Yip, M.; Bowers, P.; Noel, V.; Chandrakasan, A.; Stankovic, K.M. Energy-efficient waveform for electrical stimulation of the cochlear nerve. *Sci. Rep.* **2017**, *7*, 13582. [CrossRef]
18. Jezernik, S.; Morari, M. Energy-optimal electrical excitation of nerve fibers. *IEEE Trans. Biomed Eng.* **2005**, *52*, 740–743. [CrossRef]
19. Frijns, J.H.M.; De Snoo, S.L.; Ten Kate, J.H. Spatial selectivity in a rotationally symmetric model of the electrically stimulated cochlea. *Hear. Res.* **1996**, *95*, 33–48. [CrossRef]
20. Herrmann, D.P.; Kretzer, K.V.A.; Pieper, S.H.; Bahmer, A. Effects of electrical pulse polarity shape on intra cochlear neural responses in humans: Triphasic pulses with anodic and cathodic second phase. *Hear. Res.* **2021**, *412*, 108375. [CrossRef]
21. Undurraga, J.A.; van Wieringen, A.; Carlyon, R.P.; Macherey, O.; Wouters, J. Polarity effects on neural responses of the electrically stimulated auditory nerve at different cochlear sites. *Hear. Res.* **2010**, *269*, 146–161. [CrossRef]
22. Spitzer, E.R.; Hughes, M.L. Effect of stimulus polarity on physiological spread of excitation in cochlear implants. *J. Am. Acad. Audiol.* **2017**, *28*, 786–798. [CrossRef]
23. Macherey, O.; Carlyon, R.P.; Van Wieringen, A.; Deeks, J.M.; Wouters, J. Higher sensitivity of human auditory nerve fibers to positive electrical currents. *J. Assoc. Res. Otolaryngol.* **2008**, *9*, 241–251. [CrossRef]
24. Hughes, M.L.; Goehring, J.L.; Baudhuin, J.L. Effects of stimulus polarity and artifact reduction method on the electrically evoked compound action potential. *Ear Hear.* **2017**, *38*, 332–343. [CrossRef]
25. Kalkman, R.K.; Briaire, J.J.; Dekker, D.M.T.; Frijns, J.H.M. The relation between polarity sensitivity and neural degeneration in a computational model of cochlear implant stimulation. *Hear. Res.* **2022**, *415*, 108413. [CrossRef]

Disclaimer/Publisher's Note: The statements, opinions and data contained in all publications are solely those of the individual author(s) and contributor(s) and not of MDPI and/or the editor(s). MDPI and/or the editor(s) disclaim responsibility for any injury to people or property resulting from any ideas, methods, instructions or products referred to in the content.

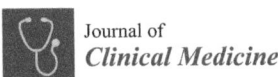

Article

The Effects of Multi-Mode Monophasic Stimulation with Capacitive Discharge on the Facial Nerve Stimulation Reduction in Young Children with Cochlear Implants: Intraoperative Recordings

Fabiana Danieli [1,2,*], Miguel Angelo Hyppolito [3], Raabid Hussain [4], Michel Hoen [5], Chadlia Karoui [5] and Ana Cláudia Mirândola Barbosa Reis [6]

1. Postgraduate Program at the Department of Health Sciences, RCS, Ribeirão Preto Medical School, University of São Paulo, Bandeirantes 3900, Ribeirão Preto 14049-900, Brazil
2. Clinical Department, Oticon Medical, Lino de Moraes Leme 883, São Paulo 04360-001, Brazil
3. Department of Ophthalmology, Otorhinolaryngology, Head and Neck Surgery, Ribeirão Preto Medical School, University of São Paulo, Bandeirantes 3900, Ribeirão Preto 14049-900, Brazil
4. Research & Technology Department, Oticon Medical, 2765 Smørum, Denmark
5. Clinical Evidence Department, Oticon Medical, 2720 Chem de Saint-Bernard, 06220 Vallauris, France
6. Department of Health Sciences, RCS, Ribeirão Preto Medical School, University of São Paulo, Bandeirantes 3900, Ribeirão Preto 14049-900, Brazil
* Correspondence: fabianadanieli@hotmail.com

Abstract: Facial nerve stimulation (FNS) is a potential complication which may affect the auditory performance of children with cochlear implants (CIs). We carried out an exploratory prospective observational study to investigate the effects of the electrical stimulation pattern on FNS reduction in young children with CI. Ten ears of seven prelingually deafened children with ages up to 6 years old who undergone a unilateral or bilateral CI surgery were included in this study. Electromyographic (EMG) action potentials from orbicularis oculi muscle were recorded using monopolar biphasic stimulation (ST1) and multi-mode monophasic stimulation with capacitive discharge (ST2). Presence of EMG responses, facial nerve stimulation thresholds (T-FNS) and EMG amplitudes were compared between ST1 and ST2. Intra-cochlear electrodes placement, cochlear-nerve and electrode-nerve distances were also estimated to investigate their effects on EMG responses. The use of ST2 significantly reduced the presence of intraoperative EMG responses compared to ST1. Higher stimulation levels were required to elicit FNS with ST2, with smaller amplitudes, compared to ST1. No and weak correlation was observed between cochlea-nerve and electrode-nerve distances and EMG responses, respectively. ST2 may reduce FNS in young children with CI. Differently from the electrical stimulation pattern, the cochlea-nerve and electrode-nerve distances seem to have limited effects on FNS in this population.

Keywords: facial nerve stimulation; cochlear implant; electromyography; stimulation strategy; image analysis; computed tomography; image segmentation; 3D model

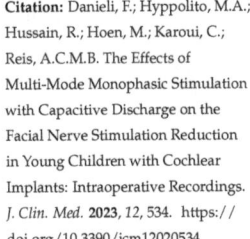

Citation: Danieli, F.; Hyppolito, M.A.; Hussain, R.; Hoen, M.; Karoui, C.; Reis, A.C.M.B. The Effects of Multi-Mode Monophasic Stimulation with Capacitive Discharge on the Facial Nerve Stimulation Reduction in Young Children with Cochlear Implants: Intraoperative Recordings. *J. Clin. Med.* **2023**, *12*, 534. https://doi.org/10.3390/jcm12020534

Academic Editor: Giuseppe Magliulo

Received: 7 December 2022
Revised: 28 December 2022
Accepted: 5 January 2023
Published: 9 January 2023

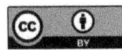

Copyright: © 2023 by the authors. Licensee MDPI, Basel, Switzerland. This article is an open access article distributed under the terms and conditions of the Creative Commons Attribution (CC BY) license (https://creativecommons.org/licenses/by/4.0/).

1. Introduction

Cochlear implant (CI) is the most effective treatment option for young children with profound sensorineural hearing loss. A longitudinal study showed that children implanted up to 2 years old scored on average above 50% on open-set speech recognition tasks after 4 years of CI experience [1]. The rate of complications with cochlear implantation has also decreased with advances in the CI field in the last years [2]. However, one potential complication that persists and affects the auditory performance of children with CI is the facial nerve stimulation (FNS).

FNS incidence was reported to range from 1.14% to 43% in children, with immediate or delayed onset [3]. Although it is known that otosclerosis, meningitis, temporal bone fractures and congenital cochlear anomalies increase the risk of FNS, some patients experience it after cochlear implantation without any of these etiologies. FNS symptoms may range from mild facial movements to severe facial spasms, painful or debilitating [4], either visually detected or self-reported by the patient. In young children, FNS has been underestimated, as they may not accurately report its symptoms. Cushing, Papsin and Gordon [5] reported a large difference in the incidence of FNS in children with CI when electrophysiological recordings are compared to their reports or even to observation of facial movements.

It is assumed that the electric current passing from the electrode to spiral ganglion cell can spread to the nearby facial nerve causing FNS [6], but the exact mechanism underlying the FNS remains unclear, as well as the relative contribution of factors to trigger the symptoms and the best treatment option to resolve it.

Some strategies have been adopted to manage FNS symptoms, including maximum comfort levels (MCL) reduction [7], pulse wide widening [8], the use of triphasic pulses [9], electrode deactivation [10] and cochlear re-implantation [11]. However, these strategies may result in auditory performance decline [7] and does not ensure to resolve FNS [8].

Recently, the use of the multi-mode monophasic stimulation was proposed as a promising strategy to manage FNS [7,12,13]. It resolved severe FNS in some adult CI recipients, after cochlear re-implantation with the Neuro Zti device (Oticon Medical, Smørum, Denmark). Most current CI devices use monopolar biphasic stimulation, and, in this CI electrical stimulation pattern, the total amount of electrical charge flows from intra-cochlear electrodes to extra-cochlear ground electrodes, and each phase of the pulse stimulates different group of neurons, increasing the spatial extent of stimulation. Using multi-mode monophasic stimulation with subsequent capacitive discharge, most of the electrical current is maintained within the cochlea, and the anodic stimulating phase of the monophasic pulse is followed by a non-stimulating cathodic phase (with reduced amplitude, compared to anodic phase). It is hypothesized that multi-mode monophasic stimulation decreases the spatial extent of electrical stimulation and reduces the amount of the current spread to the periphery structures, including the facial nerve, thereby reducing FNS.

To the best of our knowledge, the effects of multi-mode monophasic stimulation on FNS reduction in children were not previously investigated. Thus, in this study, we recorded intraoperative EMG action potentials to investigate the use of the multi-mode monophasic stimulation in young children and the effects of this stimulation pattern on the FNS reduction in this population. We also used 3D image processing techniques to estimate the CI intra-cochlear electrodes placement, as well as the distances between the basal turn of the cochlea and electrodes (based on their real intra-cochlear positioning) to the labyrinthine segment of the facial nerve, to investigate their influence on the EMG recordings.

2. Materials and Methods

This was an exploratory prospective observational study approved by the Institutional Ethics Committee under protocol 5.117.640. Parental informed consent was obtained from all subjects involved in the study.

2.1. Subjects

Ten ears from seven prelingually deafened children aged up to 6 years old who undergone either unilateral or bilateral CI surgeries were included in this study. All subjects were implanted with the Neuro Zti Evo® device associated to the Neuro 2 sound processor (Oticon Medical, Smørum, Denmark). The exclusion criteria was comprised of subjects with preoperative facial palsy or other facial nerve dysfunctions, neuromuscular diseases, and epilepsy, as they could affect the EMG responses. T demographic data of the subjects are shown in the Table 1.

Table 1. Subject demographics.

Subject	Ear	Side	Sex	Age at CI Surgery (m)	Etiology
S1	EA1	L	M	18	Congenital
	EA2	R			Congenital
S2	EA3	R	F	18	Genetics
	EA4	L			Genetics
S3	EA5	R	F	14	Idiopathic
	EA6	L			Idiopathic
S4	EA7	R	F	66	Ototoxicity
S5	EA8	L	F	47	Idiopathic
S6	EA9	R	F	45	Auditory neuropathy
S70	EA10	L	F	30	Genetics

S1–S7: subjects 1–7; EA1–EA10: implanted ears 1–10; L: left; R: right; M: male; F: female; CI: cochlear implant; m: months.

2.2. Procedure

EMG responses were recorded in all subjects during CI surgery, under general anesthesia (Propofol and Fentanyl). The duration of measurement was about 10–15 min to not prolong the surgery time, and it was carried out immediately after the insertion of the EVO® electrode array inside the cochlea of the subjects. Pre-anesthetic sedatives were not administrated to avoid muscle relaxation and their influence on the EMG recordings and facial nerve monitoring.

FNS stimulation was investigated through the EMG action potentials recorded from the orbicular oculi or oris muscles, both innervated by the facial nerve. Prior to sterile surgical preparation, bipolar needle electrodes were placed inside the orbicularis oculi and oris muscles, ipsilateral to the cochlear implantation site. Intraoperative facial nerve monitoring was initially performed to assess EMG recordings from inputs (i.e., orbicularis oculi and oris muscles) using the Nerve Integrity Monitor—NIM-2 equipment (Medtronic Xomed Inc., Jacksonville, FL, USA). After insertion of the electrode array, the experimental protocol was performed firstly using only the orbicularis oculi input channel, to limit the duration of the measurement in young children. If absent or no clear responses were recorded from this channel, the orbicularis oris input channel was then used.

2.3. Stimulation Parameters and EMG Responses

The intracochlear electrical stimulation was produced by the cochlear implant, using the eCAP tool of the Genie Medical CI fitting software, version 1.6, and CI-Link interface (Oticon Medical, Smørum, Denmark), connected to a computer and external antenna, responsible for transmitting the electrical stimuli to internal antenna via radiofrequency. Four electrodes were tested in each ear: one basal (E1), two medial (E8, E15) and one apical (E20). For the facial nerve stimulation thresholds (T-FNS) investigation purposes, current levels started from 20 SA (stimulation amplitude, 1 SA = 1/45 mA) and increased by 5 SA steps until reach 70 SA (maximum current level). The pulse duration was fixed at 30 SD (stimulation duration, 1 SD = 1 µs). The stimulation level (nC/phase) at which an EMG response was first evoked was defined as T-FNS, and no further increase in stimulus level was performed after detection of an FNS response. Peak-to-peak amplitudes of EMG responses at T-FNS were also recorded.

In order to investigate EMG responses using the two different CI stimulation patterns, the experimental protocol first employed monopolar biphasic stimulation (ST1) and then, multi-mode monophasic stimulation (ST2). Figure 1 shows the schematic of different stimulation patterns used in this study. Stimulation parameters used to record EMG responses are provided in the Table 2.

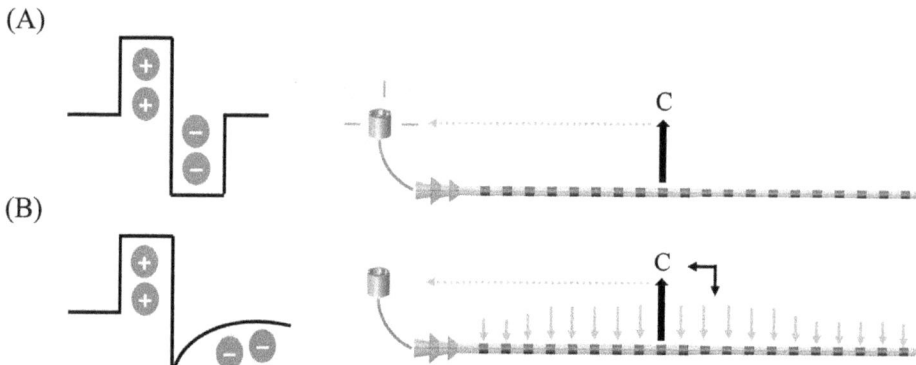

Figure 1. Schematic representation of different stimulation patterns used in this study. (**A**) Monopolar biphasic stimulation (stimulation pattern ST1) and (**B**) multi-mode monophasic stimulation with capacitive discharge (stimulation pattern ST2).

Table 2. Stimulation parameters used to record EMG responses.

Stimulation Patten	Stimulation Mode	Waveform	Polarity	Pulse Train	Coding	Pulse Amplitude Min:Step:Max (µA)	Pulse Duration (µs)	Stimulation Rate (Hz)
1 Monopolar biphasic	MP	Biphasic active symmetrical	Anodic leading	Masker probe	Amplitude	444:110:1554	30	83
2 Multi-mode Monophasic with CD	MM	Monophasic capacitive discharge	Anodic leading	Continuous	Amplitude	444:110:1554	30	250

CD: capacitive discharge; MP: monopolar; MM: multi-mode grounding; min: minimum; max: maximum.

2.4. Radiological Examination

Pre- and postoperative CT scans of the ears were performed to investigate the intra-cochlear electrodes placement and the distance between the cochlea and labyrinthine segment of the facial nerve (cochlea-nerve distance). For this purpose, postoperative CT scans were performed in all subjects three months after cochlear implantation.

The CT-scans were acquired at a resolution of $0.3 \times 0.3 \times 0.4$ mm^3. CT image reconstruction was performed using a web-based research platform Nautilus [14], which combines a convolutional neural network (CNN) approach with Bayesian joint appearance and shape inference for segmenting the cochlea and determining the trajectory of the electrode arrays. The angular positioning of the electrodes was determined automatically using Nautilus which extracts electrode position from postoperative CT-scan using a CNN approach and registers it with preoperative CT-scan for determining the electrode position with respect to the cochlear segmentation. The closest distance between the lateral wall of the cochlea and the labyrinthine segment of the facial nerve (cochlea-nerve distance) were measured on the pre-operative CT-scans. Next, the cochlea-nerve distance at each electrode's angular location (electrode-nerve distance) were also measured to estimate the electrodes placed closest to the facial nerve. The 3D cochlear view reconstruction, including scala tympani segmentation, was input to Slicer 3D and manual annotation of the facial nerve was performed (Figure 2).

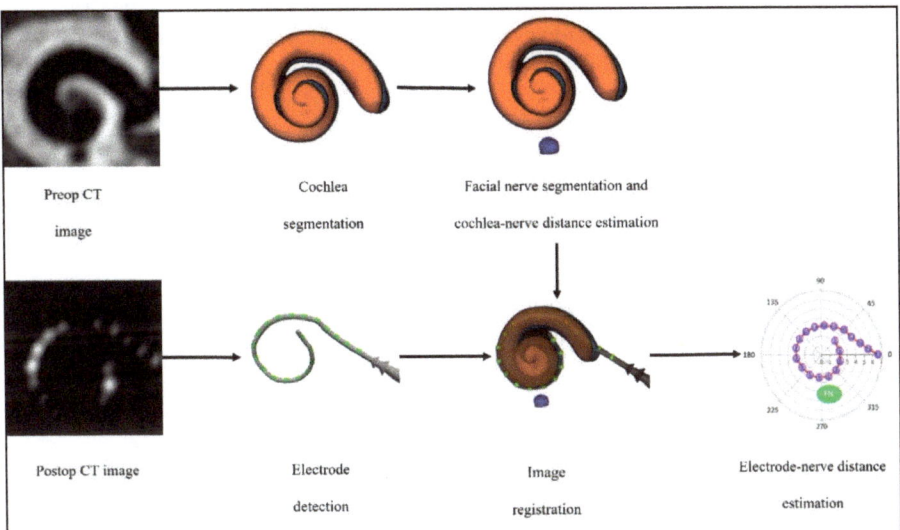

Figure 2. Model of CT image reconstruction performed by the software Nautilus in this study: cochlear segmentation, angular positioning of the electrodes and cochlear-nerve and electrode-nerve distances estimation.

2.5. Statistical Analyses

The proportion of EMG responses with ST1 and ST2 were compared using the McNemar's test. Spearman's correlation test was used to investigate associations between intraoperative EMG responses and cochlea-nerve distances estimation of the subjects. The correlation between the electrode-nerve distances estimation of the electrode E15 (placed in the range closest to the facial nerve in most subjects, from 250 to 290 degrees) and T-FNS were also investigated. The results were expressed in correlation coefficient (ρ) and p-value. A significance level of 5% was adopted.

3. Results

Table 3 shows the proportion of intraoperative EMG responses recorded on each tested electrode using the stimulation patterns ST1 and ST2. ST1 stimulation leaded to intraoperative EMG responses in at least one electrode in 9 of 10 ears while the ST2 stimulation induced EMG responses only in the most basal electrode (E1) in 1 of 10 ears (#S4). Subject #S3 (EA6) showed absent EMG recordings with both stimulation patterns ST1 and ST2 (with orbicularis oculi and oris muscles input channels). Overall, the paired analyses indicated that the use of ST2 was significantly associated to lower incidence of intraoperative EMG responses recorded on all tested electrodes compared to ST1.

Table 3. Proportion of intraoperative EMG responses recorded in each tested electrode using the stimulation patterns ST1 and ST2.

Electrode	ST1 N (%)	ST2 N (%)	p-Value
E1 (basal)	9 (90.0)	1 (10.0)	0.0143 *
E8 (medial)	8 (80.0)	0 (0.0)	0.0047 *
E15 (medial)	8 (80.0)	0 (0.0)	0.0047 *
E20 (apical)	8 (80.0)	0 (0.0)	0.0047 *

ST1: stimulation pattern 1 (monopolar biphasic stimulation); ST2: stimulation pattern 2 (multi-mode monophasic stimulation); N: number of EMG responses in each implanted ear. * Significant difference (McNemar's test, 5% of significance level).

Figure 3 shows individual T-FNS (A) and EMG amplitudes (B), when recorded, using CI stimulation patterns ST1 and ST2. Two subjects showed EMG responses only in the electrode E1 (#S5 with ST1 and #S4 with ST2), and their absence in the remaining electrodes. Higher stimulation levels were required to elicit FNS (T-FNS) with ST2 (37 nC/phase) compared to ST1 (13 nC/phase) in the subject #S4 (electrode E1). Furthermore, peak-to-peak EMG amplitudes were smaller using ST2 (15 µV) compared to ST1 (27 µV) in this electrode.

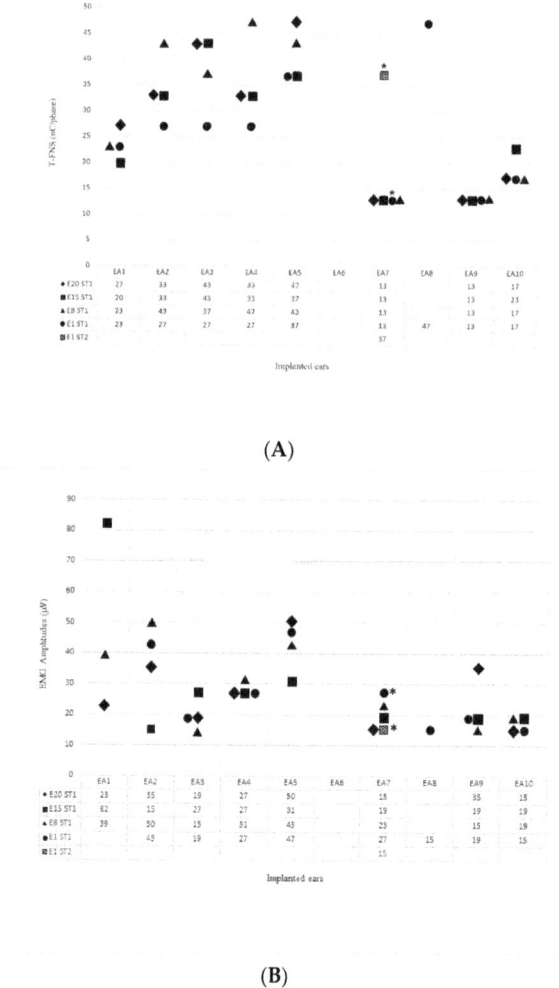

Figure 3. Individual T-FNS (**A**) and EMG amplitudes (**B**), when recorded, using CI stimulation patterns ST1 and ST2. Blank: no EMG responses. EA1–EA10: implanted ears 1–10. *Asterisks: comparison between values recorded with ST1 and ST2, in the same electrode (#Subject 4, EA7).

The intra-cochlear electrodes placement and cochlea-nerve distances estimation are provided in the Table 4. Four subjects (six ears) showed at least one extra-cochlear electrode placement (basal electrodes), including the subject #4, who showed EMG responses only in the most basal electrode with ST2 (Figure 4). The cochlea-nerve distances ranged from 0.20 to 1.00 mm (mean = 0.42 ± 0.26 mm). One subject (#S3, EA6) showed the longest cochlea-nerve distance and absent intraoperative EMG recordings with both the ST1 and

ST2, but no correlation was observed between cochlear-nerve distances and EMG responses (Table 5). E15 and E16 were the Evo® electrodes placed closest to the labyrinthine segment of the facial nerve, being recorded from 250 to 290 degrees insertion depth angle in most subjects. The electrode-nerve distance from the electrode E15 showed a weak correlation with the T-FNS recorded on this electrode ($\rho = 0.42$; p-value = 0.30).

Table 4. Intra-cochlear electrodes placement, cochlea-nerve and electrode-nerve distances estimation of the subjects.

Subject	Ear	Side	Extra-Cochlear Electrodes	Cochlear-Nerve Distance (mm)	Insertion Depth Angle (°)	Electrode Closest to the FN
S1	EA1	L	0	0.24	279	15
	EA2	R	2	0.20	281	18
S2	EA3	R	1	0.20	285	15
	EA4	L	1	0.40	290	15
S3	EA5	R	1	0.44	267	16
	EA6	L	2	1.00	270	16
S4	EA7	R	1	0.20	273	16
S5	EA8	L	0	0.32	279	14
S6	EA9	R	0	0.56	276	11
S70	EA10	L	0	0.64	250	10

S1–S7: subjects 1–7; EA1–EA10: implanted ears 1–10; L: left; R: right; cochlea-nerve distance: closest distance between basal turn of the cochlea and the labyrinthine segment of the facial nerve; mm: millimeters; Electrode closest to the facial nerve: Evo® electrode with closest electrode-nerve distance values; FN: facial nerve.

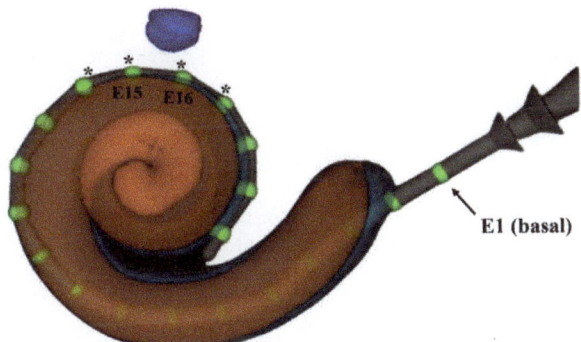

Figure 4. Example of electrodes placement estimation performed by Nautilus for the subject #S4 (EA7), who showed FNS responses with ST1 and ST2, in the electrode E1. Electrode 1 (basal) is extra-cochlear. * Blue circle and asterisks correspond to the labyrinthine segment of the facial nerve and Evo® electrodes with closest electrode-nerve distances, respectively.

Table 5. Relationship between cochlear-nerve distances and EMG responses of the subjects.

	Spearman (rho)		p-Value	
Electrode	T-FNS (nC/Phase)	EMG Amplitude (µV)	T-FNS (nC/Phase)	EMG Amplitude (µV)
E20	−0.1975	0.1605	0.6391	0.7042
E15	−0.1975	0.0881	0.6391	0.8358
E8	−0.1605	−0.2332	0.7042	0.5784
E1	−0.1384	−0.2981	0.7439	0.4732

nC: Nanocoulomb; µV: microvolt; T-FNS: facial nerve stimulation thresholds; EMG Amplitude: peak-to-peak electromyographic amplitudes. Spearman's correlation test, at a significant level of 5%.

4. Discussion

The purpose of this study was to investigate the effects of the CI electrical stimulation pattern on FNS reduction in young children. We recorded intraoperative EMG action potentials in children implanted up to 6 years old, using two different CI electrical stimulation patterns: monopolar biphasic stimulation (ST1) and multi-mode monophasic stimulation with capacitive discharge (ST2). Presence of EMG responses, T-FNS and EMG amplitudes were compared between them. Multi-mode monophasic stimulation with capacitive discharge significantly reduced the presence of EMG responses compared to monopolar biphasic stimulation using equal stimulation levels in young children with CI.

To the best of our knowledge, this is the first study comparing intraoperative EMG action potentials between ST1 and ST2 electrical stimulation patterns in CI children recipients and providing electrophysiological evidence of ST2 on FNS reduction in this population. Similar results were recently reported by Eitutis et al. [7] in three adult patients re-implanted with the Neuro Zti device due to severe FNS. Intraoperative FNS were recorded in all the three subjects with ST1, while no FNS was observed with ST2. In our study, FNS was recorded only in the most basal electrode of the subject #S4 with ST2, and the 3D image reconstruction revealed that this electrode was extra-cochlear (Table 4, Figure 4). It is known that extra-cochlear electrodes increase the risk of FNS in CI recipients [15,16], since the total amount of current spread from electrodes which lie outside the cochlea to the periphery structures, including the facial nerve. Thus, considering only the electrodes placed inside the cochlea and, therefore, excluding the extracochlear electrodes from the analysis, the FNS was not recorded with ST2 in any of the subjects included in this study. Our results reinforce those found by Eitutis et al. [7] in adults and suggest that the stimulation pattern ST2 seems to have comparable effects on FNS reduction in the first CI implantation of young children.

Higher stimulation levels were required to elicit FNS with ST2, with smaller EMG amplitudes, compared to ST1. This is also the first time that EMG input-output functions [9] (i.e., charge level required to elicit FNS versus EMG amplitude) could be compared between ST1 and ST2. The CI stimulation pattern ST2 corresponds to the combination of both, the multi-mode grounding stimulation and anodic monophasic pulse shape with capacitive discharge. The relative contribution of each of these features in FNS reducing in CI recipients has been unclear, since the software Genie Medical CI (Oticon Medical, Denmark) does not allow their dissociation for stimulation. In the multi-mode grounding stimulation, a greater amount of electrical current is maintained inside the cochlea since it flows from a stimulating intra-cochlear electrode to the remaining non-stimulating intra-cochlear electrodes. Considering that the electrode E1 (#S4) was extra-cochlear, the comparison of the EMG input-output functions between ST1 and ST2 seems to have been mainly influenced by the pulse shape, since the total amount of the electrical current was spread outside the cochlea, similarly to the monopolar stimulation mode pathway.

The distance between the basal turn of the cochlea and the labyrinthine segment of the facial nerve in the subjects ranged from 0.20 to 1.00 mm. These results are in accordance with previous studies on human temporal bones based on histological image measurements or macroscopical/microscopical analysis [17,18] and CI adult recipients based on preoperative CT scans analysis (axial and coronal orientation plan) [4]. Hatch et al. [4] also investigated the effects of the cochlea-nerve distance on FNS in 49 ears of adult CI recipients and found lower cochlea-nerve distances in subjects with FNS compared to a control group (with no FNS). They suggested that cochlea-nerve distances longest than 0.6 mm should decrease the risk of FNS in this population. In our study, no correlation was observed between cochlear-nerve distances and intraoperative EMG responses in young children with CI, but one subject (#S3, EA6) showed cochlea-nerve distance longer than 0.6 mm, and only this subject showed absent intraoperative EMG recordings with both the ST1 and ST2. The Evo® electrodes E15 and E16 were the closest to the labyrinthine segment of the facial nerve, and they were placed in the upper basal turn of the cochlea, from 250 to 290 degrees insertion depth angle, in most subjects (Figure 4). Seyyedi et al. [19] supposed that electrodes placed in the upper basal turn of cochlea should be most likely to excite the facial nerve, due to their proximity to it. Our findings may confirm the closest proximity of the electrodes placed in the upper basal turn of cochlea to the labyrinthine segment of the facial nerve, but only a weak correlation was observed between the electrode-nerve distance and intraoperative FNS responses, based on our results to the electrode E15. One limitation of this analysis was the small sample size (N = 10), nevertheless, strong correlations between these factors should be detected using the Spearman's correlation test at $p < 0.05$. Even though, further investigations with a larger number of subjects are required to explore the results of intra-cochlear electrodes positioning to better understand the relative influence of this factor on FNS reduction in this population. Anyway, the use of 3D image processing techniques allowed us to accurately estimate the CI electrodes positioning and electrode-nerve distances based on the real intra-cochlear electrodes' placement. This analysis was essential and provided better investigation on these aspects, considering the high variability in the CI electrodes positioning [20,21].

In this study, the EMG recordings were carried out under general anesthesia, and, as muscle relaxants could affect the EMG responses [9], they were not administrated, and thereby our findings may be compared to the clinical routine of non-anesthetized patients.

Finally, our results suggest that CI electrical stimulation pattern may affect the FNS in young children and multi-mode monophasic stimulation with capacitive discharge should far reduce FNS in young children with CIs. The adoption of this electrical stimulation pattern should be an effective option for patients with a higher risk of experiencing FNS after CI surgery, such as patients with otosclerosis, meningitis, temporal bone fractures and congenital cochlear anomalies, or those who have indication for cochlear re-implantation due to severe FNS.

5. Conclusions

Multi-mode monophasic stimulation with capacitive discharge may reduce FNS in young children with CIs. Differently from the CI electrical stimulation pattern, the cochlea-nerve and electrode-nerve distances seem to have limited effects on FNS reduction in this population.

Author Contributions: Design of the study, F.D., A.C.M.B.R., M.A.H. and M.H.; data acquisition, F.D. and M.A.H.; data analysis, F.D. and R.H.; data interpretation, F.D., R.H., A.C.M.B.R., M.A.H., M.H. and C.K.; manuscript drafting: F.D. and R.H.; manuscript review: F.D., A.C.M.B.R., M.A.H., R.H., M.H. and C.K.; supervision, A.C.M.B.R. and M.A.H. All authors have read and agreed to the published version of the manuscript.

Funding: This research received no external funding.

Institutional Review Board Statement: The study was conducted in accordance with the Declaration of Helsinki and approved by the Institutional Ethics Committee of Ribeirão Preto Medical School, University of São Paulo (Protocol number: 5.117.640, Date of approval: 22 November 2021).

Informed Consent Statement: Parental informed consent was obtained from all subjects involved in the study.

Data Availability Statement: The data presented in this study are available on request from the corresponding author.

Acknowledgments: The authors want to thank Denny Marcos Garcia for the review of the statistical analysis.

Conflicts of Interest: F.D. works in the clinical department and R.H., C.K. and M.H. work in the Research & Technology and Clinical Evidence Departments, at Oticon Medical, manufacturer of the Neuro Zti cochlear implant system. The remaining authors declare no conflict of interest.

References

1. Dunn, C.C.; Walker, E.A.; Oleson, J.; Kenworthy, M.; Van Voorst, T.; Tomblin, J.B.; Ji, H.; Kirk, K.I.; McMurray, B.; Hanson, M.; et al. Longitudinal speech perception and language performance in pediatric cochlear implant users: The effect of age at implantation. *Ear Hear.* **2014**, *35*, 148–160. [CrossRef] [PubMed]
2. Binnetoglu, A.; Demir, B.; Batman, C. Surgical complications of cochlear implantation: A 25-year retrospective analysis of cases in a tertiary academic center. *Eur. Arch. Otorhinolaryngol.* **2020**, *277*, 1917–1923. [CrossRef] [PubMed]
3. Van Horn, A.; Hayden, C.; Mahairas, A.D.; Leader, P.; Bush, M.L. Factors influencing aberrant facial nerve stimulation following cochlear implantation: A systematic review and metanalysis. *Otol. Neurotol.* **2020**, *41*, 1050–1059. [CrossRef]
4. Hatch, J.L.; Rizk, H.G.; Moore, M.W.; Camposeo, E.E.; Nguyen, S.A.; Lambert, P.R.; Meyer, T.A.; McRackan, T.R. Can Preoperative CT Scans Be Used to Predict Facial Nerve Stimulation Following CI? *Otol. Neurotol.* **2017**, *38*, 1112–1117. [CrossRef] [PubMed]
5. Cushing, S.L.; Papsin, B.C.; Gordon, K.A. Incidence and characteristics of facial nerve stimulation in children with cochlear implants. *Laryngoscope* **2006**, *116*, 1787–1791. [CrossRef]
6. Kelsall, D.C.; Shallop, J.K.; Brammeier, T.G.; Prenger, E.C. Facial nerve stimulation after Nucleus 22-channel cochlear implantation. *Acta Otorhinolaryngol. Ital.* **1997**, *18*, 336–341.
7. Eitutis, S.T.; Carlyon, R.P.; Tam, Y.C.; Salorio-Corbetto, M.; Vanat, Z.; Tebbutt, K.; Bardsley, R.; Powell, H.R.F.; Chowdhury, S.; Tysome, J.R.; et al. Management of Severe Facial Nerve Cross Stimulation by Cochlear Implant Replacement to Change Pulse Shape and Grounding Configuration: A Case-series. *Otol. Neurotol.* **2022**, *43*, 452–459. [CrossRef]
8. Polak, M.; Ulubil, S.A.; Hodges, A.V.; Balkany, T.J. Revision cochlear implantation for facial nerve stimulation in otosclerosis. *Arch. Otolaryngol. Head Neck Surg.* **2006**, *132*, 398–404. [CrossRef]
9. Bahmer, A.; Adel, Y.; Baumann, U. Preventing Facial Nerve Stimulation by Triphasic Pulse Stimulation in Cochlear Implant Users: Intraoperative Recordings. *Otol. Neurotol.* **2017**, *38*, 438–444. [CrossRef]
10. Broomfield, S.; Mawman, D.; Woolford, T.; O'driscoll, M.; Luff, D.; Ramsden, R. Non-auditory stimulation in adult cochlear implant users. *Cochlear Implant. Int.* **2000**, *1*, 55–66. [CrossRef]
11. Alharbi, F.A.; Spreng, M.; Issing, P.R. Facial nerve stimulation can improve after cochlear reimplantation and postoperative advanced programming techniques: Case report. *Int. J. Clin. Med.* **2012**, *3*, 62–64. [CrossRef]
12. Gärtner, L.; Lenarz, T.; Ivanauskaite, J.; Büchner, A. Facial nerve stimulation in cochlear implant users—A matter of stimulus parameters? *Cochlear Implants Int.* **2022**, *23*, 165–172. [CrossRef] [PubMed]
13. Hyppolito, M.A.; Barbosa, A.C.M.; Danieli, F.; Hussain, R.; Le Goff, N. Cochlear re-implantation with the use of multi-mode grounding associated with anodic monophasic pulses to manage abnormal facial nerve stimulation. *Cochlear Implants Int.* **2022**, *30*, 1–10. [CrossRef] [PubMed]
14. Margeta, J.; Hussain, R.; López Diez, P.; Morgenstern, A.; Demarcy, T.; Wang, Z.; Gnansia, D.; Martinez Manzanera, O.; Vandersteen, C.; Delingette, H.; et al. A Web-Based Automated Image Processing Research Platform for Cochlear Implantation-Related Studies. *J. Clin. Med.* **2022**, *11*, 6640. [CrossRef] [PubMed]
15. Maas, S.; Bance, M.; O'Driscoll, M.; Mawman, D.; Ramsden, R.T. Explantation of a nucleus multichannel cochlear implant and re-implantation into the contralateral ear. A case report of a new strategy. *J. Laryngol. Otol.* **1996**, *110*, 881–883. [CrossRef]
16. Burck, I.; Helal, R.A.; Naguib, N.N.N.; Nour-Eldin, N.A.; Scholtz, J.E.; Martin, S.; Leinung, M.; Helbig, S.; Stöver, T.; Lehn, A.; et al. Postoperative radiological assessment of the mastoid facial canal in cochlear implant patients in correlation with facial nerve stimulation. *Eur. Radiol.* **2022**, *32*, 234–242. [CrossRef]
17. Redleaf, M.I.; Blough, R.R. Distance from the labyrinthine portion of the facial nerve to the basal turn of the cochlea. Temporal bone histopathologic study. *Ann. Otol. Rhinol. Laryngol.* **1996**, *105*, 323–326. [CrossRef]
18. Kruschinski, C.; Weber, B.P.; Pabst, R. Clinical relevance of the distance between the cochlea and the facial nerve in cochlear implantation. *Otol. Neurotol.* **2003**, *24*, 823–827. [CrossRef]
19. Seyyedi, M.; Herrmann, B.S.; Eddington, D.K.; Nadol, J.B. The pathologic basis of facial nerve stimulation in otosclerosis and multi-channel cochlear implantation. *Otol. Neurotol.* **2013**, *34*, 1603–1609. [CrossRef]
20. De Seta, D.; Nguyen, Y.; Bonnard, D.; Ferrary, E.; Godey, B.; Bakhos, D.; Mondain, M.; Deguine, O.; Sterkers, O.; Bernardeschi, D.; et al. The role of electrode placement in bilateral simultaneously cochlear-implanted adult patients. *Otolaryngol. Head Neck Surg.* **2016**, *155*, 485–493. [CrossRef]
21. Danieli, F.; Dermacy, T.; do Amaral, M.S.A.; Reis, A.C.M.B.; Gnansia, D.; Hyppolito, M.A. Auditory performance of post-lingually deafened adult cochlear implant recipients using electrode deactivation based on postoperative cone beam CT images. *Eur. Arch. Otorhinolaryngol.* **2021**, *278*, 977–986. [CrossRef] [PubMed]

Disclaimer/Publisher's Note: The statements, opinions and data contained in all publications are solely those of the individual author(s) and contributor(s) and not of MDPI and/or the editor(s). MDPI and/or the editor(s) disclaim responsibility for any injury to people or property resulting from any ideas, methods, instructions or products referred to in the content.

MDPI
St. Alban-Anlage 66
4052 Basel
Switzerland
www.mdpi.com

Journal of Clinical Medicine Editorial Office
E-mail: jcm@mdpi.com
www.mdpi.com/journal/jcm

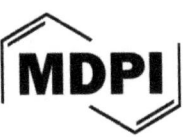

Disclaimer/Publisher's Note: The statements, opinions and data contained in all publications are solely those of the individual author(s) and contributor(s) and not of MDPI and/or the editor(s). MDPI and/or the editor(s) disclaim responsibility for any injury to people or property resulting from any ideas, methods, instructions or products referred to in the content.

www.ingramcontent.com/pod-product-compliance
Lightning Source LLC
LaVergne TN
LVHW070654100526
838202LV00013B/962

9 7 8 3 0 3 6 5 9 5 3 4 4